Textbook of
BIOCHEMISTRY AND BIOPHYSICS
for Nurses

Textbook of
BIOCHEMISTRY AND BIOPHYSICS
for Nurses

As per the Syllabus of Post Basic BSc Nursing of Indian Nursing Council (INC)

Second Edition

Suresh K Sharma MScN PhD FNRS RN (USA)
Professor and Principal
College of Nursing
All India Institute of Medical Sciences (AIIMS)
Jodhpur, Rajasthan, India

Foreword
Prof (Dr) Raj Kumar

JAYPEE BROTHERS MEDICAL PUBLISHERS
The Health Sciences Publisher
New Delhi | London

Jaypee Brothers Medical Publishers (P) Ltd

Headquarters

Jaypee Brothers Medical Publishers (P) Ltd
EMCA House, 23/23-B
Ansari Road, Daryaganj
New Delhi 110 002, India
Landline: +91-11-23272143, +91-11-23272703
+91-11-23282021, +91-11-23245672
Email: jaypee@jaypeebrothers.com

Corporate Office

Jaypee Brothers Medical Publishers (P) Ltd
4838/24, Ansari Road, Daryaganj
New Delhi 110 002, India
Phone: +91-11-43574357
Fax: +91-11-43574314
Email: jaypee@jaypeebrothers.com

Overseas Office

J.P. Medical Ltd
83 Victoria Street, London
SW1H 0HW (UK)
Phone: +44 20 3170 8910
Fax: +44 (0)20 3008 6180
Email: info@jpmedpub.com

Website: www.jaypeebrothers.com
Website: www.jaypeedigital.com

© 2023, Jaypee Brothers Medical Publishers

The views and opinions expressed in this book are solely those of the original contributor(s)/author(s) and do not necessarily represent those of editor(s) and publisher of the book.

All rights reserved. No part of this publication may be reproduced, stored or transmitted in any form or by any means, electronic, mechanical, photocopying, recording or otherwise, without the prior permission in writing of the publishers.

All brand names and product names used in this book are trade names, service marks, trademarks or registered trademarks of their respective owners. The publisher is not associated with any product or vendor mentioned in this book.

Medical knowledge and practice change constantly. This book is designed to provide accurate, authoritative information about the subject matter in question. However, readers are advised to check the most current information available on procedures included and check information from the manufacturer of each product to be administered, to verify the recommended dose, formula, method and duration of administration, adverse effects and contraindications. It is the responsibility of the practitioner to take all appropriate safety precautions. Neither the publisher nor the author(s)/editor(s) assume any liability for any injury and/or damage to persons or property arising from or related to use of material in this book.

This book is sold on the understanding that the publisher is not engaged in providing professional medical services. If such advice or services are required, the services of a competent medical professional should be sought.

Every effort has been made where necessary to contact holders of copyright to obtain permission to reproduce copyright material. If any have been inadvertently overlooked, the publisher will be pleased to make the necessary arrangements at the first opportunity.

Inquiries for bulk sales may be solicited at: jaypee@jaypeebrothers.com

Textbook of Biochemistry and Biophysics for Nurses

First Edition: **2014**

Second Edition: **2023**

ISBN: 978-93-5465-576-0

Dedicated to
My Parents

Sh Badri Narayan Sharma

and

Late Smt Bhagwati Devi Sharma

Whose unconditional love and believe in my capabilities provided me power and energy to bring this book.

Contributors

Mrs Navjot Kaur MScN
Assistant Professor
College of Nursing
All India Institute of Medical Sciences
Deoghar, Jharkhand, India

Dr Shiv Kumar Mudgal PhD
Associate Professor
College of Nursing
All India Institute of Medical Sciences
Deoghar, Jharkhand, India

Dr Rakhi Gaur PhD
Assistant Professor
College of Nursing
All India Institute of Medical Sciences
Deoghar, Jharkhand, India

Reviewers

Er Kishor Kumar Sharma M Tech
Ex-Fellow, Indian Institute of Technology (IIT)
Kharagpur, West Bengal, India

Dr Navjot Bajwa MD
Professor and Head
Department of Biochemistry
Dayanand Medical College and Hospital
Ludhiana, Punjab, India

Dr Rajeev Goyal MD
Associate Professor
Department of Biochemistry
Lady Hardinge Medical College
New Delhi, India

Ms Monika Stephen BScN
Nursing Tutor
College of Nursing
Dayanand Medical College and Hospital
Ludhiana, Punjab, India

Er Kuldeep Gautam B Tech
Ex-Fellow, KIIT University
Bhubaneswar, Odisha, India

Er Prashant S Geel B Tech
Malaviya National Institute of Technology
Jaipur, Rajasthan, India

Dr Satyaveer Rulania PhD
Tutor
College of Nursing
All India Institute of Medical Sciences
Jodhpur, Rajasthan, India

Foreword

Biochemistry and Biophysics is a growing enterprise worldwide, driven primarily by the widespread realization of the major contribution that can be made to biological and medical science including nursing. Traditionally, nurses were involved in practicing several biochemical and biophysical principles in healthcare delivery without an optimal understanding of the subjects. It is to be realized that an increased utilization of biochemical and metabolic principles as well as techniques in healthcare discipline have raised the necessity of learning the biochemistry and biophysics to the nurses. Because of it, the Indian Nursing Council, has incorporated Biochemistry and Biophysics as an integral subject in syllabus of Post Basic BSc Nursing Program in recent past. This has been done in order to enhance the learning of this subject because there has been a limited exposure in this discipline at the entry level of basic diploma nursing program.

It would be important to point out here that in an era of Critical Care Medicine and different types of ICUs in different medical specialties and sub-specialties (subserved by the nurses), they remain devoid of training related with biochemical changes of sick human body, which seems injudicious in the part of health delivery services to criticals.

This book written by *Dr Sharma et al.* includes the basic aspects of Biochemistry, such as introduction to biochemistry and cell, water and electrolytes, enzymes, food digestion and absorption, carbohydrate, protein and fat metabolism. Furthermore, Biophysics section includes basics of biophysics and their application in nursing, such as introduction to biophysics, motion, gravity, force, energy, work, heat, light, pressure, sound, atomic energy. This book also gives importance to medico-electronics and electromagnetics along with application to medical and nursing sciences.

I am sure this book would be useful for nursing students, academicians, nursing scholars and researchers as a ready reference. I wish it would be a great success.

Prof (Dr) Raj Kumar
MS, Mch, PhD, FRCS, FASET, MRCS
Professor and Head
Department of Neurosurgery
Sanjay Gandhi Postgraduate Institute of Medical Sciences
Lucknow, Uttar Pradesh, India
Formerly:
Vice Chancellor, UP University of Medical Sciences, Saifai, Uttar Pradesh, India
Director, All India Institute of Medical Sciences
Rishikesh, Uttarakhand, India

Preface to the Second Edition

Biochemistry and Biophysics is a growing enterprise worldwide, driven primarily by the widespread realization of the major contribution that can be made to biological science by a combination of truly state-of-the-art physical measurements with modern molecular biology. The field occupies a unique and central position at the intersection of the biological, chemical, physical, and medical sciences. It is a reality that this area of study is rapidly evolving and changing. Therefore, it is important to revise the content to keep a pace with development in the field.

This revised edition titled *Textbook of Biochemistry and Biophysics for Nurses* is a modest attempt to reorganize the sequence and content of chapters as per the syllabi designed by Indian Nursing Council for Post Basic BSc Nursing. The chapters are enriched with basic principles and practices of biochemistry and biophysics in simple, lucid and illustrative manner by incorporating their applications to healthcare and nursing practices.

The content in textbook is divided into two sections; Section 1 Biochemistry and Section 2 Biophysics. Section 1 includes chapters on basics of biochemistry, cell, water, electrolytes, enzymes, digestions and absorption of food. Section 2 includes chapters on basic physical principles and healthcare/nursing applications of biophysics, motions, gravity, force, energy, work, heat, light, pressure, sound, electricity, electromagnetism, atomic energy and electronics.

I believe the updated edition of this book will be able to meet the requirements of Indian nursing students and educators while also giving readers useful content planning for various competitive exams for jobs or higher education.

Suresh K Sharma

Preface to the First Edition

Biochemistry and Biophysics is a growing enterprise worldwide, driven primarily by the widespread realization of the major contribution that can be made to biological science by a combination of truly state-of-the-art physical measurements with modern molecular biology. The field occupies a unique and central position at the intersection of the biological, chemical, physical, and medical sciences.

Most of the human biological functions or healthcare practices has basis of principles of biochemistry and biophysics. Therefore, nurses involved in providing nursing care must understand the biochemical and physical principles and their applications in healthcare practices. So that, nurses can assess, plan, implement and evaluate each care intervention more effectively and scientifically.

This textbook titled *Biochemistry and Biophysics: Theory and Application in Nursing"* is a modest attempt to present the basic principles and practices of biochemistry and biophysics in simple, lucid and illustrative manner by incorporating their applications to healthcare and nursing practices. The content in text book is divided into two sections; Section 1 Biochemistry and Section 2 Biophysics. Section 1 has included basics of biochemistry, cell, water, electrolytes, enzymes, digestions and absorption of food. Furthermore, it has presented biochemical aspects and metabolism of carbohydrates, protein and fat. Section 2 has included basic physical principles and healthcare/nursing applications of biophysics, motions, gravity, force, energy, work, heat, light, pressure, sound, electricity, electromagnetism, atomic energy and electronics. The content of biophysics has been presented using non-mathematical approach by incorporating adequate examples from healthcare and nursing sciences. In addition, it has been ensured that each physical principle is simply defined and discussed with its application to nursing practices. Moreover, each topic of the content is presented in simple and lucid manner by using the illustrations and examples from healthcare and nursing practice areas. Content of this text book will fully meet the needs of the nursing students studying in *Post Basic BSc Nursing* program, since it is designed on the lines of revised syllabus of Indian Nursing Council, New Delhi. In addition, it will be also useful for the nurses planning for different competitive exams for jobs or higher studies.

Suresh K Sharma

Contents

SECTION 1: BIOCHEMISTRY

Chapter 1: Introduction to Biochemistry and Cell   3
Suresh K Sharma, Navjot Kaur
- Definitions of Biochemistry   3
- Importance of Biochemistry in Nursing   4
- Structure of a Cell   5
- Various Components of a Cell   5

Chapter 2: Water and Electrolytes   20
Suresh K Sharma, Navjot Kaur
- Water   20
- Water and Fluid Balance   25
- Electrolytes of Human Body   27
- Acids   33
- Bases   35
- Salts   36
- Buffer Action in the Human Body   37

Chapter 3: Enzymes, Digestion and Absorption   41
Suresh K Sharma, Navjot Kaur
- Characteristics of Enzymes   41
- Mechanism of Action   42
- Factors Affecting Enzyme Activity   44
- Specificity of Enzymes   45
- Naming and Classification of Enzymes   45
- Diagnostic Applications   46
- Precautions While Handling Enzyme Preparations   46
- Digestion and Absorption of Carbohydrates, Proteins and Fats   48
- Factors Influencing the Digestion and Absorption   53
- Malabsorption Syndrome   54

Chapter 4: Carbohydrates   58
Shiv Kumar Mudgal, Navjot Kaur
- Classification of Carbohydrates   59
- Functions of Carbohydrates   64
- Metabolism of Carbohydrates   64
- Glycolysis   66
- Glycogenolysis   70
- Gluconeogenesis   71
- Glycogenesis   72
- Tricarboxylic Acid Cycle   73
- Blood Glucose and its Regulation   75
- Glycemia   76
- Glucose Tolerance Test   77
- Hyperglycemia and Diabetes   79
- Hypoglycemia   81

Chapter 5: Proteins   84
Suresh K Sharma, Navjot Kaur
- Amino Acids   84
- Classification of Amino Acids   85
- Proteins   91
- Formation of Urea   102
- Gout   105
- Nitrogenous Constituents of Urine and Blood   107

Chapter 6: Lipids   111
Navjot Kaur, Suresh K Sharma
- Functions of Lipids   111
- Classification of Lipids   112
- Role of Liver in Fat Metabolism   113
- Biological Importance of Important Lipids and their Functions   113
- Alcohols Present in Lipids   117
- Cholesterol and Lipoproteins   118
- Phospholipids   122
- Glycolipids   123
- Lipoproteins and Their Functions   124
- Metabolism of Fatty Acids   125
- Ketone Bodies   129
- Interrelationship in Metabolism   130

SECTION 2: BIOPHYSICS

Chapter 7: Introduction to Biophysics   135
Suresh K Sharma, Navjot Kaur
- Meaning of Biophysics   136
- Importance of Biophysics in Nursing   136
- Concept of Units   138
- Fundamental and Derived Units   138
- Systems of Units   139
- Fundamental Units in Various Systems   140

Chapter 8: Motion — 145
Suresh K Sharma, Navjot Kaur
- Scalars and Vectors 145
- Rest and Motion 146
- Speed 147
- Velocity 148
- Acceleration 148
- Applications of Motion in Nursing 149

Chapter 9: Gravity — 151
Suresh K Sharma, Navjot Kaur
- Specific Gravity 151
- Center of Gravity 152
- Mass and Weight 153
- Principles of Gravity 155
- Applications of Archimedes' Principle 156
- Effects of Gravitational Forces on the Human Body and Application of Principles of Gravity in Nursing 157

Chapter 10: Force, Energy and Work — 161
Suresh K Sharma, Navjot Kaur
- Force 161
- Units of Measurement 162
- Newton's Law of Motion 162
- Principles of Friction 165
- Forces in the Circular Motion 166
- Work 168
- Energy 169
- Types and Transformation of Energy 169
- Energy in the Body 170
- Conservation of Energy 171
- Power 171
- Principles of Machines 172
- Efficiency and Mechanical Advantage of a Machine 172
- Body Mechanics 173
- Lever 173
- Lever Action of Jaw 175
- Lever Action of Foot 175
- Lever Action of Forearm 176
- Pulley 178
- Traction 178
- Inclined Plane 181
- Wedge 182
- Screw 182
- Application of Principles of Gravity in Nursing 182

Chapter 11: Heat — 184
Navjot Kaur, Suresh K Sharma
- Nature of Heat 184
- Measurement of Heat 185
- Transfer of Heat 186
- Effects of Heat on Matter 188
- Humidity 190
- Specific Heat 191
- Temperature Scales 192
- Regulation of Body Temperature 193
- Use of Heat for Sterilization 195
- Application of Heat Principles in Nursing 195

Chapter 12: Light — 198
Suresh K Sharma, Navjot Kaur
- Nature of Light 198
- Law of Reflection and Refraction of Light 202
- Lenses 205
- The Physics of Vision 206
- Defects of Vision and Its Corrections 208
- Biological Effects of the Light 210
- Uses of Light in Therapy 213
- Ultraviolet Radiation 216
- X-rays 216
- Photosensitivity 218
- Application of Principles of Light in Nursing 218

Chapter 13: Pressure and Fluid Mechanics — 220
Navjot Kaur, Shiv Kumar Mudgal
- Importance of Pressure in the Human Body 221
- Atmospheric Pressure 221
- Hydrostatic Pressure 224
- Pressure in Flowing Fluids 226
- Osmotic Pressure 227
- Measurement of Pressures 229
- Applications of these Pressures in Nursing 232

Chapter 14: Sound Waves — 234
Rakhi Gaur, Navjot Kaur
- Mechanism of Propagation of Waves 235
- Types of Waves 235
- Types of Wave Motion 236
- Sound Waves 237

Contents | xvii

- Some Important Terms Connected with Wave Motion 238
- Wave Phenomenon 240
- Characteristics of Sound 242
- Vocalization and Hearing 243
- Doppler Effect 244
- Applications 244
- Noise Pollution and its Prevention 249

Chapter 15: Electricity and Electromagnetism 253
Suresh K Sharma, Navjot Kaur
- Types of Electricity 254
- Sources of Electric Current 260
- Effects of Electric Current 262
- Effects of Electricity on the Human Body 265
- Magnetism 265
- Applications of the Magnet and Magnetism 268
- Electroencephalography 269
- Electrocardiography 270
- Phonocardiography 271
- Electromyography 272
- Electromyography Pattern 272
- Electrostimulation 272
- Electroconvulsive Therapy 273
- Electronic Cardiac Pacemaker 273
- Brain Pacemaker 274
- Defibrillation 275
- Automated External Defibrillator 276
- Magnetic Resonance Imaging 278
- Cat Scan 279

Chapter 16: Nuclear Physics 283
Suresh K Sharma, Navjot Kaur
- Structure of Atom 283
- Radiation and Radioisotopes 290
- Radiation Protection Limits 298
- Instruments used for Detection of Ionizing Radiation, X-rays 300

Chapter 17: Electronics in Nursing 302
Suresh K Sharma, Rakhi Gaur
- Principles of Electronics 303
- Capacitors 304
- Transistors 306
- Transducers 306
- Common Electric Equipment Used in Patient Care 307

Index 313

INC Syllabus
Biochemistry and Biophysics

Placement: First Year Post Basic BSc Nursing

Time Allotted:
Section A (Biochemistry): Theory 30 Hours
Section B (Biophysics): Theory 30 Hours

COURSE DESCRIPTION

This course introduces the basic principles of Biochemistry and Biophysics related to nursing.

OBJECTIVES

At the end of the course, the student will:
1. **Identify the basic principles of Biochemistry and Biophysics**
2. **Synthesize the knowledge of these principles in various nursing situations.**

Section 1: Biochemistry

Theory: 30 hours

COURSE CONTENTS

Chapter 1
- **Introduction:** Importance of Biochemistry in nursing
- Study of cell and its various components

Chapter 2
- **Water and Electrolytes:** Water-sources, property and functions in human body
- Water and fluid balance
- Electrolytes of human body, functions, sources

Chapter 3
- **Enzymes:**
  - Mechanism of action
  - Factors affecting enzyme activity
  - Diagnostic applications
  - Precautions for handling specimens for enzymes estimation
- Digestion and absorption of carbohydrates, proteins and fats
- Various factors influencing the digestion and absorption, malabsorption syndrome

Chapter 4

- **Carbohydrates:** Catabolism of carbohydrates for energy purposes
- Mitochondrial oxidation and oxidation phosphorylation
- Fats of glucose in the body. Storage of glucose in the body, glycogenesis, glycogenolysis and neoglucogenesis, blood glucose and its regulation
- Glucose tolerance test, hyperglycemia, hypoglycemia, glycemia

Chapter 5

- **Protein:** Amino acids, hormones
- Essential amino acids. Biosynthesis of protein in the cells
- Role of nucleic acid in protein synthesis
- Nitrogenous constituents of urine, blood, their origin-urea cycle, uric acid formation, gout
- Plasma proteins and their functions

Chapter 6

- **Fat:** Biosynthesis of fats and storage of fats in the body
- Role of liver in fat metabolism
- Biological importance of important lipids and their functions
- Cholesterol and lipoprotein
    - Sources, occurrence and distribution
    - Blood level and metabolism
    - Ketone bodies and utilization
- Inter-relationships in metabolism and cellular control of metabolic processes

Section 2: Biophysics

Theory: 30 hours

COURSE CONTENTS

Chapter 7
- **Introduction:** Concepts of unit and measurements
- Fundamental and derived units
- Units of length, weight, mass, time

Chapter 8
- Vector and scalar motion, speed, velocity and acceleration

Chapter 9
- **Gravity:** Specific gravity, center of gravity, principles of gravity
- Effect of gravitational forces on human body
- Application of principles of gravity in nursing

Chapter 10
- **Force, Work, Energy:** Their units of measurement
- Type and transformation of energy, forces of the body, static forces
- Principles of machines, friction and body mechanics
- Simple mechanics-lever and body mechanics, pulley and traction, incline plane, screw
- Application of these principles in nursing

Chapter 11
- **Heat:** Nature, measurement, transfer of heat
- Effects of heat on matter
- Relative humidity, specific heat
- Temperature scales
- Regulation of body temperature
- Use of heat for sterilization
- Application of these principles in nursing

Chapter 12
- **Light:** Laws of reflection
- Focussing elements of the eye, defective vision and its correction, use of lenses
- Relationship between energy, frequency and wavelength of light
- Biological effects of light
- Use of light in therapy
- Application of these principles in nursing

Chapter 13

- **Pressures:** Atmospheric pressure, hydrostatic pressure, osmotic pressure
- Measurements of pressures in the body:
  - Arterial and venous blood pressures
  - Ocular pressure
  - Intracranial pressure
  - Applications of these principles in nursing.

Chapter 14

- **Sound:** Frequency, velocity and intensity
- Vocalization and hearing
- Use of ultrasound. Noise pollution and its prevention
- Application of these principles in nursing.

Chapter 15

- **Electricity and Electromagnetism:** Nature of electricity. Voltage, current, resistance and their units
- Flow of electricity in solids, electrolytes, gases and vacuum
- Electricity and human body
- ECG, EEG, EMG, ECT
- Pacemakers and defibrillation
- Magnetism and electricity
- MRI scanning, CAT scan

Chapter 16

- **Atomic Energy:** Structure of atom, isotopes and isobars.
- **Radioactivity:** Use of radioactive isotopes
- Radiation protection units and limits, instruments used for detection of Ionising radiation. X-rays.

Chapter 17

- **Principles of Electronics:** Common electronic equipments used in patient care.

Practicum

- Experiments and tests should be demonstrated wherever applicable.

Section 1

Biochemistry

Section Outline

Chapter 1: Introduction to Biochemistry and Cell
Chapter 2: Water and Electrolytes
Chapter 3: Enzymes, Digestion and Absorption
Chapter 4: Carbohydrates
Chapter 5: Proteins
Chapter 6: Lipids

CHAPTER 1

Introduction to Biochemistry and Cell

Suresh K Sharma, Navjot Kaur

Chapter Outline
- Definitions of Biochemistry
- Importance of Biochemistry in Nursing
- Structure of a Cell
- Various Components of a Cell

■ INTRODUCTION

Nursing is considered as oldest art and youngest science; therefore nursing professionals base their advanced nursing knowledge on the knowledge acquired from the basic sciences such as anatomy, physiology, biochemistry, pathology and so on. Biochemistry is one of the most important basic disciplines in the formation of healthcare professionals, including for nursing. It is concerned with the composition, characterization and transformation of matter. Thus, biochemistry can be defined as a science that tells us about the chemical constituents of the living cell and the reactions and processes that they undergo. Nurses take care of sick patients who cannot care for themselves with varying levels of medical conditions. Therefore, nurses need to be equipped with basic knowledge of biochemistry so that they understand the biochemical basis of disease condition and further understand the changes that occurred in the biochemical constitution of a patient's body during the course of illness so that they can inform about the disease progression and recovery of the patient.

■ DEFINITIONS OF BIOCHEMISTRY

- Biochemistry can be defined as the science concerned with the chemical basis of life. It is the study of biochemical changes that occur within the human body, during health and disease.
- Biochemistry constitutes the study of the chemistry of biomolecules and metabolic processes which constitute our body and are essential for life.
- Biochemistry is the study of structures and physical properties of biological molecules including protein, carbohydrates, lipids and nucleic acids, the mechanism of enzyme action, the chemical regulation of metabolism, the chemistry of nutrition, the molecular basis of genetics (inherence); the chemistry of vitamins, energy utilization in the cell and the chemistry of the immune response.

IMPORTANCE OF BIOCHEMISTRY IN NURSING

Biochemistry deals with the chemical basis of living beings including human beings. Nurses are the largest group in healthcare organizations who are directly involved in promotive, preventive, curative and rehabilitative services. Biochemistry is of great use in the field of Nursing, with many practical applications that can assist in becoming a better nurse. Therefore, the study of biochemistry is significantly important for nurses and it facilitates the nurses to:

- **Understand the biochemical basis of health and illness:** With the knowledge of biochemistry, nurses understand the chemical aspects of different biological processes such as digestion, respiration, reproduction, excretion, the behavior of hormones, contraction, and relaxation of muscles, etc. Moreover, nurses will be able to understand that quite a large proportion of disorders have a biochemical basis. In addition, they will learn about:
  - Normal and abnormal biochemical processes and their regulations such as:
    - Composition and functions of fluid and electrolytes in the human body.
    - Enzymes and their role in digestion and absorption of carbohydrates, proteins and fats.
    - Metabolism, storage and catabolism of carbohydrates, proteins and fats.
  - Role of different biochemical processes in the maintenance of health or causation of illness.
  - Good or bad biochemical situations for health-illness continuum.
  - Biochemical factors playing role in an individual's health.
  - Biochemical contribution towards different diseases and disorders.
- **Interpret the biochemical diagnostics test reports:** The knowledge of clinical biochemistry will help the nurses to understand the needs of different biochemical tests and will also be able to interpret the biochemical reports of the patients with different disease conditions. The ability of nurses to interpret the biochemical diagnostic test reports will help them in early identification and prompt action during serious life-threatening situations, which may significantly affect the morbidity outcome among such patients. Therefore, it is essentially important for nurses to study biochemistry; so that they can become active resourceful members of the healthcare team. The common biochemical tests nurses generally encounter and may need to interpret in their day-to-day clinical practices are:
  - Serum electrolytes level
  - Glucose tolerance test
  - Blood sugar levels
  - Plasma protein levels
  - Renal function tests like urea, creatinine
  - Serum cholesterol and lipid profile
  - Serum enzyme levels such as amylase, lipase, etc.
  - Serum hormonal analysis such as TSH, T3, T4, and other hormones.
- **Contributes towards health promotion with biochemical aspect:** There are several biochemical tests that are carried out for screening purposes or to identify the risk of certain life-threatening illness such as cardiovascular diseases. For example, if a nurse is aware that increased level of serum cholesterol and lipid profile has a risk of cardiovascular disorders, then she may educate the people about maintaining the serum lipid level within the normal limits through dietary modification, regular exercises and medicines; so that future risk of coronary artery disease may be minimized. Thus through learning biochemistry, nurses may contribute towards health promotion with biochemical aspect.
- **Carryout effective assessment and planning for nursing needs:** It is the most essential function of a nurse to identify the priority needs of the patients. This may be further facilitated by the basic knowledge of biochemistry. For example, a nurse is assessing a diabetic patient

admitted to the medical ward, her biochemistry knowledge facilitates her to interpret biochemical test reports such as blood sugar level that will help her in the identification of the nutritional needs of the patient and plan nursing interventions accordingly.
- **Implement the health education based on biochemical rationalization:** Health education is also one of the important roles of nurses; with knowledge of biochemistry, nurses will be able to understand the biochemical basis of illness and offer health education to clients based on biochemical rationalization when and where required so that their client can be more convinced and clear about their illness, treatment and prevention.

STRUCTURE OF A CELL

Introduction

The cell, discovered by Robert Hooke in 1665, is a basic, living, structural and functional unit of the body. They are often called the building block of life. "Cell is the structural and functional unit of all living organisms". Human body cells are of different types, sizes and shapes such as muscle cells, bone and cartilage cells, nerve cells, visual cells in the eye, etc. Division of work and distribution of various functions is the hallmark of a multicellular organism. The work assignment begins at the subcellular level and extends to the organ and tissue systems.

Types of Cells

Some organisms are unicellular such as bacteria, while some are multicellular, e.g., human cells are of many types. On the basis of structural differences, cells are divided as eukaryotes and prokaryotes **(Table 1.1)**. Prokaryotes are simple and usually independent cells, while eukaryotes are often found in multicellular organisms.
- **Prokaryotic cells:** The most primitive cell structure where there is an absence of nuclear membrane, nucleolus and membrane-bound organelles. The genetic material in them is stored in the form of nucleoids, found freely distributed in the cytoplasm. Generally, this genetic material is made-up of one or more folded DNA strands without the presence of histone proteins. The bacteria, viruses and some of the fungi are good examples of prokaryotic cells, which are significant in health sciences.
- **Eukaryotic cells:** It is the most advanced cell with well-developed nucleus with nucleic membrane, nucleolus and genetic material in the form of chromosomes. These cells are found in the higher organism such as human beings. Structurally and functionally eukaryotic cells are larger in size, advanced, developed and complex **(Fig. 1.1)**.

VARIOUS COMPONENTS OF A CELL

The cells are too small to be seen with naked eyes. However, a microscope is used to view a cell and its components after staining with appropriate dyes. Cell and its components absorb the dye and their structure and size may be clearly differentiated using a microscope. A typical eukaryotic cell consists of the following components:
- **Plasma membrane:** Outer, limiting membrane separating the cell's internal components from the extracellular materials and external environment.
- **Cytosol:** The thick intracellular fluid is termed cytosol. The cytosol contains many dissolved proteins and enzymes, nutrients, ions and other small molecules, which all participate in various phases of metabolism. Organelles and inclusions are suspended in the cytosol.
  - The term cytoplasm includes cytosol, all organelles (except nucleus) and inclusions.
- **Organelles:** Highly organized structures with characteristic shapes that are specialized for specific cellular activities. The organelle with the largest volume is the nucleus, which contains

SECTION 1: Biochemistry

Table 1.1: Difference between prokaryotic and eukaryotic cells.

Features	Prokaryotic cells	Eukaryotic cells
Cell size	Size of prokaryotic cell varies between 0.1 and 10 micron in diameter	Typically eukaryotic cell is between 10 and 100 micron in diameter
Cell membrane	Prokaryotic cells are covered by a cell envelop, which generally is made-up of muramic acid.	Eukaryotic cells are covered with a complex structure cell wall made-up of phospholipids, glycolipid, cholesterol and proteins.
Cell wall appendages	Simple structured flagella are present on cell envelop, which are not differentiated into axoneme and sheath.	Complex structure flagella, cilia and microvilli are present on cell wall. Flagella if present are differentiated into axoneme and sheath.
Nucleus	Nucleus is not present, no nucleic membrane and nucleolus; simple chromosomes are directly suspended in cytoplasm.	Most of the cells have a nucleus, which is covered with double layered nucleic membrane, complex-structured chromosomes and nucleolus is present in nucleus.
Genetic material	Simple structure chromosomes without presence of histone proteins.	Complex structure chromosomes are presented associated with histone proteins.
Cytoplasm and cell components	Cytoplasm is present without major cell components such as mitochondria, endoplasmic reticulum, etc.	Cytoplasm is present and most of the cells contain major cell components such as mitochondria, endoplasmic reticulum, etc.
Ribosomes	Cell contains ribosomes of only one size.	Cell contains two types of ribosomes, one in cytoplasm and smaller type is in mitochondria.
Cell division	Cell division does not involve meiosis; reproduce sexually by the transfer of DNA fragments through conjugation. They are generally fast-multiplying cells	Cell division involves mitosis and meiosis and relatively slow multiplying but versatile

Fig. 1.1: Basic structure and components of an eukaryotic cell.

most of the cell genetic material. The other major organelles are mitochondria, endoplasmic reticulum, golgi apparatus, lysosomes, ribosomes and vacuoles and peroxisomes.
* **Inclusions:** These are the temporary structures in the cytoplasm that contain secretions and storage products of the cell.

Plasma Membrane

The plasma membrane is the gatekeeper that regulates the passage of substances into and out of the cell. In other words, the plasma membrane is a lipid bilayer of phospholipids that separate the cytoplasm from the environment. Within the phospholipid bilayer, cholesterol, glycolipids, proteins and glycoproteins are interseparated **(Fig. 1.2)**. The structure of the plasma membrane can be explained with the help of *Fluid Mosaic Model.*

The **fluid mosaic model** of membrane structure describes the molecular arrangement of the plasma membrane and other membranes in living organisms. A mosaic is a pattern of many small pieces fitted together. According to this model, the membrane is a mosaic of proteins floating like icebergs in a sea of lipids.

Plasma membrane like the other membranes is composed of lipids and proteins. These two major components arrange themselves in a manner to form plasma membrane. There are the following three *types of lipids* involved in the formation of the plasma membrane.
* **Phospholipids:** About 75% of the lipids are phospholipids that contain phosphorus.
    * Phospholipids are arranged in two parallel layers forming a phospholipid bilayer. So, this model is also known as the phospholipid bilayer model. This arrangement occurs because phospholipids are amphipathic in nature, each molecule consisting of polar and nonpolar regions. The polar part is the phosphate-containing "head", which is hydrophilic and the nonpolar parts are two fatty acid "tails", which are hydrophobic. The head faces outward on either side, towards the watery cytosol and extracellular fluid.
* **Glycolipid:** About 5% of lipids are gycolipids with attached sugar groups. Glycolipids are also amphipathic in nature. They only appear in the layer that faces extracellular fluid (ECF).
* **Cholesterol:** The remaining 20% of plasma membrane lipids are cholesterol molecules, which are located among the phospholipid in animal cells. However, plant cells lack cholesterol in the cell membrane.

Fig. 1.2: Basic structure of plasma membrane.

The plasma membrane also contains two types of proteins; which are discussed as follows:
- **Integral proteins:** These are extended across the phospholipid bilayer among the fatty acids tails. The most integral proteins are glycoproteins, which are proteins with attached sugar groups.
- **Peripheral proteins:** These are proteins that do not extend across the phospholipid bilayer. They are loosely attached to the inner and outer surfaces of the membrane and are easily separated.

The molecular composition of plasma membranes also differs from tissue to tissue and this change in the composition is partly, responsible for the functional differences in the tissues.

Appendages of Plasma Membrane

Following are the main appendages of a plasma membrane, i.e., cilia, flagellum and microvilli, etc.
- **Cilia:** These are the extensions of the plasma membrane containing parallel microtubules, 10 micrometers in length. The main function of the cilia is to move materials over the surface of the cells.
- **Flagellum:** These are the extensions of the plasma membrane containing parallel microtubules, 55 micrometers in length. In human cells, flagella are responsible for the movement of spermatozoa.
- **Microvilli:** These are the extensions of the plasma membrane containing microfilaments. The main functions of the microvilli are to increase the surface area of the plasma membrane for absorption and secretion and modified to form sensory receptors.

Functions of Plasma Membrane

Following are the major functions of the plasma membrane of a cell:
- **Semipermeable:** The plasma membrane regulates the entry and exit of materials inside the cell. It permits the passage of certain substances and restricts the passage of others. This property of membrane is known as "selective permeability."
- **Receptor:** The plasma membrane proteins can identify and attach to a specific molecule such as hormones, neurotransmitters or a nutrient that is important for some cellular function.
- **Communication:** The plasma membrane functions in cellular communication. This includes interactions with the other body cells, foreign cells, hormones, neurotransmitters, enzymes, nutrients and antibodies in extracellular fluid.
- **Electrochemical gradient:** The membrane maintains an electrical and chemical gradient, called an electrochemical gradient, between the inside and outside the cell. The electrochemical gradient and the resulting membrane potential are important for the proper functioning of most cells.
- **Physical barrier:** The plasma membrane surrounds all cells and physically separates the cytoplasm, from the extracellular fluid outside the cell. This protects all the components of the cell from the outside environment and allows separate activities to occur inside and outside the cell. The plasma membrane provides structural support to the cell. It tethers the cytoskeleton, which is a network of protein filaments inside the cell that hold all the parts of the cell in place. This gives the cell its shape.
- **Endocytosis and exocytosis:** Endocytosis is when a cell ingests relatively larger contents than the single ions or molecules that pass through channels. Through endocytosis, a cell can take in large quantities of molecules or even whole bacteria from the extracellular fluid. Exocytosis is when the cell releases these materials. The cell membrane plays an important role in both of these processes. The shape of the membrane itself changes to allow molecules to enter or exit the cell.

Cytosol

Chemically, cytosol is 75–90% water plus solid components. Proteins, carbohydrates, lipids and inorganic substances comprise most of the solids. Inorganic substances and smaller organic substances, such as simple sugars and amino acids are soluble in water and are present as solutes. Larger organic compounds like proteins, polysaccharides, glycogen, are found as colloid particles that remain suspended in the surrounding medium although they are not dissolved. The colloids bear electrical charges that repel each other and thus remain suspended and separated.

The cytosol contains enzymes that catalyze catabolic and anabolic reactions, ATP is produced in glycolysis reactions.

Organelles

The main organelles present in the cell are nucleus, endoplasmic reticulum, Golgi complex, mitochondria, ribosomes, lysosomes, peroxisomes, centrioles, and spindle fibers, etc.

1. Nucleus

It occupies a central position in the cell. It is spherical or oval and much denser than the cytoplasm. It is the governing organelle of the cell that controls the functions, growth, and multiplication of the cell. It is generally situated in center of the cell, covered with a double-layered membrane called a nuclear membrane and contains chromosomes, nucleoplasm and nucleolus. Chromosomes carry the genetic material of the cell and nucleolus serves as a site for ribosome synthesis.

Most of the cells contain a single nucleus, but few may have more such as some of the liver cells have more than one nucleus and long muscle cells do have hundreds of nuclei. However, red cell during their maturation lose their nucleus.

The main parts of the nucleus are (**Fig. 1.3**):
- **Nuclear membrane:** It is a double membrane enclosing the nucleus. The outer membrane is continuous with the endoplasmic reticulum; nuclear pores extend through the nuclear envelope. The nuclear membrane helps to maintain the shape of the nucleus and assists in regulating the flow of molecule including RNA into and out of the nucleus through nuclear pores.
- **Chromatin:** The mass of DNA and proteins inside a chromosome is referred to as chromatin. Thin strands of DNA, histones and other proteins condenses to form chromosomes during cell division.

Fig. 1.3: Structure of nucleus.

- **Nucleolus:** When a nucleus is not dividing, a structure called a nucleolus becomes visible which is the most prominent structure within the nucleus. Usually there is only a single nucleolus present, but some nuclei have multiple nucleoli. It is a mass of granules and fibers attached to chromatin. It consists of ribosomal RNA and proteins and the nucleolus serves as a site for ribosome synthesis.

Functions of Nucleus
Following are the main functions of the nucleus in a cell:
- It is the seat of all metabolic activities of the cell.
- The nuclear membrane helps in separating the nucleus from the cytoplasm and regulates the movement of material into and out of the nucleus.
- All cells in the human body contain a nucleus except mature RBCs in circulation.
- The nucleus contains DNA, the chemical basis of the genes, which governs all the functions of the cell. It contains the cell's hereditary information and controls the cell's growth and reproduction.
- DNA replication and RNA synthesis are taking place inside the nucleus.
- The nucleolus is the area for RNA processing and ribosome synthesis.

2. Endoplasmic Reticulum

It is a network of tubular channels traversing the cytosol. The individual tubules are called as cisterns which vary in size, shape and connectivity with various subcellular organelles. Endoplasmic reticulum is connected to the plasma membrane and surrounds the nucleus and other organelles **(Fig. 1.4)**. On the basis of appearance as well as function, the endoplasmic recticulum can be divided into:
- **Rough endoplasmic reticulum:** It is also known as granular endoplasmic reticulum. These are studded with ribosomes on its outer surface. The rough endoplasmic reticulum is involved in active protein synthesis with the help of ribosomes, synthesizes secretory proteins like digestive enzymes, protein sorting and initial post-translational modification such as glycosylation, sulfation, phosphorylation and hydroxylation of proteins and also

Fig. 1. 4: Structure of endoplasmic reticulum.

the synthesis of phospholipids. Protein sorting involves several factors and a sequence of events.
- **Smooth endoplasmic reticulum:** It is also known as the agranular endoplasmic reticulum. These are not studded with ribosomes on their outer surface. The smooth endoplasmic reticulum is found abundant in cells. The smooth ER has a wide range of functions including carbohydrate and lipid synthesis. It serves as a transitional area for vesicles that transport ER products to various destinations. In liver cells, the smooth ER produces enzymes that help to detoxify certain compounds and foreign substances like drugs and toxins and glycogen metabolism. In muscle cells, it stores calcium that assists in the contraction of muscle cells. In the adrenal cortex and gonad cells, it synthesizes steroid hormones. It is also involved in lipid metabolism and membrane formation. It carries enzymes for the modification of proteins synthesized in the rough endoplasmic reticulum.

Functions of Endoplasmic Reticulum
Following are the main functions of endoplasmic reticulum:
- Ribosomes associated with the rough ER synthesize proteins destined for insertion into the plasma or export from the cell.
- Rough ER serves as a temporary storage area for newly synthesized molecules and may add sugar groups to certain proteins, thus forming glycoproteins.
  Smooth ER is the site of fatty acid, phospholipid and steroid synthesis. It is also responsible for the metabolism of carbohydrates.
- Also within certain cells, enzymes within the smooth ER can inactivate or detoxify a variety of chemicals, including alcohol, pesticides and carcinogens. The endoplasmic reticulum is also considered a cell skeletal system and helps to keep cell organelle in position. The smooth ER stores and releases calcium ions. These are quite important for the nervous system and muscular systems.
- The endoplasmic reticulum also helps in the formation of vacuoles.

3. Golgi Complex
It is derived from endoplasmic reticulum. It is an organelle located near the nucleus. It consists of flattened sacs called cisterns. Associated with the cisterns are small golgi visicles, which cluster along the expanded edges of cisterns **(Fig. 1.5)**. The golgi complex can be divided into three regions:-
a. **Proximal or cis region:** This is the immediate extension of the endoplsmic reticulum and receives proteins synthesized from it.
b. **Medial region:** Most of the post-translational modifications of synthesized proteins take place in this region.
c. **Distal or trans region:** This region of the golgi apparatus is primarily associated with secretory activity.

Functions of Golgi Complex
- Golgi complex processes, sorts, packages and delivers proteins and lipids to the plasma membrane and forms lysosomes and secretory vesicles.
- As mentioned above the primary function of golgi complex is the formation of secretory vesicles and lysosomes.
- Golgi complex helps the endocrine cells in the secretion of hormones.
- It is also involved in the formation of acrosomes, during the maturation of sperms.
- Golgi complex also activates mitochondria to produce ATP.
- It also helps in the modification of proteins by adding certain prosthetic groups.

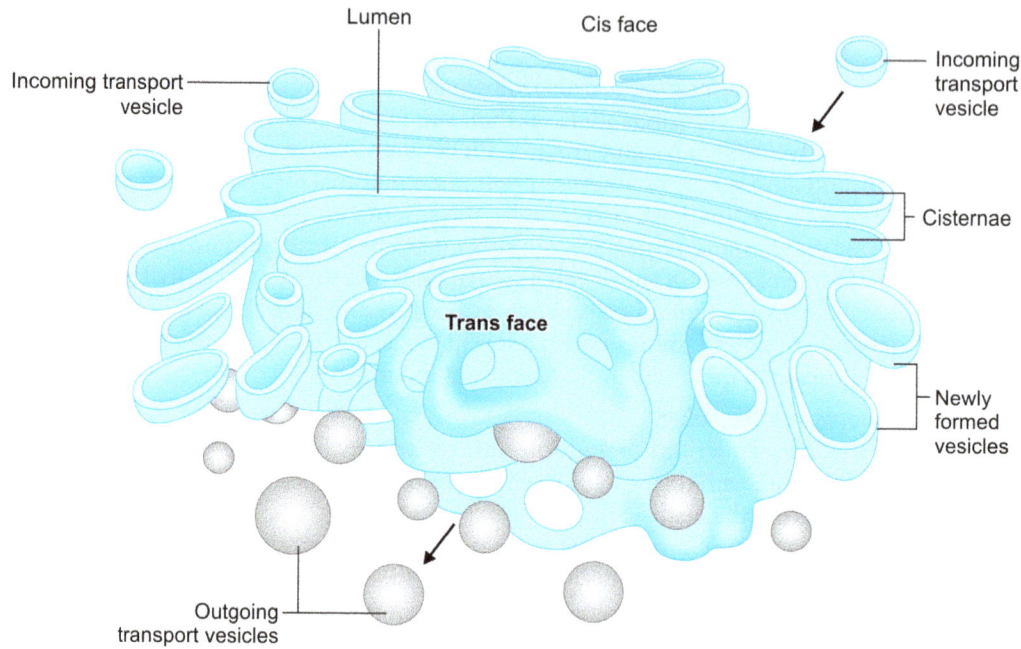

Fig. 1.5: Structure of golgi complex.

- Golgi complex also helps in the regulation of cellular fluid balance by expelling extra fluid from the cell.

4. Mitochondria

It is known as the "powerhouse" of the cell. A typical mammalian cell carries between 800 and 2500 mitochondria. The highest number of mitochondria is found in neurons and muscle cells. About 10% of body weight of a human adult is mitochondria. Mitochondria consist of two membranes, each of which is similar in structure to plasma membrane: (a) outer mitochondrial membrane which is smooth and (b) inner mitochondrial membrane which is arranged in series of folds called cristae. The central cavity of mitochondria, enclosed by the inner membrane and cristae is called the matrix. The mitochondrial membrane divides the mitochondria into two chambers **(Fig. 1.6)**:

- **Outer chamber:** The outer chamber is formed between outer smooth membrane and inner mitochondrial membrane, which is arranged in series of folds. It is lipid-rich membrane composed of phospholipids and cholesterol.
- **Inner chamber:** The inner chamber is formed by the inner membrane, which is arranged in a series of folds named as matrix. This inner chamber contains semifluid matrix. It is a protein-rich membrane with a protein: lipid ratio is about 3.7: 1. The matrix has protein particles, ribosomes, RNA, DNA, enzymes of Krebs cycle, amino acid synthesis and fatty acid metabolism, etc.

Functions of Mitochondria

Following are the main functions of the mitochondria:
- It is the main site for the generation of ATP.

Fig. 1.6: Structure of mitochondria.

- The elaborated folds of the cristae provide an enormous surface area for a series of chemical reactions, known as "cellular respiration", which provides most of a cell's ATP. Enzymes that catalyze these reactions are located in the matrix and on the cristae.
- Active cells such as muscles, liver and renal tubule, have a large number of mitochondria and use ATP at a high rate.
- Mitochondria self-replicate, they divide to increase in number. Their replication is controlled by the genes within the mitochondria. Self-replication usually occurs in response to the increased cellular need for ATP and at the time of cell division.
- Mitochondrial matrix contains various enzymes for the synthesis of fatty acids.
- Cell death, also called apoptosis, is an essential part of life. As cells become old or broken, they have cleared away and destroyed. Mitochondria help decide which cells are destroyed.
- Mitochondria help in storing calcium by quickly absorbing calcium ions and holding them until they are needed.
- Mitochondria can generate heat to keep the body warm through non-shivering thermogenesis.

5. Ribosomes

Ribosomes are tiny granules that contain ribosomal RNA (rRNA) and many ribosomal proteins. Structurally, ribosome consists of two subunits, one about half the size of the other (**Fig. 1.7**). They are made up of ribonucleic acid and protein, so-called ribonucleoprotein particles. Ribosomes are popularly known as 'protein factories'. They produce proteins from amino acids through the process called 'translation'. Ribosomes have four sites that help in protein synthesis, i.e., (a) mRNA-binding site, (b) A (Aminoacyl) site, (c) P (Peptidyl) site (d) E (Exit) site.

Some ribosomes called 'Free Ribosomes' float in the cytosol, they have no attachments to other organelles. The free ribosomes occur singly or in clusters. Other ribosomes attach to a cellular structure called the endoplasmic reticulum. Further ribosomes may occur singly as monosomes or in groups named polyribosomes.

Types of Ribosomes

Based on the size and sedimentation coefficient, ribosomes are classified into two main types:
1. **70S Ribosomes:** These are smaller in size and found in prokaryotic cells, mitochondria and chloroplast of eukaryotic cells. 70S ribosome consists of large (50S) and smaller (30S) subunits.
2. **80S Ribosomes:** These ribosomes are larger in size and found in eukaryotic cells. They consist of larger (60S) and smaller (40S) subunits. A tunnel occurs between the larger and smaller subunit for the passage of mRNA during protein synthesis.

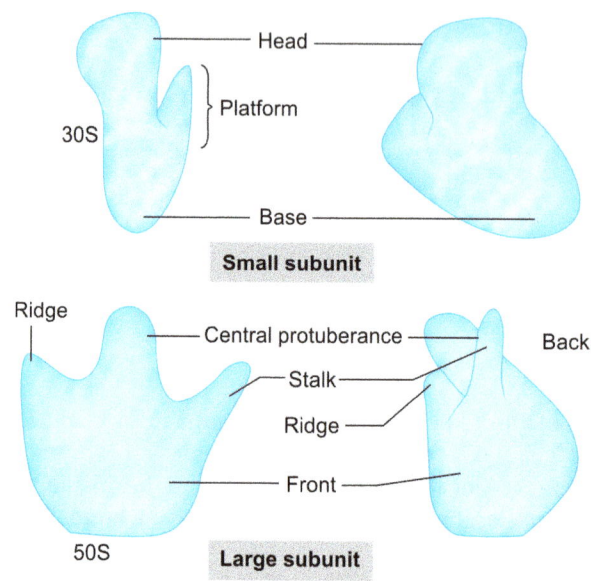

Fig. 1.7: Structure of ribosome.

Functions of Ribosome
- The main function of the ribosomes is the sites of protein synthesis. They assemble amino acids to form proteins that are essential to carry out cellular functions.
- The ribosomes contain rRNAs for providing attaching points to mRNA and tRNAs.

6. Lysosomes

They are membrane-enclosed vesicles that form in the golgi complex. They originate by budding off from the membrane of the trans-golgi network. They are tiny sac-like granules bounded by a single membrane containing hydrolytic enzymes in it. They are also known as 'Suicide Bags' because of a number of digestive enzymes in them. Lysosomes contain as many as 40 kinds of powerful digestive enzymes capable of breaking down a wide variety of molecules. The structure and functions of the lysosome are depicted in **Fig. 1.8**.

Functional Polymorphism of Lysososome
On functional basis lysosomes at different stages present with polymorphism and these functional stages of polymorphism are of three types, i.e., primary lysosomes, secondary lysosomes and residual bodies.
- *The primary lysosome:* They are small size tiny sac-like bodies bounded by a single membrane containing many hydrolytic enzymes and popularly known as storage granules. They are present in silent form but ready to act whenever the need for autodigestion within the cell is desired.
- *The secondary lysosomes:* They are active digestive vacuoles containing the foreign material and enzymes within the membrane for the auto-digestion. When a liquid foreign material is ingested in these vacuoles for the auto-digestion process of cells, they are known as pinosomes and the process is called pinocytosis or cell drinking. On another hand when a solid foreign material is ingested in these vacuoles for the auto-digestion process of the cell, they are known as phagosomes and the process is called phagocytosis or cell eating.

CHAPTER 1: Introduction to Biochemistry and Cell

Fig. 1.8: Illustration depicting structure and functions of lysosome.

❖ *The residual body:* After the process of pinocytosis or phagocytosis, an undigested material is left in the cell. A residual body of lysosomes is formed which attach to the plasma membrane and are thrown out of the cell by ephagy.

Functions of Lysosomes
❖ Lysosomal enzymes digest bacteria and other substances that enter the cell in phagocytic vesicles during phagocytosis, pinocytic vesicles during pinocytosis.
❖ Lysosomes take part in the natural defence of the body.
❖ They also help in breaking down of the aging cells and dead cells. Therefore, they are involved in programmed cell death.
❖ Lysosomes also help in intracellular scavenging by removing old or useless organelles.

7. Peroxisomes

These are single membrane-bound organelles found free in the cytosol. They are similar in structure to lysosomes but smaller in size. They are so named because they usually contain one or more enzymes that use molecular oxygen to oxidize (remove hydrogen atoms from) various organic substances. Perxisomes are minute, somewhat spherical and single unit membrane particles with diameter varying from 0.5 to 1.0 μm **(Fig. 1.9)**. The shape and size is variable from cell to cell. They are present in abundant numbers in parenchyma of liver and kidney.

Fig. 1.9: Structure of peroxisomes.

Functions of Peroxisomes
- They detoxify harmful molecules such as ethanol, phenols, formic acid, etc.
- They contain oxidase and catalase that helps in oxidation and removal of hydrogen peroxide.
- The chief function is to help in the metabolism of glycolate during photosynthesis.
- The long-chain and branched fatty acids are catabolized by peroxisomes.
- The substances which cannot be catabolized by normal enzymes are generally catabolized by peroxisomes.

8. Centrioles

These are the pair of cylindrical organelles in the centrosome, consisting of triplets of parallel microtubules **(Fig. 1.10)**. These are made of tubulin protein. These are located very close to the nucleus of the cell.

Functions of Centrioles
Following are the main functions of the centrioles:
- It is the center for microtubule formation.
- The main function of centriole is to help with cell division. It determines cell polarity during cell division.
- The centrioles also help in the formation of the spindle fibers that separate the chromosomes during cell division (mitosis).
- It forms the basal bodies of cilia and flagella.

9. Spindle Fibers

These are the microtubules extending between the two centrosomes, where chromosomes are arranged at middle of the cell during a cell division, which are called spindle fibers **(Fig. 1.11)**. Spindle fibers only appear during cell division; therefore, they cannot be seen during time other than cell division. Spindle fibers form a protein structure that divides the genetic material in a cell. The spindle is necessary to equally divide the chromosomes in a parental cell into two daughter cells during both types of nuclear division: mitosis and meiosis. During mitosis, the

Fig. 1.10: Structure of centrioles.

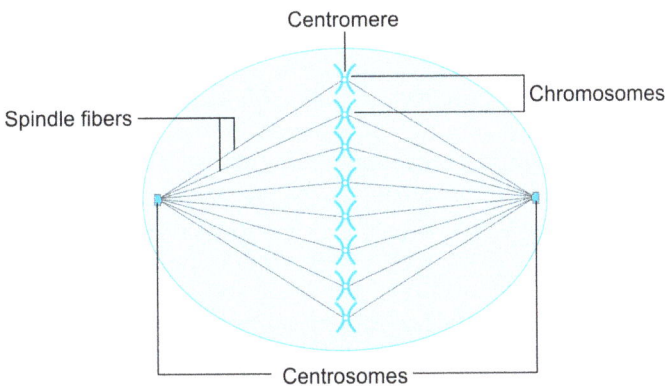

Fig. 1.11: A cell division depicting appearance of spindle fibers.

spindle fibers are called the mitotic spindle. Meanwhile, during meiosis, the spindle fibers are referred to as the meiotic spindle.

Functions of Spindle Fibers
- These assist in the separation of chromosomes during cell division. Spindle fibers help in the division of genetic component of the cell during division.
- Spindle fibers get attached to kinetochores and arms of chromosomes and help in the segregation and movement of chromatids.
- During metaphase, chromosomes get aligned in the middle with the help of the spindle and then move to the opposite poles during the anaphase stage.

10. Cytoskeleton

Organization of the cells into tissues requires them to stick to and interact with each other for the coordinated metabolic responses to various stimuli. Most of these features of the tissues are derived from a set of structural proteins that form a meshwork of fine filament within the cells, known as the cytoskeleton.

Functions of the cytoskeleton:
- Giving specific shapes to cells
- Binding the cells together to form the tissues, for example, cell-cell adhesion
- Providing high tensile strength

The cytoskeleton is divided into three levels of organization:
- Microfilaments
- Intermediate filaments
- Microtubules

11. Cytoplasm

The organelle-free sap of cells is called cytoplasm. The cytoplasm is a protein-rich fluid that harbors a number of enzymes and is the site of a number of metabolic reactions.

Cell Inclusion

Inclusions are considered to be nonliving components of the cell that do not possess the metabolic activity and are not bound by membranes. The most common inclusions are glycogen, lipid droplets, crystals and pigments.
- ***Glycogen:*** Glycogen is the most common form of glucose in animals and is especially abundant in cells of muscles and liver. It appears in electron micrographs as clusters, or rosettes of beta particles that resemble ribosomes, located near the smooth endoplasmic reticulum. Glycogen is an important energy source of the cell. Therefore, it will be available on demand. The enzymes responsible for glycogenolysis degrade glycogen into individual molecules of glucose and can be utilized by multiple organs of the body.
- ***Lipids:*** Triglycerides are the storage form of lipids, it is not only stored in specialized cells (adipocytes) but also located as individual droplets in various cell type especially hepatocytes. These are fluid at body temperature and appear in living cells as refractile spherical droplets. Lipid yields more than twice as many calories per gram as does carbohydrate. On-demand, they serve as a local store of energy and a potential source of short carbon chains that are used by the cell in its synthesis of membranes and other lipid-containing structural components or secretory products.
- ***Crystals:*** Crystalline inclusions have long been recognized as normal constituents of certain cell types such as sertolli cells and Leydig cells of the human testis, and occasionally in macrophages. It is believed that these structures are crystalline forms of certain proteins which are located everywhere in the cell such as in the nucleus, mitochondria, endoplasmic reticulum, golgi body, and free in cytoplasmic matrix.
- ***Pigments:*** The most common pigment in the body, besides hemoglobin of red blood cells is melanin, manufactured by melanocytes of the skin and hair, pigment cells of the retina and specialized nerve cells in the substantia nigra of the brain. These pigments have protective functions in the skin and aid in the sense of sight in the retina but their functions in neurons are not understood completely. Furthermore, cardiac tissue and central nervous system neurons show yellow to brown pigment called lipofuscin, some believed that they have lysosomal activity.

CHAPTER 1: Introduction to Biochemistry and Cell

■ QUESTION

Q.1: Explain the structure and functions of 'Golgi apparatus' in a cell.

■ BIBLIOGRAPHY

1. Amenta PS. Histology: from normal microanatomy to pathology. PICCIN; 1997: 17.
2. Campbell NA, Williamson B, Heyden RJ. Biology: Exploring Life. Boston, Massachusetts: Pearson Prentice Hall; 2006.
3. Cooper GM. The cell: a molecular approach, 2nd edition. Washington DC: ASM Press, 2000.
4. Coper GM. The Cell. A molecular approach. 8th edition. Oxford University Press. New York. 2019; 1–10
5. Gartner LP, Hiatt JL. Textbook of Histology, 3rd edition WB Saunders Company;1997.
6. Griffiths G. Cell evolution and the problem of membrane topology. Nature reviews. Molecular cell biology. 2007; 8(12):1018–24.
7. Iwara J & Marshall W. Karp's Cell biology. John Wiley & Sons. Singapore. 2016; 1–4
8. Lal Harbans, Sachdeva Ashuma. Textbook of Biochemistry. 4th edition. CBS Publishers and distributors. New Delhi. 2017; 1–17.
9. Lodish H, Berk A, Matsudaira P, et al. Molecular Cell Biology 5th edition. New York, NY: WH Freeman; 2004.
10. Maton, Johnson J, LaHart S, et al. Cells Building Blocks of Life. New Jersey: Prentice Hall; 1997.
11. Sterrer W. "On the origin of sex as vaccination". Journal of Theoretical Biology. 2002; 216: 387–96.

CHAPTER 2

Water and Electrolytes

Suresh K Sharma, Navjot Kaur

Chapter Outline
- Water
- Water and Fluid Balance
- Electrolytes of Human Body
- Acids and Bases
- Salts
- Buffer Action in the Human Body

■ INTRODUCTION

Water and electrolytes are an important components of the human body, which play a central role in the metabolic activities of an organism. Homeostasis of water and electrolyte in the body fluids is very essential to normal cellular functions. Water and electrolyte are present in different compartments in the human body, i.e., intracellular and extracellular compartments. The extracellular compartment consists of intravascular, interstitial, and transcellular space. The most common electrolytes present in the human body are cations and anions. The common cations present in the human body are sodium, potassium, calcium, magnesium and hydrogen ions. The common anions present in the human body are chlorides and bicarbonates, etc.

■ WATER

Water is the most abundant of all chemical compounds and it exists in the form of solid, liquid and gas. Water is the very essence of life of almost all plants, animals and human beings. Water is a universal solvent that dissolves many substances forming solutions.

Life is possible on earth due to the presence of water. Nearly three-fourths of the earth's surface is covered with water. Water is also found below the earth's surface. It is present in air in the form of water vapor. The bodies of all plants and animals contain water.

One cannot imagine a life without water. For example, in absence of water in human body: muscles will refuse to function, food will not be digested, elimination of waste and the building of new tissue would stop and regulation of body temperature will be disturbed. Therefore, water is the most essential component of the human life. About 2–2.5 liters of water is lost daily by excretion, respiration and perspiration and equal amount of water is required by the human body to avoid fluid imbalance. This requirement must be met through about 1.5 liters of beverages and fluids and 0.8 liters of water obtained from food substances.

Sources of Water

The natural sources of the water are rainwater, oceans, rivers, lakes, streams, ponds and springs. Dams, wells, tube wells, hand-pumps, canals, etc. are man-made sources of water.

- **Rainwater:** Rainwater collects on the earth in the form of surface water and underground water.
- **Surface water:** Water present on the surface of the earth in the form of oceans, rivers, lakes, ponds and streams is called surface water. The water in rivers and lakes comes from rain and melting of snow on mountains.
- **Underground water:** Some of the rainwater seeps through the soil on to the non-porous rocks below. This is underground water. Sometimes due to high pressure, this water sprouts out in the form of springs. It can be obtained by digging wells, sinking tube wells, etc.

  The main sources of water for a human being are drinking water and beverages like tea, coffee and alcohol drinks. Water is also present in many other foods like meat and fish. Fruits, green vegetables are rich in water. Almost all the foods contain water except those high in fat content like butter and dry foods like flour, sugar, etc.
- *Ice glacier:* Snowfalls when accumulated over time form glaciers. Over time, glaciers advance and retreat. Glaciers are perennial ice features that temporarily store freshwater at the higher altitudes and latitudes of Earth. Glacier meltwater and runoff contribute to and module downstream water flow.

Properties of Water

The importance and practical applicability of any compound is naturally dependent on its properties. The role played by water as liquid water, ice, and water vapor in living organisms is of such immense importance that it is essential to know its properties.

Physical properties: Following are the basic physical properties of the water:

- *Nature:* Pure water is a colorless, tasteless and odorless liquid. Distilled water is pure. Drinking water has a pleasant taste because dissolved minerals and air in water make it taste better.
- *States:* Pure water exists in all three states as solid (ice), liquid (water), and gaseous (steam or water vapor).
- *Freezing point of water:* Pure water freezes to solid ice at 0°C (at 760 mm of mercury pressure). If water contains impurities, it freezes at a temperature less than 0°C. The presence of impurities lowers the freezing point. Also, at a higher pressure, water freezes at a temperature slightly less than 0°C. That is why, on mountains (at a lower atmospheric pressure), water freezes at a temperature slightly higher than 0°C.
- *Boiling point of water:* Pure water boils at 100°C (at 760 mm of mercury pressure). At high pressure, the boiling point is more than 100°C. When pressure is high, molecules of water vapor cannot escape easily from the surface. This is why food cooks faster in a pressure cooker. At low pressures (or on high mountains), water boils at a temperature slightly less than 100°C. This is so because water molecules are free to escape from the water surface.
- *Stable substance:* Water is a stable substance. It is broken into its components H_2 and O_2 when we heat water beyond 500°C. Alternatively, electrolysis breaks molecules of water into H_2 and O_2. During freezing and boiling, the molecules of water are not broken down.

- *Anomalous expansion:* Normally, a substance expands on heating and contracts on freezing but with water, it is just the opposite, when heated or cooled between 4°C and 0°C.
  - On cooling below 4°C, water expands and hence its volume increases. So, the volume of ice at 0°C is greater than the volume of water at 0°C. Water contracts from 0°C to 4°C and then expands as usual with rise in temperature.
  - On heating water at 0°C, water contracts, and hence its volume decreases. This happens up to 4°C. On freezing water, its volume increases by about 10%.
- *Density:* The density of solid water, i.e., ice is lower than the density of liquid water at room temperature. That is why ice cubes float in water. Hence, it is lighter than water. The density of a substance is defined as its mass per unit volume mathematically; pure water has the maximum density at 4°C and minimum density at 0°C. Ice is lighter and floats on water.
  - Hence, pure water has a minimum volume at 4°C and maximum volume at 0°C. Very cool water at around 4°C is the most packed arrangement.
  - It means that for the same mass of ice and water, the volume of ice is more than that of water. In other words, the size of water increases on solidification while mass remains the same.
  - Therefore, water expands in volume when it is solidified to ice. But with ghee or oil, it is just the opposite; they expand on heating and contract on freezing. Normally 1 cm^3 (c.c.) of water has a mass of 1 gram. That is, the density of water is 1 gram/cm^3.
- *Heat capacity of water:* The heat capacity of a substance is the heat required to raise its temperature by one degree. The heat capacity of water is the highest among all liquids.
- *A good solvent:* Water is an excellent solvent. It dissolves many substances forming aqueous solutions. Therefore, it is known as a 'universal' solvent. A solution of a substance in water is known as an aqueous solution [aqueous means watery].
- *Poor conductor of heat and electricity:* water does not conduct heat and electricity well.
- Regulating the temperature of the surroundings is yet another function served by a large body of water such as lake or pond. Water has unique ability to absorb large amounts of heat from its surroundings during summer and yet dose not allow its temperature to rise very much. Similarly, in the winters, it releases stored heat to the surroundings to keep it warm. Thus, water may be said to function as nature's air conditioner.

Chemical properties: Following are the basic chemical properties of the water:
- Water is a very stable compound. Even on heating to a temperature of 250°C, only a small amount of steam is split into oxygen and hydrogen molecules. The covalent bonding in water molecules is not easily disrupted. However, on passing an electric current through water (a process known as electrolysis), to which few drops of an acid are added, it is readily broken down to molecules of oxygen and hydrogen.
- Metals that are very reactive, such as sodium, potassium, and calcium, combine with water, even at room temperature (25°C), and displace hydrogen from it. Less reactive metals, magnesium, zinc, iron, etc. displace hydrogen on reacting with steam. However, silver and gold do not react even with steam.
- Water is an essential participant (as a reactant) in an important chemical reaction on hydrolysis (hydrolysis means breakage of a substance using water).
  - Hydrolysis is of extreme importance in living cells, where many complex substances are broken down into simpler substances with the help of water. For example, a reaction involving the breakdown of cane sugar by acid or digestive enzyme.

- Digestion of major food components such as carbohydrates, proteins, and fats occurs through hydrolysis with the help of different enzymes.

❖ Water reacts with oxides (compound formed by a metal or nonmetal on combining with oxygen) of metals and nonmetals to give bases and acids.

Types of Water

Basically water is classified under two broad categories, i.e., hard water and soft water; details are discussed as follows:

❖ **Hard water:** Water is rarely pure since many types of substances are dissolved in it. The presence of certain inorganic salts renders the water hard. Hard water does not give lather readily with soap, whereas soft water readily forms leather with soap. Inorganic salts responsible for hardness of water are bicarbonates of calcium and magnesium; sulfates of calcium and magnesium and chlorides of calcium and magnesium. Use of hard water results in:
  - Deposition of insoluble inorganic compounds formed with soap on utensils and clothes.
  - Deposition of inorganic impurities inside pipes and boilers in which it is heated.
  - Toughening of food cooked in it.
  - Consumption of more food for leather formation.

❖ **Soft water:** Soft water is the water without presence of any dissolved impurity also called as pure water. The soft water is considered good for drinking if it is potable. However, practically, it is generally not possible to get the soft water readily available for drinking purpose. Therefore, available hard water is converted to soft water for drinking purposes. The temporary hard water is converted to soft water by just simple boiling because calcium/magnesium bicarbonates are precipitated as insoluble carbonates. However, permanent hard water is softened by adding washing soda (sodium carbonate), lime (calcium hydroxide) and washing soda mixture, ammonia, sodium hydroxide, sodium tetraborate (borax) and trisodium phosphate, etc **(Table 2.1)**.

Table 2.1: Difference between hard water and soft water.

Hard water	Soft water
It is rich in minerals	Contains very few elements
Soap is not so effective	Soap is easily effective
No foam and lather from soaps	Bubbly lather from soaps
Leaves spots on the washed dishes after they are dried	Does not leave any spots on dishes after they are dried
Contains minerals like magnesium and calcium	Contains sodium ion
Sometimes preferred drinking water	Sometimes not preferred drinking water
Example: Groundwater like deep wells	Example: Rainwater
Hair and skin become dry	Hair and skin become soft

Body Water Distribution

Approximately 60% of lean human body mass in man, 50% in women and 80% in newborn is water **(Fig. 2.1)**: two thirds of total body water is located inside the cell as intracellular fluid (ICF) and one third is extracellular fluid (ECF). The ECF is further divided into and 25% intravascular fluid and 75% interstitial fluid **(Fig. 2.2)**.

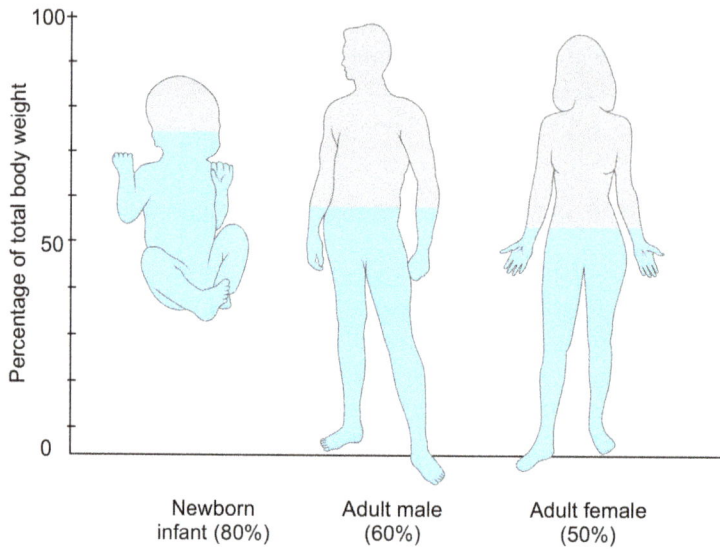

Fig. 2.1: Proportion of water in human body.

Fig. 2.2: Body fluid distribution in human body.

Body Fluid Compartments

Body fluid is present in different compartments as discussed below **(Figs. 2.2 and 2.3)**:
- **Intracellular fluids:** The amount of water present inside the cell is called as intracellular fluid. It forms about two-thirds of total body water and thus contributes nearly 40% of the total body weight.

Fig. 2.3: Distribution of total body fluid.

- **Extracellular fluid:** The extracellular fluid is the amount of water present outside the cell. It forms about one-third of the total body fluid and 20% of the total body weight. Extracellular fluid is further categorized in following subtypes:
  - *Interstitial fluid:* The fluid circulating between the cells is called as intracellular fluid. It forms about two-thirds of the total extracellular fluid and 15% of the total body weight.
  - *Plasma:* The amount of the fluid circulating in the blood vessels; popularly it is also known as intravascular fluid; which constitutes 25% of the total extracellular fluid and 5% of the total body weight.
- **Lymph:** Lymphatic fluid is the amount of fluid which is circulated in the lymphatic circulation. Generally, it is also categorized under intravascular fluid.
- **Transcellular fluid:** The transcellular fluid is that which represents all those body fluids, which are formed by the secretion of the epithelial cells. This fluid is contained within epithelial lined space and includes cerebrospinal, pleural, pericardial, peritoneal, intraocular, synovial, and gastrointestinal fluids.

Functions of Water in Human Body

Functions of water are very important and diverse too, both to nature and to the living organisms. These include:
- Maintaining the body temperature by repeated sweating, evaporation, and condensation.
- Keeping the protoplasm (cell contents) in a solution state to aid chemical changes.
- Providing a proper degree of dilution to the fluids that bathe the cells.
- Transporting food components into the cell and waste products out of it in a fluid medium, i.e., through blood and urine.
- Regulating the body temperature through respiration.
- Lubricating the mucous membranes and joints.
- Being the major component of the digestive juices secreted by different glands.
- Carrying out hydrolysis of complex food components.
- Dissolving a large number of chemical components (acting as universal solvent).

WATER AND FLUID BALANCE

Fluid balance is the concept of human homeostasis in that the amount of fluid lost from the body is equal to the amount of fluid taken in. Humans can survive for 4 to 6 weeks without food, but for only a few days without water. A proper balance between its consumption and excretion is vital to prevent dehydration of living organisms.

The amount of water consumption varies with the individual, as it depends on the condition of the subject, the amount of physical exercise, and on the environmental temperature and

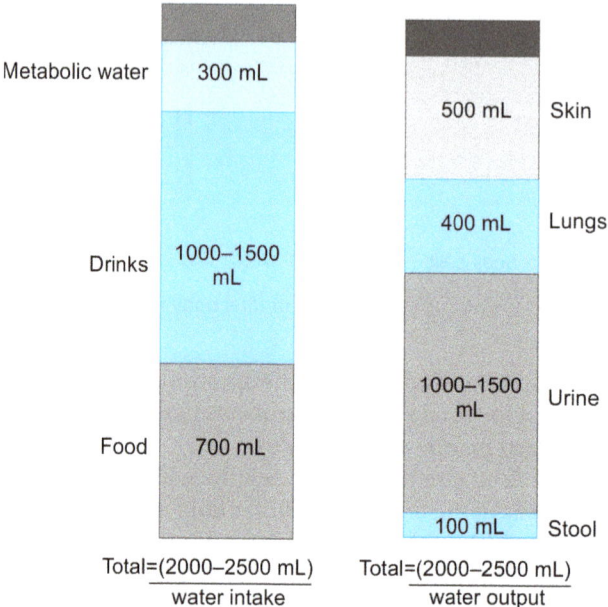

Fig. 2.4: Water and fluid balance: daily average adult water intake and output.

humidity. In the US, the reference daily intake (RDI) for water is 3.7 liters per day for human males older than 18, and 2.7 liters per day for human females older than 18 including water contained in food, beverages, and drinking water.

An adult human maintains the daily water balance through average intake and output maintained between 2000 and 2500 mL through different channels. The most common sources of intake are food (about 700 mL), fluid drinks (1000-1500 mL), and water generated in the body through metabolic activities (300 mL). Similarly, daily output is maintained through urine (1000-1500 mL), stool (100 mL), sweats through the skin (500 mL), and exhalation of water vapors through lungs (400 mL) **(Fig. 2.4)**.

Sources of Water Intake

An individual approximately ingests a total of 2000-2500 mL water per day.
- Water through ingested fluids is approximately 1000-1500 mL/day.
- Water from ingested foods 700 mL/day.
- Water from metabolic activities of the body during oxidation 300 mL/day.

Regulation of Water Input

The input of water is regulated mainly through ingested fluids, which, in turn, depends on thirst. An insufficiency of water results in an increased osmolarity in the extracellular fluid. This is sensed by osmoreceptors in the organum vasculosum of the lamina terminalis, which triggers thirst. Thirst can, to some degree, be voluntarily resisted, as during fluid restriction.

Sources of Water Loss

- The majority of fluid output occurs via the urine, approximately 1000-1500 mL/day in the normal adult resting state.

- Some fluid is lost through perspiration (part of the body's temperature control mechanism) and as water vapor in expired air. These are termed "insensible fluid losses" as they cannot be easily measured. Some sources say insensible losses account for 500 mL through skin and about 400 mL water through lungs in adults. In children, one calculation used for insensible fluid loss is 400 mL/m² body surface area.
- In addition, an adult loses approximately 100 mL/day of fluid through feces.
- These outputs are in balance with the input of 2000–2500 mL/day.

Regulation of Water Output

The body's homeostatic control mechanisms, which maintain a constant internal environment, ensure that a balance between fluid gain and fluid loss is maintained. The hormones ADH (Antidiuretic hormone, also known as vasopressin) and aldosterone play a major role in this.
- If the body becomes fluid-deficient, there will be an increase in the secretion of these hormones, causing fluid to be retained by the kidneys and urine output to be reduced.
- Conversely, if fluid levels are excessive, secretion of these hormones is suppressed, resulting in less retention of fluid by the kidneys and a subsequent increase in the volume of urine produced.
- **Antidiuretic hormone:** If the body is becoming fluid-deficient, this will be sensed by osmoreceptors in the organum vasculosum of the lamina terminalis and subfornical organ. These areas project to the supraoptic nucleus and paraventricular nucleus, which contain neurons that secrete the antidiuretic hormone, vasopressin, from their nerve endings in the posterior pituitary. Thus, there will be an increase in the secretion of antidiuretic hormone, causing fluid to be retained by the kidneys and urine output to be reduced.
- **Aldosterone:** Fluid-insufficiency causes decreased perfusion of the juxtaglomerular apparatus in the kidneys. This activates the renin-angiotensin system. Among other actions, it causes renal tubules (i.e., the distal convoluted tubules and the cortical collecting ducts) to reabsorb more sodium and water from the urine. Potassium is secreted into the tubule in exchange for the sodium, which is reabsorbed. The activated renin-angiotensin system stimulates zona glomerulosa of the adrenal cortex which in turn secretes the hormone aldosterone. This hormone stimulates the reabsorption of sodium ions from distal tubules and collecting ducts. Water in the tubular lumen follows the sodium reabsorption osmotically.

■ ELECTROLYTES OF HUMAN BODY

Electrolytes are the substances that are dissolved in solution and some of their molecules split or dissociate into electrically charged atoms or ions. Chemically, electrolytes are substances that become ions in solution and acquire the capability to conduct electricity. Electrolytes are present in the human body and the balance of electrolytes in the human body is essential for the normal functioning of body cells and organs. The common electrolytes in the human body considered medically important are sodium, potassium, chloride and bicarbonates. The positively charged ions such as Na^+ and K^+ are called cations and negatively charged ions such as Cl^- and HCO_3^- are called anions. The normal levels of the essential electrolytes, i.e., sodium, potassium, calcium, magnesium, phosphorus, chlorides, and bicarbonates are depicted in **Table 2.2**.

Sodium

About 50% of the total sodium present in the human body is found in the extracellular fluids and the fluids within the blood vessels. The remaining little amount is distributed in the intracellular fluids. Sodium can be easily interchanged between bones and the extracellular fluid. Some of it

Table 2.2: Type of electrolytes with their normal values in human body.

Positively charged ions cations(+)		Negatively charged ions anions(−)	
Electrolyte	Normal plasma levels	Electrolyte	Normal plasma levels
Sodium (Na$^+$)	135–145 mEq/L	Chlorides (Cl$^-$)	98–107 mEq/L
Potassium (K$^+$)	3.5–5.1 mEq/L	Bicarbonates (HCO$_3^-$)	22–29 mEq/L
Calcium (Ca$_2^+$)	8.6–10 mg/dL	Phosphorus (HPO$_4^-$)	2.7–4.5 mg/dL
Magnesium (Mg$_2^+$)	1.6–2.6 mg/dL		

is also found in the deep regions of the long bones. Sodium is commonly available from common salt or sodium chloride. A normal blood sodium level is 135–145 milliequivalents/liter (mEq/L) or in international units, 135–145 millimoles/liter (mmol/L). Sodium regulation occurs in the kidneys. The proximal tubule is where the majority of sodium reabsorption takes place. In the distal convoluted tubule, sodium undergoes reabsorption. Sodium transport takes place via sodium-chloride symporters, which are by the action of the hormone aldosterone.

Functions of Sodium

- Sodium is the main determinant of osmolality (tonicity) since it is the major extracellular fluid cation.
- Sodium maintains normal osmotic pressure and water balance of the body as it is the principal electrolyte in extracellular fluid.
- Sodium accounts for 90% of the basic ions in the extracellular fluids and helps to maintain body neutrality by counteracting the effect of the acid-forming elements.
- Many processes in the body, especially in the brain, nervous system and muscles require electrical signals for communication. The movements are critical in generation of these electrical signals. In the transmission of nerve impulses, sodium balance is absolutely necessary within the cell and outside the cell.
- Sodium is also essential for the absorption of glucose and in the transport of other nutrients across membranes.

Daily Allowance

Sodium chloride requirements depend on climate, occupation and physical activity. On an average, 5–10 gms of salt is sufficient for an adult in a day. However, salt intake is restricted in the case of patients having high blood pressure, cardiac failure, acute and chronic renal failure.

Sources of Sodium

Sodium is found in milk, eggs, meat, fish, poultry and in vegetables such as spinach, fenugreek, pulses and cereals. The common sources of sodium are given in **Table 2.3**.

Table 2.3: Common sources of the sodium.

• Bacon	• Milk
• Butter	• Mustard
• Canned food	• Processed food, snack food
• Cheese such as cottage cheese	• Soy sauce
• Frankfurter	• Table salt
• Lunch meat	• White and whole-wheat bread

Among the electrolyte disorders, hyponatremia is the most frequent. Diagnosis is when the serum sodium level is less than 135 mmol/L. Hyponatremia has neurological manifestations. Patients may present with headaches, confusion, nausea, delirium. Hypernatremia presents when the serum sodium levels are greater than 145 mmol/L. Symptoms of hypernatremia include tachypnea, sleeping difficulty, and feeling restless. Rapid sodium corrections can have serious consequences like cerebral edema and osmotic demyelination syndrome.

Potassium

Potassium is the one of major intracellular cations (positive ion). The optimum level of potassium is essential for normal cellular function. The normal blood potassium level is 3.5–5.1 milliequivalent/liter (mEq/L) or in international units, 3.5–5.1 millimoles/liters (mmol/L). The sodium-potassium adenosine triphosphatase pump has the primary responsibility for regulating the homeostasis between sodium and potassium, which pumps out sodium in exchange for potassium, which moves into the cells. In the kidneys, the filtration of potassium takes place at the glomerulus. Potassium has wide variety of functions in human; however, the major functions includes regulation of the heartbeats and the function of the muscles. A seriously abnormal increased level of potassium (hyperkalemia) or decreased level of potassium (hypokalemia) can profoundly affect the neuromuscular system and can be potential for arrhythmia (irregularities in heartbeat), which may be extremely life-threatening.

Functions of Potassium

- Potassium is a very important mineral for the proper function of all cells, tissues, and organs in the human body.
- It is also an electrolyte, a substance that conducts electricity in the body, along with sodium, chloride, calcium, and magnesium.
- Potassium acts as cofactor for several enzymatic reactions.
- Potassium is crucial to heart function and plays a key role in skeletal and smooth muscle contraction, making it important for normal digestive and muscular function.
- Potassium also plays an important role in regulation of blood pH.

Daily Allowance

- **Adults and older:** 4.7 grams/day
- **Pregnant women:** 4.7 grams/day
- **Breastfeeding women:** 5.1 grams/day

Sources of Potassium

Many foods contain potassium, including all meat, some types of fish such as salmon, cod, and flounder, and many fruits, vegetables, and legumes. Dairy products are also good sources of potassium. The sources of potassium are deputed in **Table 2.4**.

Table 2.4: Common sources of the potassium.

Avocado	Orange
Bananas	Potatoes
Cantaloupe	Pork, beef and veal
Carrot	Raisins and spinach
Fish	Strawberries
Mushrooms	Tomatoes

Calcium

Calcium has a significant physiological role in the body. Calcium (Ca^{2+}) levels in human body are regulated, with bone acting as the major storage site. Calcium ions are released from bone into the bloodstream under controlled conditions. Calcium is transported through the bloodstream as dissolved ions or bound to proteins such as serum albumin. Parathyroid hormone secreted by the parathyroid gland regulates the reabsorption of Ca^{2+} from bone, reabsorption from the kidney and back into circulation, and increases in the activation of vitamin D_3 to calcitriol. Calcitriol, the active form of vitamin D_3, promotes absorption of calcium from the intestines and the mobilization of calcium ions from bone matrix. Calcitonin secreted from the parafollicular cells of the thyroid gland also affects calcium levels by opposing parathyroid hormone; however, its physiological significance in humans is dubious. Calcium is stored in intracellular organelles that constantly accumulate Ca^{2+} ions and release them during certain cellular events. Intracellular Ca^{2+} storages include mitochondria and the endoplasmic reticulum.

Functions of Calcium

- Calcium (Ca^{2+}) plays a important role in the physiology and biochemistry of organisms and the cell. It plays an important role in signal transduction pathways, where it acts as a second messenger, during neurotransmitter release from neurons, contraction of all muscle cell types, and fertilization.
- Many enzymes require calcium ions as a cofactor. Those of the blood-clotting cascade being notable examples.
- Calcium is required to regulate permeability of capillary walls and excitability of the nerve fibers.
- Extracellular calcium is also important for maintaining the potential difference across excitable cell membranes, as well as proper bone formation.

Daily Allowance

An adult requires about 800–1200 mg/day calcium for the normal body functioning. Age-wise requirement of the calcium is given in **Table 2.5**.

Sources of Calcium

The main sources of calcium are depicted in **Table 2.6**.

Magnesium

Magnesium is the second most abundant element inside human cells and the fourth most abundant positively charged ion in the human body. Within the body's cells, it serves literally

Table 2.5: Age-group-wise requirement of calcium.

Age	Daily requirement of calcium (mg/day)
1–3 years	700
4-8 years	1000
9–18 years	1300
19–50 years (female)	1000
20–70 years (male)	1000
Over 50 years (female)	1200
Over 70 years (male)	1200

Table 2.6: Common sources of the calcium.	
Dairy foods	Milk, cheese, soya milk, yogurt and other dairy products
Leafy green vegetables	Broccoli, kale, spinach
Fruits	Oranges
Beans and peas	Tofu, peanuts, peas, black beans, baked beans
Fish	Salmon, sardines
Miscellaneous	Sesame seeds, blackstrap molasses, corn tortillas, almonds, brown sugar

hundreds of functions. Magnesium is an intracellular cation. Magnesium is mainly involved in ATP metabolism, contraction and relaxation of muscles, proper neurological functioning, and neurotransmitter release.

Magnesium is a macromineral, which, unlike trace minerals, is needed by the body in large amounts; calcium, sodium, and potassium are also macrominerals. The average human body contains about 25 grams of magnesium, one of the six essential minerals that must be supplied in the diet.

Once magnesium enters the body through food, supplements, or topical applications, it is broken down and released to form independent magnesium atoms, or "ions". In its ionic form, magnesium has a positive charge, commonly noted as Mg^{2+}.

Magnesium cations function as a part of the structure of the body through their presence in bone. But arguably more important is their function as cell regulators in hundreds of chemical reactions throughout the body.

Functions of Magnesium

- Magnesium's role is primarily regulatory. It allows enzymes to function properly, which in turn enable a vast majority of the body's chemical reactions.
- Magnesium is an essential ingredient of the energy-production process that occurs inside the tiny structures within cells.
- DNA stability is dependent in part on magnesium. Magnesium not only stabilizes DNA structures, it also functions as a cofactor in the repair of DNA damage by environmental mutagens. Combined with ATP, magnesium also assists in the healthy production of RNA, responsible for "reading" DNA and manufacturing the proteins used in our body.
- Magnesium's role in homeostasis of important minerals such as calcium, sodium and potassium affects the conduction of nerve impulses, muscle contraction, and heart rhythms.
- The effect of magnesium on blood vessels is one of dilation, whereas calcium promotes contraction.
- Magnesium is also thought to antagonize calcium promotion of blood clotting.

Daily Allowance

An adult requires about 300–400 mg/day magnesium for the normal body functioning.

Sources of Magnesium

Spinach, broccoli, almonds, cashews, and peanuts, barley, oat bran, and brown rice, whole wheat grain, skimmed milk and yogurt, bananas, raisins, fish, kidney beans and soybeans, cocoa and coffee are good sources of magnesium.

Phosphorus

Phosphorus is a mineral that is part of every cell in our body. It is an extracellular fluid cation. It is found mainly in bones and teeth. Phosphate (HPO_4) is obtained from phosphorus (HPO_3) in two forms, i.e., as inorganic phosphorus and organic phosphorus. Inorganic phosphorus in the form of the phosphate PO^{3-} is required for all known forms of life playing a major role in biological molecules such as DNA and RNA where it forms part of the structural framework of these molecules. Living cells also use phosphate to transport cellular energy in the form of adenosine triphosphate (ATP).

Phosphorus imbalance may result due to three processes: dietary intake, gastrointestinal disorders, and excretion by the kidneys

Functions of Phosphorus

- Phosphorus is needed for healthy bones and teeth, energy metabolism, and acid-base balance in the body.
- Inorganic phosphate as well as organic esters of phosphate such as ADP, glucose-6 phosphate are necessary for metabolism of carbohydrates.
- Phosphorus works with calcium and other nutrients to build healthy bones and teeth.
- Phosphorus also helps maintain normal acid/base balance, supports growth, and is involved in the storage and use of energy.

Daily Allowance

An adult requires about 800–1200 mg/day phosphorus for the normal body functioning.

Sources of Phosphorus

The main food sources for phosphorus are foods containing protein, although proteins do not contain phosphorus. For example, milk, meat, and soya typically also have phosphorus. Milk, grains, lean meats and food additives are rich source of phosphorus.

Chloride

Chloride is an anion found predominantly in the extracellular fluid. Chloride plays a role in helping the body maintain a normal balance of fluids. The balance of chloride ion is closely regulated by the body. Significant increase or decrease in chloride can have deleterious or even fatal consequences. The normal serum range of chloride is 98–107 mEq/L. Chloride is to found in many chemicals and other substances in the body. It is an important part of the salt found in many foods and used in cooking. Chloride is needed to keep the proper balance of body fluids. It is an essential part of digestive (stomach) juices. The kidneys predominantly regulate serum chloride levels. Most of the chloride, which is filtered by the glomerulus, is reabsorbed by both proximal and distal tubules (majorly by proximal tubule) by both active and passive transport. Hyperchloremia can occur due to gastrointestinal bicarbonate loss. Hypochloremia presents in gastrointestinal losses like vomiting or excess water gain like congestive heart failure.

Functions of Chloride

- Chloride is essential for the proper fluid balance in the body through maintaining osmotic pressure.
- It is also an important component of the HCl of gastric juices.
- Chloride is also essentially important in maintaining the acid-base balance of the body.

Daily Allowance

Infants
- **0–6 months:** 0.18 grams/day
- **7–12 months:** 0.57 grams/day

Children
- **1–3 years:** 1.5 grams/day
- **4–8 years:** 1.9 grams/day
- **9–13 years:** 2.3 grams/day

Adolescents and Adults
- **Males and females age 14–50 years:** 2.3 grams/day
- **Males and females 51–70:** 2.0 grams/day
- **Males and females 71 and over:** 1.8 grams/day

Sources of Chloride

Chloride is found in table salt or sea salt as sodium chloride. It is also found in many vegetables. Foods with higher amounts of chloride include seaweed, rye, tomatoes, lettuce, celery, and olives.

Some of the common causes of electrolyte disorders seen in clinical practices are:
- **Hyponatremia:** Low dietary sodium intake, primary polydipsia, SIADH, congestive heart failure, hepatic cirrhosis, failure of adrenal glands, hyperglycemia, dyslipidemia
- **Hypernatremia:** Unreplaced fluid loss through the skin and gastrointestinal tract, osmotic diuresis, hypertonic saline administration
- **Hypokalemia:** Hyperaldosteronism, loop diuretics
- **Hyperkalemia:** Increases release from cells as in metabolic acidosis, insulin deficiency, beta-blocker or decreased potassium excretion as in acute or chronic kidney disease, aldosterone deficiency or resistance
- **Hypercalcemia:** Malignancy, hyperparathyroidism, chronic granulomatous disease
- **Hypocalcemia:** Acute pancreatitis, parathyroid hormone deficiency after thyroidectomy, neck dissection, resistance to parathormone, hypomagnesemia, sepsis
- **Hypermagnesemia:** Increases oral magnesium intake
- **Hypomagnesemia:** Renal losses as in diuretics, alcohol use disorder, or GI losses as in diarrhea
- **Bicarbonate level:** Increases in primary metabolic alkalosis or compensation to primary respiratory acidosis—decreases in primary metabolic acidosis or compensation to primary respiratory alkalosis.
- **Hyperchloremia:** Normal saline infusion
- **Hypochloremia:** GI loss as in diarrhea, renal losses with diuretics
- **Hypophosphatemia:** Refeeding syndrome, vitamin D deficiency, hyperparathyroidism
- **Hyperphosphatemia:** Hypoparathyroidism, chronic kidney disease

ACIDS

Acids are compounds made-up of hydrogen and a nonmetal. All water-soluble acids give hydrogen ions. Many of our foods contain acids and they are constantly forming in the body. The gastric juice and the urine are acid fluids.

Table 2.7: Types of organic and inorganic acids.

Inorganic acids	Organic acids
Hydrochloric acid (HCl)	Acetic acid in vinegar
Nitric acid	Citric acid in lemons
Sulfuric acid	Lactic acid in sour milk
Carbonic acid	Tartaric acid in sour grapes
Boric acid	

Classification of Acids

- These are organic and inorganic **(Table 2.7)**. All of the organic compounds contain carbon and they are often derived from plant and animal sources. Organic acids are weak.
- The important inorganic acids are known as mineral acids.
- Hydrogen is an essential constituent of all acids.

Properties of Acids

Following are the basic properties of the acids:
- **Sour taste:** When acids dissolve in water, they impart a sour taste to the water. For example, sour taste of lemons, oranges, grapes is due to citric acid.
- **Action on indicators:** Many colored compounds change color in the presence of acids. So these are used as a indicator for detecting acids, e.g. blue litmus dye which changes to red color in the presence of an acid.
- **Action on certain metals:** When active metals such as Na, Mg or Zn placed in acid solutions, they react chemically and hydrogen gas is usually liberated. Because of this corrosive action the acids are kept in glass containers.
- **Action on oxides and hydroxides:** Many acids react with the oxides and hydroxides of metals. Neutralization is a useful reaction for counteracting the action of an acid or a base.
- **Action on carbonates and bicarbonates:** Whenever an acid solution comes into contact with a carbonate or a bicarbonate, effervescence comes out due to evolution of carbon dioxide gas.
- **Action on tissues:** The physiological action of strong concentrated acids upon the tissue is to destroy the tissue through corrosive action. But very diluted acids only extract water from tissues.

Antidotes for Acids

- Mild alkaline substances liking baking soda, lime water, milk of magnesia may be used as effective antidotes for mineral acid poisoning.
- To counteract the action of an acid spilled upon the clothing or skin is to remove the acid by use of running water.
- The remaining acid may be neutralized by very dilute ammonium hydroxide.

Functions and Importance of Acids to Nurses

Inorganic Acids

- **Hydrochloric acid:** Antiseptic by destroying fermentation of bacteria in intestinal tract.
- **Nitric acid:** Coagulant in testing for albumin in the urine.

- **Hypochlorus:** Disinfectant, antiseptic, and bleaching agent.
- **Boric acid:** Antiseptic for inflamed mucous membrane in eyes, nose, or mouth.

Organic Acid
- **Acetic acid:** Removes insoluble soaps and nits from the hair.
- **Citric acid:** In form of citrate of magnesia, as a laxative.
- **Lactic acid:** Checks growth of putrefying bacteria in the large intestine.
- **Salicyclic acid:** In form of salicylate, as an antiseptic.
- **Tartaric acid:** As salt in some effervescent salts and baking powder.

BASES
- Bases are compounds madeup of a metallic element and a hydroxyl radical (OH). The stronger bases are referred to as alkalis or as caustics. The chemical behavior of bases is the opposite of acids.
- A base is a compound that furnishes hydroxyl ions as the only negative ions in water solution.

Properties of Bases
Following are the basic properties of the bases:
- **Soapy feeling:** Whenever a strong base is dissolved in water, the solution feels slippery or soapy.
- **Bitter taste:** Bases generally have bitter test, when touched to the tongue.
- **Action on indicators:** Bases reverse the color change that acids produce with indicators. Bases turn red litmus paper blue.
- **Reaction with acids:** Reaction with acids to form salts. This is a very important function in the body, for maintaining the alkaline reaction in the blood.
- **Action on tissues:** Bases react with fats to form soaps. Strong bases destroy tissues by attracting the water, dissolving the albumin, and reacting with the fats. Bacteria are destroyed in the same matter.
- They are given to dilute the concentrated hydrochloric acid found in the stomach. For example, gastric ulcer, duodenal ulcer, and sometimes in carcinoma cases.
- They are used for removing certain stains.
- The property of dissolving albumin and reacting with fats makes basic acting substances very useful as cleansing agents, e.g. ammonia and washing soda.

Examples of Bases
Examples of bases are given in **Table 2.8**.

Table 2.8: Examples of bases.

Chemical name	Formula	Common name
Sodium hydroxide	NaOH	Caustic soda
Potassium hydroxide	KOH	Caustic potash
Ammonium hydroxide	NH_4OH	Ammonia water
Calcium hydroxide	$Ca(OH)_2$	Lime water
Magnesium hydroxide	$Mg(OH)_2$	Milk of magnesia

Antidotes for Bases

- To neutralize strong bases, taken internally, weak acids like those present in citrus juices, sour milk are used.
- Lime water and a solution of baking soda are used internally to combat hyperacidity.
- As in the cases of acids, when strong bases are spilled on clothing or skin, they should be removed immediately by washing in running water before attempting to neutralize it with any dilute acid.

Functions of Bases

- **NaOH:** It is used as a household article as a drastic cleanser because it reacts with grease to make soap. Commercially, it is used in the manufacturing of hard soaps.
- **Ca(OH)$_2$:** Lime water is used in medicine to overcome high acidity in the stomach.
  - Lime water is used in the diet for building bones and teeth.
  - It serves as a special antidote for oxalic acid poisoning.
- **NH$_4$OH:** It has weekly basic properties. In medicine, ammonium hydroxide is used as a heart respiratory stimulant.
- **Mg(OH)$_2$:** In medicine, a thick suspension known as milk of magnesia is used as an antacid. Magnesium compound is a laxative in its physiological action.

SALTS

Salts play a far more important part in our bodies than either bases or acids. They are essential for both animal and plant tissues. Salts are also of great importance in the household and in industry.

Neutralization

The reaction between an acid and a salt, where salt and water are formed, is known as neutralization.

$$NaOH + HCl \longrightarrow NaCl + H_2O$$

Salt is a compound containing the negative radical of an acid and the positive radical of a base.

Incompatibility of Salts

It is seen by the precipitation or by a change in color or anything which shows a chemical change has taken place.
- For example, two soluble salts may react to form an insoluble salt.

$$AgNO_3 + NaCl \longrightarrow AgCl + NaNO_3$$

  - Silver chloride is an insoluble salt. Silver nitrate is used in bladder infections. The germicidal action of the silver nitrate is stopped, since the sodium chloride in the urine reacts with silver nitrate to form insoluble silver chloride.
- Two salts may react to form new salts with different properties causing harm.
  - Never give two medicines together if they form a precipitate.

BUFFER ACTION IN THE HUMAN BODY

The process of digestion and cell activity produces numerous substances which enter the bloodstream. These substances may be acidic, some alkaline and other neutral, the blood maintains a remarkably constant pH, which ranges normally from 7.35 to 7.45. This constancy of hydrogen ion concentration is possible because of the presence of certain molecules and related ions in the blood, which act as buffers, i.e., shock absorbers.

Proper physiological functioning depends on the balance between the concentrations of acids and bases in the blood. A variety of buffering systems permits blood and other bodily fluids to maintain a narrow pH range, even in the face of perturbations. A buffer is a chemical system that prevents a radical change in fluid pH by dampening the change in hydrogen ion concentrations in the case of excess acid or base. Most commonly, the substance that absorbs the ions is either a weak acid, which takes up hydroxyl ions, or a weak base, which takes up hydrogen ions.

Buffers in the Body

Buffers are the fast-acting regulatory systems that function only to keep the pH within narrow limits of stability when too much acid or base is released into the system. The different buffer systems acting in our body are:

Primary Buffer Systems

- **Hemoglobin system:** The red blood cells in the human body contain hemoglobin. Hemoglobin is the principal protein inside of red blood cells and accounts for one-third of the mass of the cell. During the conversion of CO_2 into bicarbonate, hydrogen ions liberated in the reaction are buffered by hemoglobin, which is reduced by the dissociation of oxygen. This system works on the phenomenon of 'chloride shift'. Chloride shifts in response to changes in the level of oxygen in the blood. For each chloride ion that enters the cell, a bicarbonate ion leaves, and vice versa.
- **Plasma proteins system:** Nearly all proteins can function as buffers. Proteins are made up of amino acids, which contain positively charged amino groups and negatively charged carboxyl groups. The system works along with the liver to vary the number of hydrogen ions in the chemical structure of the protein. In acidic pH, proteins act as a base, NH_2 group accepts hydrogen ions and becomes NH_3. While during alkalinity reverse happens. ^-COOH group of proteins dissociates and forms H^+ and COO^-. H^+ combines with ^-OH to produce water.
- **Bicarbonate system:** Bicarbonate is the main buffer system in ECF such as blood plasma. The system maintains pH of 7.4 with a ratio of 20 parts of bicarbonate and 1 part carbonic acid. This ratio determines the hydrogen ion concentration of body fluid. Carbonic ion concentration is controlled by the excretion of carbon dioxide by the lungs, the rate and depth of respiration changes in response to changes in carbon dioxide. The kidney controls the bicarbonate concentration and selectively retains or secrete bicarbonates in response to body needs.

$$NaHCO_3 + HCl \rightarrow H_2CO_3 + NaCl$$
(sodium bicarbonate) + (strong acid) → (weak acid) + (salt)

$$H_2CO_3 + NaOH \rightarrow HCO_{3^-} + H_2O$$
(weak acid) + (strong base) → (bicarbonate) + (water)

- **Phosphate buffer system:** The phosphate buffer has a far higher concentration in intracellular fluids than in extracellular fluids and has a high buffering capacity inside the cells. This system is especially active in the kidneys. The system acts like bicarbonate and clears spare hydrogen ions. When a strong acid enters the blood, it is reacted with Na_2HPO_4, as follows:

$$Na_2HPO_4 + HCl \longrightarrow NaH_2PO_4 + NaCl$$

- The end product thus produced is excreted in the urine.
- When alkali enters, it reacts with Na_2HPO_4, as follows:

$$Na_2HPO_4 + NaOH \longrightarrow NaH_2PO_4 + H_2O$$

The end product thus produced is excreted in the urine.

Lungs

- The lungs are the second defense of the body and interact with the buffer system to maintain acid–base balance (*refer* **Fig. 2.1**).
- In acidosis, the pH decreases and respiratory rate and depth increase in an attempt to exhale acids, the carbonic acid created by the neutralization action of bicarbonate can be carried to the lungs, where it is reduced to carbon dioxide and water and exhaled, thus hydrogen ions are inactivated and excreted.
- In alkalosis the pH increases and respiratory rate and depth decrease, the carbon dioxide is retained and carbonic acid builds to neutralize and decrease the strength of excess bicarbonate.

Flowchart 2.1: Role of lungs in maintaining the acid-base balance.

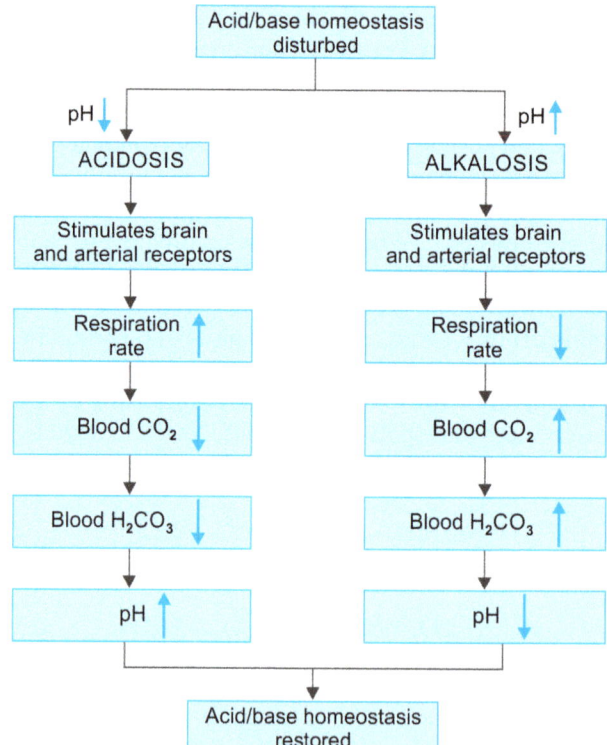

Kidneys

The pH of blood plasma is kept within normal limits by controlling the excretion of H^+ ions in the urine and the reabsorption of bicarbonate into the blood plasma. If acid is excreted in the urine, it is in effect removed from the blood when an equal quantity of bicarbonate is added to the blood. Bicarbonate (as a base) neutralizes hydrogen ions in the blood. If the blood is too acidic, more hydrogen ions are excreted; if the blood is too basic, then fewer hydrogen ions are excreted.

$$HCO_3^- + H^+ \rightarrow H_2CO_3 \rightarrow CO_2 + H_2O$$

The renal tubules excrete hydrogen ions by an unknown series of reactions into the tubular urine. The amount of hydrogen ions excreted is controlled by the concentration of H^+ (pH), bicarbonate, and the partial pressure of CO_2 (pCO_2) in the blood plasma and by the amount of Na^+ and bicarbonate in the developing urine.

Hydrogen ions and sodium ions exchange take place throughout the formation of urine. For every H^+ which enters the urine, one sodium ion is reabsorbed from the urine into the blood and is conserved. For every H^+ ion excreted and every Na^+ ion conserved, one bicarbonate ion is also reabsorbed into the blood. The charges on sodium and bicarbonate are thus always balanced **(Fig. 2.5)**.

Normally phosphate is the only buffer in urine, although carbonic acid/bicarbonate is also present. The developing urine contains NaH_2PO_4/Na_2HPO_4 in the same concentration as present in blood plasma. Na_2HPO_4 is actually the "salt" in the following dissociation reaction:

$$H_2PO_4^- \longleftrightarrow H^+ + HPO_4^{-2}$$

In the developing urine the ratio of $H_2PO_4^-/HPO_4^{-2}$ is l:4, therefore the right side of the equilibrium is favored.

When the urine is acidified (hydrogen ions added), the increase in H^+ ion causes the equilibrium to shift left to form $H_2P_4O^-$.

Fig. 2.5: Sodium hydrogen ion exchange channel.

QUESTIONS

Q.1. Name three important chemical properties and three physical properties of water and explain how these properties affect its usefulness?
Q.2: What precautions should be taken in handling concentrated solutions of acids and bases and why?
Q.3: Write three important chemical and physical properties of water.
Q.4: What is difference between acid and base?
Q.5: Write the properties of acid and base. Write an example of acid-base neutralization on reaction.
Q.6: Discuss briefly the physiological importance of electrolytes and salts.
Q.7: What are the acids and bases? Give examples.
Q.8: What are electrolytes? What are the differences between weak electrolytes and strong electrolyte?
Q.9: What are various biologically important properties of water?
Q.10: Important blood buffers and their actions.
Q.11: What are the important physiological uses of water?
Q.12: Discuss the importance of hydrogen bounding in water.
Q.13: Write sources, properties and functions of water.

BIBLIOGRAPHY

1. Boron WF, Boulpaep EL. Medical Physiology: A Cellular and Molecular Approach. Elsevier/Saunders; 2003:867.
2. Boron WF, Boulpaep EL. The Parathyroid Glands and Vitamin D. Medical Physiology: A Cellular and Molecular Approach. Elsevier/Saunders; 2003:1094.
3. Escott-Stump S. Nutrition and Diagnosis-Related Care. 6th edition, Philadelphia, Pa: Lippincott Williams & Wilkins; 2008.
4. Institute of Medicine. Food and Nutrition Board. Dietary Reference Intakes for Water, Potassium, Sodium, Chloride, and Sulfate. Washington DC, National Academy Press;2004.
5. Larsson L, Ohman S. Serum ionized calcium and corrected total calcium in borderline hyperparathyroidism. Clin. Chem; 1978; 24 (11):1962-5.
6. Levinson W. Review of Medical Microbiology and Immunology. McGraw-Hill Medical; 2008:414.
7. National Water Commission. Australian environmental water management report. NWC, Canberra; 2000.
8. Sarubin FA, Thomson C. The Health Professional's Guide to Popular Dietary Supplements. 3rd edition. Chicago, Il: American Dietetic Association;2007.
9. Wolf AT. Water and Human Security. Journal of Contemporary Water Research and Education. 2001; 118:29.
10. Shrimanker I, Bhattarai S. Electrolytes. [Updated 2021 Jul 26]. In: StatPearls [Internet]. Treasure Island (FL): StatPearls Publishing; 2022 Jan-. Available from: https://www.ncbi.nlm.nih.gov/books/NBK541123/

CHAPTER 3

Enzymes, Digestion and Absorption

Suresh K Sharma, Navjot Kaur

Chapter Outline
- Enzymes
- Digestion and Absorption of Carbohydrates, Proteins and Fats
- Factors Influencing the Digestion and Absorption
- Malabsorption Syndrome

INTRODUCTION

The term 'enzymes' means 'in yeast'. These substances were first isolated from yeast. Much later, their chemical nature was determined. Enzymes are organic compounds produced in living organisms to speed up and regulate the rate of spontaneous biochemical reactions in and outside the cells, without themselves being used. They are also known as biocatalysts. Enzymes or biocatalyst are substances that can influence the rate of a chemical reaction but which themselves remain unchanged in quantity and chemical composition. The actual process of chemical transformation at enhanced rate is known as catalysis. The substance upon which an enzyme acts is known as substrate. The function of an enzyme is to bring about various chemical transformations at very high speeds. Usually, 1 molecule of an enzyme can act upon about 1,000 molecules of the substrate per minute. The enzyme will convert the substrate into the product.

In living systems, most chemical reactions are carried out with the help of enzymes; only a few reactions proceed spontaneously without the need of any enzyme.

CHARACTERISTICS OF ENZYMES

Some important characteristics of enzymes are:
- The enzymes remain unchanged in amount and chemical composition at the end of the reaction.
- Only a small quantity of enzyme is generally needed.
- Enzymes do not alter the position of equilibrium in a reversible reaction, it only hastens the approach to equilibrium.
- Almost all enzymes are proteins. They follow the physical and chemical properties of proteins.
- Enzymes do not initiate or begin the reaction.
- Enzymes are specific in their action.
- Enzymes usually cannot alter the nature of the product of the reaction.

- Enzymes may be poisoned by certain substances (Inhibitors).
- Enzymes are heat liable and water-soluble.
- Enzymes can be precipitated by protein-precipitating reagents (like ammonia sulfate).

MECHANISM OF ACTION

- An enzyme-catalyzed reaction is initiated when the enzyme binds to its specific substrate. This binding leads to the formation of an enzyme-substrate complex, which represents the intermediate stage in the overall reaction.
- The further reaction then occurs in this complex, which transforms the substrate into the specific product, depending on the reaction specificity of the enzyme. In the final step, the product is released and the enzyme is available for binding another molecule of the substrate, to begin the same reaction overall again.
- Globular proteins possess a highly folded three-dimensional structure. One of the major reasons why polypeptide chains fold is to generate a small region, in the form of a pocket or pouch, in which the substrate molecule can bind. This small region is called the 'active site' (**Fig. 3.1**).
- It is generally composed of a few specific amino acids having charged groups. It is these charged groups that interact with groups on the substrate molecule and help in the substrate binding.

The following theories explain the mechanism of action for the enzymes:

Lowering of Activation Energy

Enzymes lower the energy of activation. Activation energy is defined as the energy required to convert all molecules of a reacting substance from the ground state to the transition state. Substrates are remaining in an energy trough and are to be placed at the higher energy level, whereupon spontaneous degradation can occur.

Lock and Key Theory

This theory is also called Fischer's template theory as it was postulated in 1894 by Emil Fischer. The specific action of an enzyme with a single substrate can be explained using a Lock and Key analogy. In this analogy, the lock is the enzyme and the key is the substrate. This theory states that the three-dimensional structure of the active site of the enzyme is complementary to the substrate. Only the correctly sized key (substrate) fits into the keyhole (active site) of the lock (enzyme) (**Fig. 3.2**).

Fig. 3.1: Mechanism of enzyme action.

Fig. 3.2: Key and lock theory of enzyme action.

Smaller keys, larger keys, or incorrectly positioned teeth on keys (incorrectly shaped or sized substrate molecules) do not fit into the lock (enzyme). Only the correctly shaped key opens a particular lock. However, Fischer explained rigid structure for enzymes, which could not explain the flexibility shown by enzymes.

Induced Fit Theory

* Not all experimental evidence can be adequately explained by using the so-called rigid enzyme model assumed by the lock and key theory. For this reason, a modification called the induced-fit theory has been proposed. In 1958, Koshland put forward the induced fit theory.
* The induced-fit theory assumes that the substrate plays a role in determining the final shape of the enzyme and that the enzyme is partially flexible. This explains why certain compounds can bind to the enzyme but do not react because the enzyme has been distorted too much. Other molecules may be too small to induce the proper alignment and therefore cannot react. Only the proper substrate is capable of inducing the proper alignment of the active site.
* In the figure given below (**Fig. 3.3**), the substrate is represented by the magenta molecule, B^1 and B^2 the enzyme protein is represented by the A^1. The cyan-colored protein is used to more sharply define the active site. The protein chains are flexible and fit around the substrate.

Fig. 3.3: Induced fit theory of enzyme action.

FACTORS AFFECTING ENZYME ACTIVITY

Factors that influence the activity status of an enzyme are:

- **Substrate concentration:** In an enzyme-catalyzed reaction, the substrate molecules are always in excess of the enzyme molecules. The reason is enzymes being catalysts, can be used over and over again, as they are not consumed in the reaction. The rate of reaction increases with an increase in substrate concentration, reaches a maximum value and thereafter remains constant. At a lower concentration of substrate, some enzyme molecules are remaining idle. As the substrate is increased, more and more enzyme molecules are working. At half-maximal velocity, 50% of enzymes are attached to the substrate. As more substrate is added, all enzyme molecules are saturated. Further increase in the substrate cannot make any effect on reaction velocity.
- **Enzyme concentration:** The reaction rate or velocity is directly proportional to the concentration of the enzyme when sufficient substrate is present. It happens so up to a particular concentration of the enzyme which is enough to bind all the available substrate and convert it into the product. Any further increase in the concentration of the enzyme does not alter the reaction rate.
- **Temperature:** At a very low temperature, the enzyme is not very active. Hence the rate of reaction is not high. However, as the temperature is raised, the rate of reaction also shows an upward trend. It reaches a maximum and then begins to fall rapidly. Enzymes in the human body are optimally active at 37°C.
- **pH of the medium:** The rate of a reaction increases slowly with an increase in pH, reaches a maximum and finally declines again slowly. The optimum pH for many enzymes is 7.0 to 9.0. Optimum pH may vary depending on the temperature, concentration of substrate, presence of ions, etc.
- **Effect of water:** The enzyme activity will be suppressed in the absence of water. Water is necessary for enzyme activity, because (a) water provides a medium for enzyme activity to take place (b) in many cases, it is one of the reactants.
- **Effect of radiation:** UV radiation either destroys or modifies the action of enzymes. Purified enzymes are more easily destroyed by light rays than the same enzymes in less purified preparations.
- **Effect of metals:** The enzyme activity may increase or sometimes may be dependent on certain metal and inorganic ions. Certain enzymes are activated by metallic ions, e.g., Mg, Mn, etc.
- **Effect of heavy metals:** Many enzymes are inactivated by heavy metals such as silver, copper and mercury. The inactivated enzymes may be reactivated by treatment with hydrogen sulfide to precipitate the metals.
- **Effect of inhibitors:** The presence of inhibitors in the reaction mixture inhibits the activity of the enzymes partially or completely depending upon the nature of inhibitors. Inhibitors are less effective when the concentration of the enzyme and the substrate is higher. Inhibitors are of three types:
    a. *Competitive inhibitors* have structural similarities with the substrate both of which compete for the same active site of the enzyme. The effective concentration of enzymes is reduced, the reaction velocity is decreased. This inhibition is reversible when the inhibitor is removed or substrate concentration is increased.
    b. *Non-competitive inhibitors* are usually poisons like heavy metals (lead, mercury) that destroy the structure of the enzyme and cause irreversible inhibition of enzyme activity.

c. *Allosteric inhibitors* bind to the enzyme at a site other than the active site and can either enhance the activity of enzymes (allosteric activation) or reduce the activity of the enzyme (allosteric inhibition).

SPECIFICITY OF ENZYMES

One of the properties of enzymes that makes them so important as diagnostic and research tools is the specificity they exhibit relative to the reactions they catalyze. A few enzymes exhibit absolute specificity; that is, they will catalyze only one particular reaction. Other enzymes will be specific for a particular type of chemical bond or functional group. In general, there are four distinct types of specificity:

a. **Absolute specificity:** The enzyme will catalyze only one reaction. For example, hydrolysis of urea to ammonia and carbon dioxide is catalyzed by urease. Urea is the only substrate to urease.
b. **Group specificity:** The enzyme will act only on molecules that have specific functional groups, such as amino, phosphate and methyl groups, e.g., hexokinase can catalyze the phosphorylation of glucose, galactose and mannose.
c. **Linkage specificity:** The enzyme will act on a particular type of chemical bond regardless of the rest of the molecular structure. It is also called bond specificity.
d. **Stereochemical specificity:** The enzyme will act on a particular steric or optical isomer. Though enzymes exhibit great degrees of specificity, cofactors may serve many apoenzymes. For example, nicotinamide adenine dinucleotide (NAD) is a coenzyme for a great number of dehydrogenase reactions in which it acts as a hydrogen acceptor. Among them are the alcohol dehydrogenase, malate dehydrogenase and lactate dehydrogenase reactions.
e. **Chirality:** Enzymes can also recognize specific chiral centers. For example, glycerol kinase phosphorylates glycerol only at the 3rd carbon and never at the first carbon.

NAMING AND CLASSIFICATION OF ENZYMES

When enzymes were isolated initially, they were given whimsical names like Pepsin, trypsin, chymotrypsin, etc. and are still in use. Later it was agreed to call enzymes by adding the suffix–"ase" to the substrate, e.g., Lactase acts on lactose and the products formed are glucose and galactose. Enzymes that hydrolyze starch (amylose) are called amylase. These are known as trivial names of enzymes.

According to the International Union of Biochemistry and molecular biology (IUBMB), there are six classes of enzymes:

Class 1: Oxidoreductases: This type of enzymes will catalyze oxidation of one substrate with simultaneous reduction of another substrate or coenzyme.

Class 2: Transferases: This class of enzymes transfers one group from the substrate to the another substrate.

Class 3: Hydrolases: This class of enzymes can hydrolyze ester, ether, peptide or glycosidic bonds by adding water and then breaking the bond.

Class 4: Lyases: These enzymes can remove groups from substrates or break bonds by mechanisms other than hydrolysis.

Class 5: Isomerases: These enzymes can produce optical, geometric or positional isomers of substrates.

Class 6: Ligases: These enzymes link two substrates together, usually with the simultaneous hydrolysis of ATP.

DIAGNOSTIC APPLICATIONS

Enzymes are synthesized in the cells, where many of them perform their catalytic function. However, some enzymes are also released into circulating blood. Enzymes in the blood are of two types:

1. **Functional enzymes:** These enzymes take part in blood clotting and clot dissolution, etc. carryout their normal functions, as their substrates are present. These enzymes are in circulation at all times in normal individuals and in comparable concentration to those in cells.
2. **Nonfunctional enzymes:** They occur in extremely low level (usually not detectable) in blood in normal individuals. They have no known function in blood and their substrates are usually absent.
   - However, on damage to a particular organ or tissue (where it is synthesized), these enzymes leak out to the circulating blood. Thus their levels are raised. This is the basis for estimating the levels of such enzymes in blood and using them as a diagnostic tool in clinical situations.
   - Some of the common enzymes estimated for diagnostic purposes:
     - *Liver enzymes:* The most sensitive and widely used of these liver enzymes are the aminotransferases. They include aspartate aminotransferase (AST or SGOT) and alanine aminotransferase (ALT or SGPT). These enzymes are normally contained within liver cells. If the liver is injured, the liver cells spill the enzymes into the blood, raising the enzyme levels in the blood and signalling the liver damage.
     - *Cardiac enzymes:* Current clinical practice is to measure cardiac enzymes when an MI is suspected: creatine kinase (CK). CK is released into the bloodstream 4–6 hours after heart cell damage occurs, and peak blood levels of CK are seen after 24 hours. Elevated CK levels usually, but not always, indicate heart muscle damage. CK levels sometimes can be increased with damage to other kinds of cells as well.
     - *Gastric enzymes:* Serum amylase and lipase are estimated to diagnose pancreatic diseases.

Enzymes in Other Body Fluids

Adenosine deaminase in pleural fluid: Elevated in tuberculous pleural effusion

Lactate dehydrogenase in CSF, pleural fluid, ascitic fluid: Elevated levels indicate the presence of a malignant tumor. But not diagnostic, as the enzyme is not tissue-specific.

PRECAUTIONS WHILE HANDLING ENZYME PREPARATIONS

Following safety measures are essential while handling enzyme preparations:
- **Training:** All employees and contractors working with enzyme preparations should have proper training in the safe use and handling procedures and contingency measures such as spill clean-up and equipment maintenance.
- **Safe handling practices:** Safe handling of enzyme preparations can be accomplished through proper work practices, engineering controls, and the use of protective equipment. When working with these preparations, it is important to use work practices that do not generate aerosols or that result in direct skin contact. For each work operation, careful consideration must be given to minimizing aerosol formation and skin or eye contact.
- Aerosols are formed through high-energy operations such as mixing, grinding, and washing with high water pressure or steam and using compressed air for clean-up operations. Sweeping, blowing, splashing, steam cleaning, and high-pressure water flushing must be avoided. Mixing and grinding operations should be contained as much as possible, and the areas in which they take place should be provided with adequate local exhaust ventilation.

- When handling enzyme preparations or enzyme contaminated equipment, avoid direct skin contact. Wear appropriate gloves when there is a potential for skin contact with enzymes. Wash enzyme-contaminated surfaces thoroughly before handling.
- **Use of personal protective equipment:** Following personal protection equipment are used while handling the enzyme specimens:
    - *Respiratory protection:* Under most operating conditions involving enzymes, respiratory protection is not normally necessary. There are some operations, such as spill clean-up, equipment cleaning, and equipment repairing, that may generate aerosols. In these instances, respiratory protection may be necessary. The use of respiratory protection is usually necessary when working with powdered enzymes. Respiratory protection should also be used when indicated by a supervisor, safety professional or medical personnel. The Occupational Safety and Health Administration (OSHA) respiratory protection standard must be followed in the selection, training and use of respirators. Use only National Institute of Occupational Safety and Health (NIOSH)-approved respiratory protection.
    - *Protective clothing and gloves:* Protective clothing should be worn when there is a potential for skin or eye contact. This clothing may include gloves, aprons, safety glasses, and outer garments, such as overalls or lab coats. Protective clothing is particularly important when working with proteolytic enzymes, which are known to cause skin irritation. Operations that may require the use of protective clothing include spill clean-up, equipment maintenance, and equipment cleaning. Gloves should be worn when there is a potential for skin contact with any enzyme material. Cotton liners or cotton-lined gloves are recommended to absorb perspiration. Protective clothing should be removed prior to leaving the work area and should not be worn into other areas of the facility (i.e. lunchroom, offices) or to the home.
- **Maintenance and spillage:** Whenever maintenance is to be performed on equipment that has been in contact with enzymes, the equipment should be cleaned before the work is begun. Use wet washing (flooding, wiping) or a vacuum system equipped with a high-efficiency particulate air filter (HEPA) to clean equipment or spills. High-pressure cleaning (steam, air, or water) must be avoided since these operations are known to cause aerosol formation. Personal protective equipment (gloves, respirators, eye protection) may be required during some maintenance operations.
- **Spill clean-up:** Spilled enzymes must be removed immediately by a central vacuum system, vacuum equipped with a HEPA filter, mopping, or washing. To prevent dust or aerosol formation during clean-up, do not sweep or use high water pressure, steam, or compressed air on spills. Use plenty of water in wet washing to flush all enzyme material away to prevent enzyme dust generation from dried material. Dependent upon the place and extent of the spill, respiratory protection and protective clothing may be required during clean-up. Disposal of spilt material should be in compliance with national, state and local regulations.
- **Personal cleanliness:** Personal cleanliness is essential to prevent irritation from proteolytic enzymes to skin and mucous membranes. The irritation response on the skin is increased in the presence of moisture and when the natural oils of the skin are removed.

    The following procedures are recommended to prevent irritation:
    - Hands should be washed with water and mild soap before leaving the work area and immediately after coming into contact with enzyme materials.
    - Change work clothes daily and whenever they are soiled with enzyme material. Do not wear work clothing home.
    - Avoid touching your face and eyes with enzyme-contaminated clothing or gloves.
    - Wear cotton-lined gloves to absorb perspiration.

- **Measuring enzyme levels in air:** There is air monitoring techniques available to measure the level of enzyme dust or mist in the air. The American Conference of Governmental Industrial Hygienists (ACGIH) has established a threshold limit value (TLV) for only one class of enzymes, subtilisin, of 60 ng/m^3 as a ceiling limit. Both low-flow and high-flow air sampling methods are available for some enzymes. Contact the enzyme manufacturer for additional information.
- **First aid treatment:** Following first aid treatment interventions may be done on the body while handling them:
  - *Skin contact:* Most enzyme materials are water-soluble; therefore, the exposed skin should first be thoroughly flushed with water and then washed with mild soap and water. If clothes are contaminated, remove them, shower and change into clean clothes. Immerse the contaminated clothes in water and wash them as usual.
  - *Inhalation:* Remove the individual from exposure and monitor for irritation or allergic symptoms. If symptoms occur, consult a physician. Symptoms may occur as late as 2 or more hours after exposure.
  - *Eye contact:* Rinse the eyes thoroughly with water for at least 15 minutes and then consult a physician.
  - *Consumer exposure assessment:* Prior to introducing an enzyme preparation into a consumer product, the potential for consumer exposure to the enzyme and possible health effects should be assessed. Since enzymes are respiratory allergens and some enzymes are irritants, both the potential for inhaling the enzyme preparation and for skin contact should be evaluated. Important factors that need to be considered include the following: Product use, potential misuses, enzyme concentration, product form (liquid, powder, granule, foam), duration and frequency of exposure, potential exposure level and the no-effect level of enzyme exposure.

DIGESTION AND ABSORPTION OF CARBOHYDRATES, PROTEINS AND FATS

The ingested food is in the form of fairly large molecules, and so, requires prior processing steps, before it can be metabolized. Digestion and absorption are the two processing steps. Carbohydrates, proteins, fats and nucleic acids need to be first digested into suitable forms for their subsequent absorption. Minor food components such as vitamins and minerals do not require digestion; they can be absorbed as such. Cooking makes the digestion process easier.
- Digestion refers to the process of the breakdown of large and complex organic molecules into simpler forms that are able to diffuse across cellular membranes.
- Digestion of food is a long process that involves the gradual breakdown of the food components in several stages and in different organs of the digestive tract.
- The major organs of the human digestive system include the mouth, stomach, liver, pancreas, and small intestine.
- The digestive process is accomplished with the help of the secretions of these organs, which may contain many enzymes and inorganic ions.
  - While the ions help to maintain the proper pH of the fluids secreted, it is the enzymes that actually split the chemical bonds in large molecules so as to convert them into simpler forms.

Digestion of Carbohydrates

Carbohydrates in the diet provide the major exogenous source for glucose, which is the primary energy source for cells. Each gram of carbohydrate provides 4 calories. Dietary carbohydrates are mainly of three types, i.e., polysaccharides (starch and glycogen), disaccharides (sucrose, lactose, maltose) and monosaccharides (glucose and fructose). The monosaccharide is absorbed without any change while polysaccharides and disaccharides need the digestion process to be converted into monosaccharides. The goal of carbohydrate digestion is to break down all disaccharides and complex carbohydrates into monosaccharides for absorption, although not all are completely absorbed in the small intestine (e.g., fiber). Digestion happens at different levels in the gastrointestinal tract with the help of different digestive enzymes **(Table 3.1)**. The combined action of various enzymes converts the carbohydrates into simple forms that are easily absorbed **(Fig. 3.4)**.

Table 3.1: Description of carbohydrates digestion.

Location of digestion	Digestion activity
Mouth	Salivary α-amylase (ptyalin) converts polysaccharides (starch, glycogen and dextrins) into simple carbohydrates (glucose, maltose and maltotriose)
Stomach	As such no carbohydrate digestion occurs in stomach, except some dietary sucrose may be hydrolyzed to equimolar amounts of glucose and fructose by HCl.
Small intestine	Pancreatic amylase (amylopsin) converts complex carbohydrates (starch, glycogen and dextrins into simple carbohydrates (glucose, maltose, isomaltose and α-dextrins).
	Intestinal juice contains intestinal amylase, maltase, isomaltase, sucrase, lactase and α-dextrinase, which converts partially complex sugars into simple carbohydrates as follows:
	Maltose $\xrightarrow{\text{Maltase}}$ Glucose
	Isomaltose $\xrightarrow{\text{Isomaltase}}$ 2 Glucose
	Sucrose $\xrightarrow{\text{Sucrase}}$ Glucose + Fructose
	Lactose $\xrightarrow{\text{Lactase}}$ Glucose + Galactose
	α-Dextrins $\xrightarrow{\alpha\text{ Dextrinase}}$ Glucose

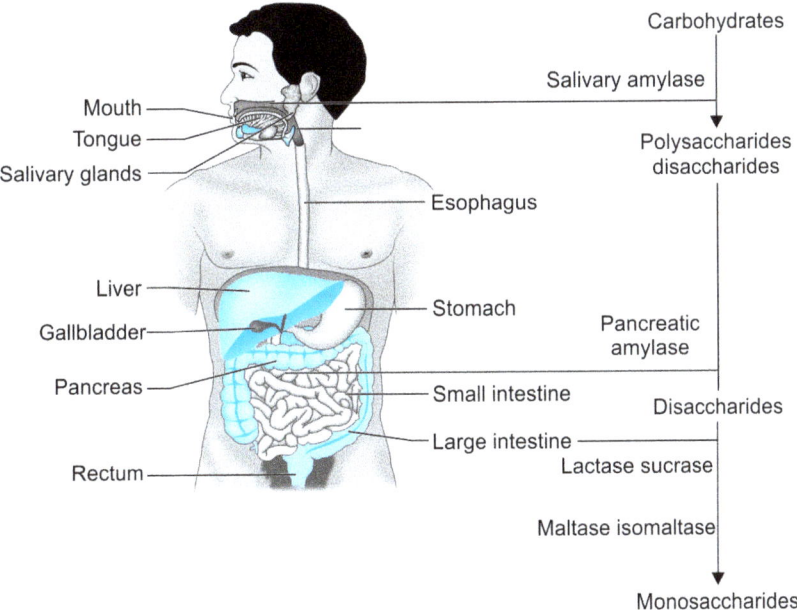

Fig. 3.4: Digestion process of carbohydrates.

Absorption of Carbohydrates

The simplest form of carbohydrates, monosaccharides, i.e., glucose, fructose and mannose are absorbed in jejunum. Fructose is absorbed more slowly than glucose and galactose. However, the monosaccharide is absorbed through the following three mechanisms:

- **Facilitative transport (with the concentration gradient):** Generally all the monosaccharide, fructose, glucose and galactose are absorbed by the diffusion with the concentration gradient by means of sodium-dependent facilitative transporter (GLUT-5). Facilitative transportation is possible when the concentration gradient is favorable. Fructose is mainly transported by GLUT-5.
- **Active transportation (Against the concentration gradient):** When concentration fall and is not favorable, then absorption of glucose is powered by active transportation. Active transportation happens by the help of sodium-linked glucose transporter (SLGT-1). This transporter binds both glucose and sodium at separate sites and transported across the plasma membrane. Active transpiration needs energy, which is provided from the hydrolysis of ATPs.
- **Glucose transporter 4:** The glucose transporter type 4: The glucose transporter type 4 (GluT4) is major glucose transporter in skeletal muscle and adipose tissue. GluT4 is under the control of insulin. But other glucose transporters are not under the control of insulin.

Digestion of Protein

Dietary proteins are obtained from vegetable and animal sources. The principal sources are pulses, cereals, peas, beans and nuts and the principal animal sources are milk, its products, meat, fish, liver, eggs, etc. Proteins are sequences of amino acids (AA) linked by peptide bonds. There are twenty amino acids; of which nine are essential and eleven are non-essential. Adults require 0.75 g/kg body weight of protein daily. Primarily proteins are hydrolyzed from polypeptides to dipeptides and then finally they are converted in amino acids and absorbed in the gut. Digestion of protein begins in the stomach and happens at different levels in the gastrointestinal tract by the help of different digestive enzymes as depicted in **Table 3.2** and **Fig. 3.5**:

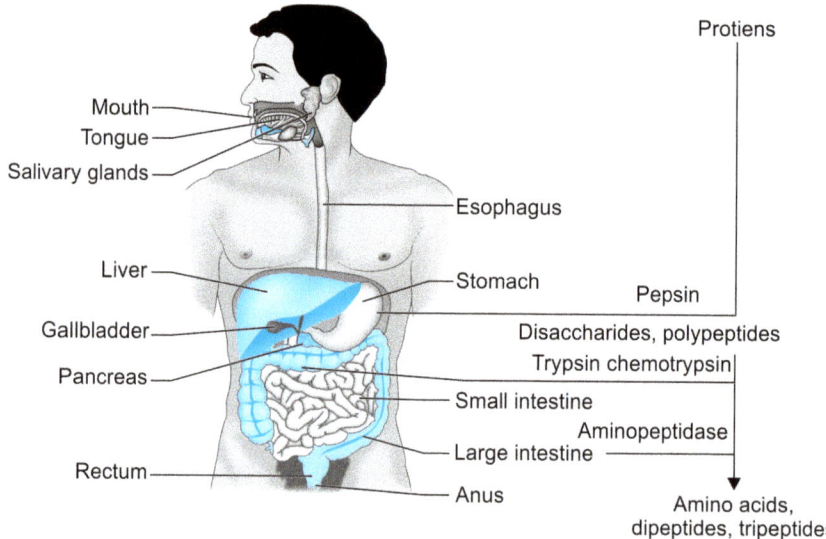

Fig. 3.5: Digestive process of proteins.

Table 3.2: Description of protein digestion.

Location of digestion	Digestion activity
Mouth	As such no protein digestion takes place in the mouth.
Stomach	Gastric juice contains a number of proteolytic enzymes such as pepsin, rennin, gastriscsin, gelatinase, etc. and these enzymes ensure the protein digestion as follows: • The pepsin is produced by the chief cells in stomach in an inactive form, i.e., pepsinogen. The pepsinogen is activated to pepsin by a hydrogen ion. The active pepsin rapidly activates further molecules of pepsinogen and continues the hydrolysis of peptide bonds of polypeptides resulting in the generation of individual amino acids. • The infants also contain one more enzyme renin, which is secreted by zymogen cells of the stomach in the form of prorenin, which is activated into renin by a hydrogen ion. The presence of calcium renin act upon a milk protein casein to convert into paracasein, which is later acted by pepsin. • Gastricsin acts as proteinase. • Gelatinase hydrolyzes gelatin in acid medium to form polypeptides.
Small intestine	• From stomach semidigested food enters into small intestine, where food comes in contact with pancreatic and intestinal enzymes, which hydrolyze the polypeptides into amino acids. Trypsin, chymotrypsin, elastase, carboxypeptidase, collagenases, enterokinase, aminopeptidase, prolidase, tripeptidase and dipeptidase are essential proteolytic enzymes which are helpful in conversion of polypeptides in dipeptides and finally free amino acids, which are absorbed in body to produce energy. • Pancreas secretes trypsinogen, which is converted into active form trypsin by the help of enteropeptidase. Once trypsin is activated, it also activates other proenzymes in pancreatic secretion, i.e., chymotrypsinogen, proelastase and procarboxypeptidase, liberating chymotrypsin, elastase and carboxypeptidase. • Among these enzymes trypsin, chymotrypsin and elastase are endopeptidases, whereas caboxypeptidase is an exopeptidase. Trypsin is specific for peptide bounds of basic amino acids, therefore bringing hydrolysis of protein into proteoses, peptones, tri and dipeptides. Proteins $\xrightarrow{\text{Trypsin}}$ Proteoses + Peptones • Chymotrypsin specifically brings the hydrolysis of peptide bond containing uncharged amino acids such as aromatic acids and converts proteoses, peptones and peptides into smaller peptides and amino acids. Proteoses, peptones $\xrightarrow{\text{Chymotrypsin}}$ Amino acids + peptides • Elastase, rather has broad specificity in attacking bonds next to small amino acids residues such as glycine, alanine and serine. They further attack on the polypeptides produced by the action of endopeptidases carried on by the exopeptidase, carboxypeptidase, which attacks the carboxy terminal peptide bonds and liberates single amino acids. • Finally, intestinal secretions complete the digestion of proteins as it contains aminopeptidase and dipeptidase. Aminopeptidase is an exopeptidase and hydrolyzes terminal peptide bond, changing the peptide stepwise into dipeptides. Dipeptides are then acted upon by dipeptidases, which complete the digestion of dipeptides to free amino acids. Finally amino acids are absorbed in intestine.

Absorption of Proteins

In adults, essentially all protein is absorbed as tripeptides, dipeptides or amino acids and this process occurs in the duodenum or proximal jejunum of the small intestine. The peptides and/or amino acids pass through the interstitial brush border by facilitative diffusion or active transport. The amino acids are of mainly two types L-isomer and D-isomer and the absorption of these end products of proteins takes place through following two mechanisms:

❖ ***Simple passive diffusion:*** Absorption of D-isomers takes place through simple passive diffusion.

❖ **Active transportation:** However, L-isomers are actively transported across the intestine by the sodium-dependent process; both L-amino acid and sodium attach to a carrier protein that is present on the mucosal surface of microvilli and forms amino acids carrier, i.e., sodium complex. The complex passes into the inner surface of the membrane and dissociates to liberate amino acids and sodium. Then sodium is actively pumped out of the cell. The energy required for this active transportation is acquired from the hydrolysis of ATPs.

Digestion of Lipids

The average normal Indian diet contains about 20–30 g of lipids. The optimum pH is 2.5–5. Lipids such as triglycerides and phospholipids are converted into glycerol and fatty acids with the help of enzymes such as lipase and esterase in the gastrointestinal tract. Digestion of triglycerides begins in the oral cavity, happens at different levels in the gastrointestinal tract with the help of different digestive enzymes as depicted in **Table 3.3** and **Fig. 3.6**.

Table 3.3: Description of lipid digestion.	
Location of digestion	Digestion activity
Mouth	◆ A small amount of emulsification of phospholipids takes place with help of lingual lipase.
Stomach	◆ A small amount of dietary triglycerides are broken down into diglycerides by the help of gastric lipase.
Small intestine	◆ In small intestine bile helps in the emulsification of the lipids and then pancreatic lipase, phospholipase, and cholesterol esterase. Pancreatic lipase is the principle fat-digesting enzyme and hydrolyzes fats in three stages. In the first stage, lipase separates one fatty acid molecule changing the triglyceride into a diglyceride. The diglyceride is broken down into another fatty acid molecule and a monoglyceride. In third stage the monoglyceride is finally hydrolyzed into fatty acids and a glycerol molecule. Thus hydrolyzing a fat molecule into fatty acid and glycerol. Triglyceride $\xrightarrow{\text{Pancreatic lipase}}$ 3 Fatty acids + Glycerol ◆ Phospholipase hydrolyzes phospholipids to liberate fatty acids and cholesterol esterase hydrolyzes cholesterol esters to liberate free cholesterol and fatty acids. ◆ In small intestine, intestine lipase also helps in the digestion of lipids, where it hydrolyzes triglycerides, diglycerides and monoglycerides into fatty acids and glycerol.

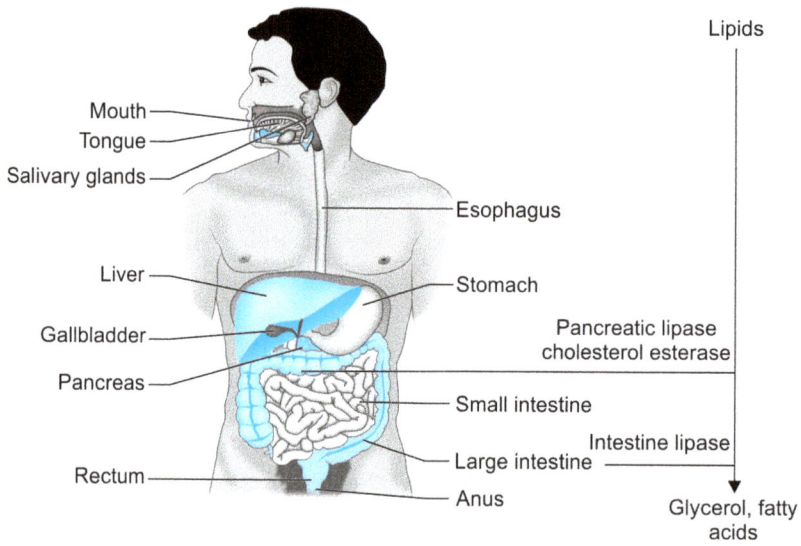

Fig. 3.6: Digestive process of lipids.

Absorption of Lipids

Most of the fat absorption takes place in the duodenum and jejunum of the small intestine. The fats can readily absorbed from the micelles by microvilli or brush border of intestinal epithelium. The end products of the fat digestion, i.e., free fatty acids, α- and β-monoglycerides mainly enter microvilli by simple diffusion through the cell membrane. The short-chain and unsaturated fatty acids are absorbed more rapidly than long-chain fatty acids, even cholesterol is also absorbed in the free form through simple diffusion. Long-chain fatty acids (chain length more than 14 carbons) are absorbed into the lymph and not directly to the blood. Short-chain fatty acids directly enter into blood vessels, then to the portal vein, finally to the liver where they are immediately utilized for energy.

Basics of Carbohydrates, Proteins and Lipids Absorption

The digested food, though inside the gastrointestinal tract, is biochemically outside the body. To reach the various parts of the body, the end product of digestion of food must enter the circulatory system. Absorption is the process of digested food entering the circulatory system. Absorption of food occurs through 2 routes.
- **Blood route:** Through the blood route simple sugars, short chain fatty acids (up to 10 carbons), amino acids, glycerol, etc. are absorbed and carried to the liver by the portal system.
- **Lymphatic route:** Substances such as long chain fatty acids, unhydrated fat, phospholipids and cholesterol are absorbed through the lymphatic route and carried through the thoracic system to venous circulation.

The small intestine is responsible for the absorption of the bulk of digested food. For this purpose, the organ has a long canal-like structure with a very absorptive surface. For absorption, two main mechanisms operate in the body. These are:
- **Simple diffusion:** This means transfer of molecules from a higher concentration region to lower concentration region. Such a flow is said to occur under a concentration gradient and it does not require the expenditure of energy. It is similar to the flow of water from a place of higher altitude to a place of lower altitude which can happen without any external aid.
  - Also during simple diffusion, ions of a particular charge flow towards ions of opposite charge due to attraction between ions. Such a flow is said to arise due to charge gradient.
- **Active transport:** It involves the transfer of:
  - Molecules from a region of lower concentration to a region of higher concentration against concentration gradient.
  - Ions of particular type move towards ions of the same type against charge gradient.

Active transport of ions and molecules across the membranes is an energy-demanding process. It is driven by chemical energy in the form of ATP.

■ FACTORS INFLUENCING THE DIGESTION AND ABSORPTION

The digestion and absorption of the nutrients is a complex and highly coordinated activity, which is influenced by variety of factors. Following are some of the main factors influencing the digestion and absorption of food.
- **Age:** Older people have relatively decreased absorption than younger people; because with advancing age gastrointestinal structure, functions and secretions get altered. Therefore, they experience decreased digestion and absorption process.
- **Disease conditions:** Several disease conditions such as gastrointestinal infections, bowel diseases, pancreatitis, gastritis, celiac disease, diabetes. Even various surgical conditions may

alter the digestion and absorption such as short bowel syndrome, ileostomy or colostomy. Furthermore, diseases of kidney, liver, gallbladder and septicemia may also affect the digestion and absorption of nutrients.

- **Eating habits:** Regular eating and well-chewing habits contribute to better food digestion and absorption. However, irregular eating habits, poor chewing, and rapid eating habits significantly contribute to the poor digestion and absorption of nutrients.
- **Exocrine functions of digestive organs:** Normal secretions of digestive juices from stomach, small intestine, pancreas, liver and gallbladder are required for effective digestion and absorption of nutrients.
- **Secretion of enzyme activators:** Some of the digestive enzymes are secreted in non-active form; but secretion of digestive enzyme activator such as secretion, cholecystokinin is essential for the proper digestion and absorption of nutrients.
- **Endocrine functions of the body:** Normal secretion of hormones from the pituitary, thyroid and adrenal gland is essential for the proper digestion and absorption of nutrients.
- **Psychological factors:** Digestion and absorption of nutrients primarily depends on the coordinated activity of the gastrointestinal tract, nervous system and endocrine system. However, psychological factors proved to be important determinants in digestion and absorption of nutrients.
- **Lack of digestive enzymes:** A fault in the digestive process may result from failure of the body to produce the enzymes needed to digest certain foods.
- **Anatomical defect in gastrointestinal organs:** Congenital or acquired structural defects or diseases of the pancreas, gallbladder, or liver may alter the digestive process.
- **Certain lifestyle factors:** Lack of sleep, alcohol intake, overeating and lack of sleep decrease the rate of digestion.
- **Psychological influences:** The taste, smell and presentation of the food can have a positive effect on digestion. Just the thought of food can trigger the saliva production and peristalsis. Stressful emotions like depression can have the reverse effect.
- **Chemical influences:** The type of protein we eat and the way it is prepared also effect the digestion. Plant proteins tend to be less digestible as compared to animal proteins. Cooking food also denatures the protein and made easily digestible.

MALABSORPTION SYNDROME

Malabsorption syndrome is an alteration in the ability of the intestine to absorb nutrients adequately into the bloodstream. Malabsorption may be due to an abnormality of the gut wall, failure to produce enzymes or bile to aid digestion, or there may be abnormalities of the flora of the gut.

Malabsorption may occur for many nutrients or for specific carbohydrates, fats, or micronutrients. "Malabsorption is a state arising from an abnormality in absorption of food nutrients across the gastrointestinal tract. Impairment can be of single or multiple nutrients depending on the abnormality. This may lead to malnutrition and a variety of anemias". Malabsorption constitutes the pathological interference with the normal physiological sequence of the body such as:
- Digestion (intraluminal process)
- Absorption (Mucosal process)
- Transport (postmucosal events) of nutrients.

Causes
Intestinal malabsorption can be due to:
- **Digestive failure caused by enzymes:** A fault in the digestive process may result from the failure of the body to produce the enzymes needed to digest certain foods
  - *Pancreatic insufficiency:* It includes—cystic fibrosis, chronic pancreatitis, carcinoma of pancreas
  - *Bile salt insufficiency:* It includes—obstructive jaundice, bacterial overgrowth
- **Structural defects:** Congenital or acquired structural defects or diseases of the pancreas, gallbladder, or liver may alter the digestive process, e.g., Chron's disease, gastrectomy and gastrojejunostomy, fistulae, diverticulae and strictures, infiltrative conditions such as amyloidosis, lymphoma and eosinophilic gastroenteropathy.
- **Musocal abnormality:** It includes—celiac disease
- **Infective agents:** It includes—Whipple's disease, intestinal tuberculosis, intestinal parasites like Giardia lamblia.
- **Systematic diseases affecting GIT:** It includes—diabetes mellitus, hyper/hypoparathyroidism, hyper/hypothyroidism, malnutrition, etc.
  - Inflammation, infection, injury, or surgical removal of portions of the intestine may inhibit absorption abilities. Reduced length or surface area of the intestine available for fluid and nutrient absorption can also result in malabsorption.
  - Radiation therapy may injure the mucosal lining of the intestine, resulting in diarrhea that may not become evident until several years later. Furthermore, the use of some antibiotics can also affect the bacteria that normally live in the intestine, thus affecting intestinal function.

Clinical Manifestations
The most common symptoms of malabsorption include:
- Anemia, with weakness and fatigue due to inadequate absorption of vitamin B12, iron, and folic acid.
- Diarrhea, steatorrhea (an excessive amount of fat in the stool), and abdominal distention with cramps bloating, and gas due to impaired water and carbohydrate absorption and irritation from unabsorbed fatty acids. The individual may also report explosive diarrhea with greasy, foul-smelling stools.
- Edema from decreased protein absorption
- Malnutrition and weight loss due to decreased fat, carbohydrate, and protein absorption
- Muscle cramping from decreased vitamin D, calcium, and potassium levels
- Muscle wasting and atrophy due to decreased protein absorption and metabolism
- Perianal skin burning, itching, or soreness due to frequent loose stools
- Irregular heart rhythms may also result from inadequate levels of potassium and other electrolytes. Blood clotting disorders may occur due to a vitamin K deficiency.

Diagnosis
- Diagnosis typically clinically apparent from a detailed patient history.
- For steatorrhea diagnosis is done with the help of 72 hour stool collection to measure the levels of fat in the stool. Where there is an excess of fat in feces, it indicates malabsorption. More than 6 grams per day is pathological.
- The next essential step is to set the basis of differentiation between absorptive abnormality and digestive abnormality. This is done with the help of the D-xylose test. D-xylose is a sugar

that is thrown out through urine and does not need to be digested to be absorbed. When the excretion of D-xylose is low, it suggests absorptive normality. Factors such as bacterial growth are responsible for this and it is confirmed by a breath test or jejunal biopsy.
- Measurement of elastase and chymotrypsin in the stool can also help differentiate pancreatic and intestinal causes of malabsorption; both are decreased in pancreatic exocrine insufficiency, whereas both are normal in intestinal causes.
- Other tests such as barium enema, CT scan, MRI scan, ultrasound, and X-rays are also required to identify abnormalities of the gastrointestinal tract.
- Sweat test: Studying a sample of sweat can help diagnose cystic fibrosis.

Management

- The treatment for malabsorption syndrome should include nutrient and fluid replacement of the patient concerned.
- Provide advice for nutritional support and meal planning. The patient should avoid fruits and fluids that are responsible for causing diarrhea. He should eat small frequent meals instead of large ones throughout the day.
- Diminishing levels of protein in the blood may also give rise to excess fluid volume. Restrictions on the intake of fluid are advised in such cases.
- In some cases, vitamin B injections may also be required in addition to oral iron supplements.
- Missing intestinal enzymes may be replaced by enzyme supplements. Pancreatic supplements become necessary in the case of patients suffering from chronic pancreatitis and cystic fibrosis.
- Abdominal cramping can be reduced by the use of antispasmodic drugs.
- Antibiotics therapy to treat small bowel bacterial overgrowth.
- Diet modifications are required in case of patients suffering from lactose intolerance and avoid foods that are not easily digestible.
- Gluten-free diet in celiac disease

QUESTIONS

Q.1: What is meant by term digestion? Describe in brief the digestion of protein, carbohydrate and lipids.
Q.2: What are enzymes? Discuss their mechanism of action.
Q.3: Define enzymes. Describe factors affecting enzyme activity.
Q.4: What are enzymes? What is meant by enzyme specificity?
Q.5: What are enzymes? Discuss the role of various enzymes in digestion.
Q.6: List three precautions which are importantly required to handle specimens for enzyme estimations.
Q.7: Describe the process of digestion and absorption of fats.

BIBLIOGRAPHY

1. Alpers DH, Solin M. The characterization of rat intestinal amylase. Gastroenterology, 1970; 58(6):833-42.
2. Bairoch A. "The Enzyme database in 2000. Nucleic Acids Res, 2000; 28(1): 304-5.
3. Blake CC, Koenig DF, Mair GA, et al. Structure of hen egg-white lysozyme. A three-dimensional Fourier synthesis at 2 Angstrom resolution. Nature, 1965; 206(4986):757-61.
4. Borgstrom B, Dahlqvist A, Lundh G, et al. Studies of intestinal digestion and absorption in the human. J Clin Invest, 1957; 36(10):1521-36.
5. Cech T. Structural biology. The ribosome is a ribozyme. Science, 2000; 289(5481):878-9.

6. Chen LH, Kenyon GL, Curtin F. 4-Oxalocrotonate tautomerase, an enzyme composed of 62 amino acid residues per monomer. J Biol Chem, 1992; 267(25):17716-21.
7. Crane RK. Na^+-dependent transport in the intestine and other animal tissues. Fed Proc, 1965;24(5): 1000-6
8. Dahlqvist A, Borgstrom B. Digestion and absorption of disaccharides in man. Biochem J, 1961;81:411-8.
9. Fridhandler L, Quastel JH. Absorption of sugars from isolated surviving intestine. Arch Biochem Biophys, 1955;56(2):412-23.
10. Gracey M, Burke V, Oshin A. Intestinal transport of fructose. Lancet, 1970;2(7677):827-8.
11. Gray GM. Carbohydrate digestion and absorption. Gastroenterology. 1970;58(1):96-107.
12. Grisham, Charles M, Garrett RH. Biochemistry. Philadelphia: Saunders College Pub, 1999: 426-7.
13. Groves JT "Artificial enzymes. The importance of being selective". Nature, 1997; 389, (6649): 329-30.
14. Holdsworth CD, Dawson AM. The Absorption of Monosaccharides in Man. Clin Sci, 1964:371-9.
15. Johnson CF. Disaccharidase: localization in hamster intestine brush borders. Science. 1967;155(3770): 1670-2.
16. Johnson FR, Kugler JH. The distribution of alkaline phosphatase in the mucosal cells of the small intestine of the rat, cat and dog. J Anat, 1953;87(3):247-56.
17. Lilley D. Structure, folding and mechanisms of ribozymes. Curr Opin Struct Biol, 2005; 15(3): 313-23.
18. Miller D, Crane RK. The digestive function of the epithelium of the small intestine. I. An intracellular locus of disaccharide and sugar phosphate ester hydrolysis. Biochim Biophys Acta, 1961;52:281-293.
19. Miller D, Crane RK. The digestive function of the epithelium of the small intestine. II. Localization of disaccharide hydrolysis in the isolated brush border portion of intestinal epithelial cells. Biochim Biophys Acta, 1961;52:293-8.
20. Nachlas MM, Monis B, Rosenbatt D, et al. Improvement in the histochemical localization of leucine aminopeptidase with a new substrate, L-leucyl-4-methoxy-2-naphthylamide. J Biophys Biochem Cytol, 1960:261-4.
21. Newey H, Sanford PA, Smyth DH. Location of function in the intestinal epithelial cell in relation to carbohydrate absorption. J Physiol, 1963;168:423-34.
22. Olsen WA, Ingelfinger FJ. The role of sodium in intestinal glucose absorption in man. J Clin Invest, 1968;47(5):1133-42.
23. Plimmer RH. On the presence of lactase in the intestines of animals and on the adaptation of the intestine to lactose. J Physiol, 1906; 35(1-2):20-31.
24. Roberts PJ, Whelan WJ. The mechanism of carbohydrase action. 5. Action of human salivary alpha-amylase on amylopectin and glycogen. Biochem J, 1960;76:246-53.
25. Schedl HP, Clifton JA. Solute and water absorption by the human small intestine. Nature, 1963;199: 1264-7.
26. Smith AL. Oxford Dictionary of Biochemistry and Molecular Biology. Oxford: Oxford University Press; 1997.
27. Vasudevan DM, S Sreekumari, Vaidyanathan Kannan. Textbook of Biochemistry for Medical Students. 9th edn. New Delhi:Jaypee Brothers Medical Publishers;2019.
28. Essential Medical Physiology edited by Leonard R. Johnson. 3rd edition.California USA:Elseviers;2003
29. Human Physiology edited by Nitin Ashok John.13th edition. Delhi India:CBS Publishers;2020.

CHAPTER 4

Carbohydrates

Shiv Kumar Mudgal, Navjot Kaur

Chapter Outline
- Classification of Carbohydrates
- Functions of Carbohydrates
- Metabolism of Carbohydrates
- Glycolysis
- Glycogenolysis
- Gluconeogenesis
- Glycogenesis
- Tricarboxylic Acid (TCA) Cycle
- Blood Glucose and its Regulation
- Glycemia
- Glucose Tolerance Test (GTT)
- Hyperglycemia and Diabetes
- Hypoglycemia

■ INTRODUCTION

Carbohydrates play a vital role in our everyday life. Carbohydrates are an ideal source of energy for the body. Carbohydrates are the most abundant biomolecules found in living organisms. Carbohydrate is an organic compound that consists only of carbon (C), hydrogen (H), and oxygen (O), usually with hydrogen: oxygen atom ratio of 2:1. The primary function of carbohydrates is to provide energy for the body, especially the brain and the nervous system. An enzyme called amylase helps breakdown carbohydrates into glucose, which is used for energy by the body. Carbohydrates are called simple or complex, depending on their chemical structure.

- *Simple carbohydrates* have one or two sugar molecules. These are broken down quickly by the body to be used as energy. They also include sugar added during food processing and refining (**Fig. 4.1**).
- *Complex carbohydrates* have three or more sugar molecules. These are madeup of sugar molecules that are strung together in long, complex chains. Many of the complex carbohydrates are good sources of fiber (**Fig. 4.2**).

Biomedical Importance of Carbohydrates
- Carbohydrates are the most abundant organic molecules in nature.
- They have a wide range of functions, including: Providing a significant fraction of the dietary calories for most organisms.
- Acting as a storage form of energy in the body.

Simple carbohydrates are found in foods such as fruits, milk and vegetables

Cake, candy, and other refined sugar products are simple sugars which also provide energy but lack vitamins, minerals, and fiber

Fig. 4.1: Simple carbohydrates.

Complex carbohydrates provide vitamins, minerals, and fiber

Food such as breads, legumes, rice, pasta, and starchy vegetables contain complex carbohydrates

Fig. 4.2: Complex carbohydrates.

❖ Serving as cell membrane components that mediate some forms of intercellular communication.

■ CLASSIFICATION OF CARBOHYDRATES

Carbohydrates or saccharides are classified into four major groups:
1. Monosaccharides
2. Disaccharides
3. Oligosaccharides
4. Polysaccharides
   This classification is based on number of saccharides units of which one molecule of carbohydrate is madeup of.

Monosaccharides

Monosaccharides, also called simple sugars, are those having only one actual or potential sugar group and cannot be hydrolyzed into a simpler form. Most monosaccharides have general formula $C_nH_{2n}O_n$. These are further categorized depending upon their functional group (**Table 4.1**). Furthermore, **Table 4.2** depicts the common monosaccharides under functional group, i.e., aldose and ketose.

Table 4.1: Primary categories of monosaccharides.

Aldoses	Ketoses
Monosaccharide having an aldehyde group (CHO) as the functional group. For example, glyceraldehyde, glucose, galactose, etc.	Monosaccharides having keto group (C = O) as the functional group. For example, ribulose, fructose, etc.

$$\begin{array}{c} H \quad O \\ | \quad \| \\ C - C - H \\ | \\ OH \end{array} \quad \text{Aldehyde group} \qquad \begin{array}{c} H \quad O \\ | \quad \| \\ C - C \\ | \\ OH \end{array} \quad \text{Keto group}$$

Table 4.2: Common monosaccharides.

No. of carbon atoms	Generic name	Aldose	Ketose
1	Trioses	Glyceraldehydes	Dihydroxyacetone
2	Tetroses	Erythrose	Erythrulose
3	Pentoses	Ribose	Ribulose
4	Hexoses	Glucose	Fructose
5	Heptoses	Glucoheptose	Sedoheptulose

Isomerism

Isomers are compounds with the same molecular formula but different structural formula.

Stereoisomers: These are compounds which have same structural formula or identical in composition and different in spatial configurations. While writing the molecular formula of monosaccharides, the spatial arrangement of H and OH groups is important, since they contain asymmetric carbon atoms. Asymmetric carbon means that four different groups are attached to the same carbon. By convention, one of these two forms is designated as the D-isomer, the other L-isomer (The absolute configurations of sugars are known from X-ray crystallography). The D and L- designation is based on the configuration of single asymmetric carbon in glyceraldehyde. When the hydroxyl group on the reference carbon is on the right in the projection formula, the sugar is the D-isomer; when on the left, it is the L-isomer. Those in which the configuration at this reference carbon is the same as that of D-glyceraldehyde, are designated D-isomers; and those with the same configuration as L-glyceraldehyde, are L isomers **(Fig. 4.3)**.

Functional isomers: These are monosaccharides which have the same molecular formula but have different functional groups. For example, glucose and fructose both have the same

Fig. 4.3: Chemical structure of D-isomer and L-isomer.

```
        H   O
         \ //
          C
          |
        H-C-OH                CH₂OH
          |                    |
       HO-C-H                  C=O
          |                    |
        H-C-OH              HO-C-H
          |                    |
        H-C-OH               H-C-OH
          |                    |
         CH₂OH               H-C-OH
                               |
                              CH₂OH
        Glucose              Fructose
```

Fig. 4.4: Functional isomers.

molecular formula ($C_6H_{12}O_6$) but have different structural formulas. Glucose has an aldehyde group and fructose has a ketone group **(Fig. 4.4)**.

Stereoisomers
1. **Optical isomers:** These are isomers which are optically active and have non-superimposable mirror images. The presence of an asymmetrical carbon atom causes optical activity. When polarized light is passed through these isomers they either rotate the plane of polarized light to the right and are called dextrorotatory or to the left are called levorotatory. The isomer which rotates the plane of light to the right is designated by small 'd' and the one to the left is designated by small 'l'. Hence D-glucose can be dextrorotatory or levorotatory. When equal amounts of dextro-and levorotatory isomers are present, then the resultant mixture has no optical activity, since the activity of each isomer cancels each other out. Such mixtures are called racemic mixtures.
2. **Epimers:** If monosaccharides differ only in one position with regard to a single carbon atom other than the reference carbon atom, then they are called epimers. They are a kind of positional isomers. For example, glucose, galactose and mannose **(Fig. 4.5)**.
3. **Anomers:** Anomers are cyclic monosaccharides which differ from each other in configuration only around anomeric carbon atom. α-D-glucopyranose and β-D-glucopyranose are anomers.

Chemical Reactions of Monosaccharides

Because of the presence of several functional OH groups in a ring structure and the potential for the existence of a free —CH=O (aldehyde) or C=O (ketone) group, monosaccharides can

Fig. 4.5: Chemical structure of D-glucose, D-galactose and D-mannose.

undergo reactions that are common to alcohols (especially those of polyhydroxy ring structures), aldehydes, and ketones. The scope of our consideration is limited to only a few of these, with a focus on reactions of biological significance.

- **Oxidation:** Three different acid derivatives of aldoses can be produced by oxidizing terminal groups to —COOH groups. Acids arising from the oxidation of the terminal —CH=O group are called aldonic acids. If the terminal —CH$_2$OH group is oxidized, an uronic acid is produced and if both terminal groups are oxidized, the product is a saccharic acid.
- **Reduction:** Two important reduced forms of sugars are polyhydroxy alcohols (e.g., alditols, i.e., reduced aldoses) and deoxy sugars.
- **Glycosides:** When a hemiacetal (ROH) reacts with an alcohol, sterol or phenol (R'OH), the product is glycosides. The newly formed linkage of anomeric-OR' is called a glycosidic bond. The monosaccharide portion of the glycoside is termed as the glycone, the R'-group a-aglycone (except when the R' group is another sugar).
- **Esterification:** Alcohols readily form esters when reacted with acids, anhydrides, or acyl halides. The most important types of sugar esters that occur in nature are:
  1. Phosphate esters (including diphosphate esters)
  2. Acyl esters (with acetic acid or fatty acids), and
  3. Sulfate esters.
- **Mutarotation:** The interconversion of the α and β anomeric forms of a monosaccharide occurs as the hemiacetal ring opens and recloses, yielding the opposite anomeric configuration. This process, which is catalyzed by dilute acid, involves the "open chain" structure with the free aldehyde or ketone group as intermediate.
  - Mutarotation refers to the rapid change of the optical rotation (denoted $[\alpha]_d$) of a freshly prepared aqueous solution of a single, pure anomeric form of a monosaccharide. α and β forms of d-glucopyranose are stereoisomers and thus, by definition, rotate the plane of plane-polarized light an equal amount but in opposite directions. B-d-glucopyranose shows an initial rotation of 19° (in water). The initial $[\alpha]_d$ of α-d-glucopyranose (+112° in water) changes upon dissolution, until it reaches a constant value of +52.5°. Mutarotation arises from the complex equilibria set-up on dissolution of monosaccharides.

Important Monosaccharides

- **Trioses:** Glyceraldehyde 3-phosphate and dihydroxyacetone phosphate are intermediates during glucose oxidation in living cells.
- **Tetroses:** Erythrose 4-phosphate is formed during glucose oxidation in living cells.
- **Pentoses:** D-ribose is a component of many nucleosides and nucleotides and ribonucleic acids (RNA). 2-deoxyribose is a component of deoxyribonucleic acid (DNA).
- **Hexoses:** D-glucose (grape sugar) is the main sugar present in blood and is present in all animal and plant cells, honey and fruits. It enters in the formation of many disaccharides and polysaccharides. It is also termed as dextrose because it is dextrorotatory. D-fructose (fruit sugar) is present in honey, fruits and semen. It is a component of sucrose and inulin. It is also termed as levulose because it is levorotatory. D-galactose is a component of lactose that is present in milk. It is also found in glycosaminoglycans (GAGS), glycolipids, and glycoproteins.

Disaccharides

The disaccharides are carbohydrates that can be hydrolyzed into two units of monosaccharides. The description and components of disaccharides is presented in **Table 4.3**. Disaccharides consist of two monosaccharides united together by glycosidic linkage. If the glycosidic linkage involves the carbonyl group of both sugars (e.g., sucrose), the resulting disaccharide is non-reducing.

Table 4.3: Description and components of disaccharides.

Disaccharide	Description	Component monosaccharides
Sucrose	Common table sugar	Glucose 1α → 2 fructose
Maltose	Product of starch hydrolysis	Glucose 1α → 4 glucose
Trehalose	Found in fungi	Glucose 1α → 1 glucose
Lactose	Main sugar in milk	Galactose 1β → 4 glucose
Melibiose	Found in legumes	Galactose 1α → 6 glucose

On the other hand, if the glycosidic linkage involves the carbonyl group of one of its two sugars (e.g., lactose and maltose), the resulting disaccharide is reducing.

a. **Maltose:** Maltose consists of two molecules of D-glucose joined by glycosidic linkage. It is produced while digestion of starch by an amylase enzyme.

Maltose

Properties of maltose
- It is a reducing sugar.
- It gives sunflower-shaped osazone crystals.
- It is water-soluble disaccharides.

b. **Lactose:** Lactose consists of one molecule of D-galactose and one of D-glucose joined together by glycosidic linkage.

Galactose ——— Glucose

Properties of lactose:
- It is a reducing sugar.
- It is a water-soluble disaccharide.
- It forms hedgehog-shaped osazones.

c. **Sucrose:** Sucrose is made-up of glucose and fructose joined together by glycosidic linkage.

Properties of sucrose:
- It is a non-reducing sugar.
- It cannot form osazones.
- It is water soluble.

Oligosaccharides

❖ They yield 2–10 monosaccharides molecule on hydrolysis. They are not an important source of carbohydrates in the diet for humans as most of them are nondigestible.
❖ Oligosaccharides are often found as a component of glycoproteins or glycolipids and as such are often used as cell surface chemical markers, often for cell recognition.
  - An example is ABO blood type specificity. Fructose, Mannose, Glucose and NAGlu residues attached on RBC cell surface contribute to the antigenicity of ABO blood groups.

Polysaccharides

Polysaccharides are composed of more than 10 monosaccharide units linked by glycosidic bonds. Since the condensation of the monosaccharide units involves the carbonyl groups of the sugars, leaving only one free carbonyl group at the end of a big molecule, polysaccharides are nonreducing. Polysaccharides include homopolysaccharides and heteropolysaccharides and depicted in **Table 4.4**.

■ FUNCTIONS OF CARBOHYDRATES

❖ Carbohydrates are the main source of energy in the body. When carbohydrates are oxidized, they liberate CO_2, water and energy.
❖ They serve as storage form of energy (glycogen).
❖ Certain carbohydrates are the starting materials for the biological synthesis of fatty acids and amino acids.
❖ Certain products of carbohydrate metabolism acts as catalyst to promote oxidation of food stuffs.
❖ Carbohydrates like glycoproteins and glycolipids participate in the structure of the cell membrane.
❖ Carbohydrates are the structural components of many organisms. Example, cellulose of plants, cell wall of microorganisms.
❖ Carbohydrates save proteins from being used in the production of energy.

■ METABOLISM OF CARBOHYDRATES

The digestion process converts all carbohydrates like polysaccharides and disaccharides to monosaccharides into gut. Then these monosaccharides are converted to glucose in the liver.

Table 4.4: Description about types of polysaccharides.

Homopolysaccharides	Heteropolysaccharides
These are made up of same type of monosaccharides.	These are made up of different types of monosaccharides.
1. Starch: Starch is the main storage form of carbohydrates in plants. – Starch consists of 2 polysaccharides components water-soluble amylase and water-insoluble amylopectin. – They are present in cord and ovum, potatoes, rice, – wheat and other food grains.	These are the essential components of tissue structure. Collagen embedded in the matrix or ground substance is predominantly composed of mucopolysaccharides. **1. Hyaluronic acid:** – It is present in vitreous humor, skin, synovial fluid, umbilical cord and ovum. – It acts as a lubricant and a shock absorber in joints and further acts as a cementing substance and contributes semi-permeability to membrane.
2. Dextran: – Dextran is a polysaccharide, closely related to starch and glycogen. – It is synthesized from sucrose by certain bacterias. – It is used as a blood substitute in extensive blood loss.	**2. Heparin:** – It occurs in the liver, lungs, thymus, blood, etc. – It acts as an anticoagulant.
3. Inulin: – It is a polysaccharide, each molecule of which is composed of 80-D fructose units. – It occurs in dahlia, onion, garlic, etc. – It is clinically used to find renal clearance value of and glomerular filtration rate.	
4. Glycogen: – It is the reserve carbohydrate in animals and often referred to as animal starch. – It is stored in the liver and muscles. – It is composed of glucose units	
5. Cellulose: – It is the chief carbohydrate in plants. – It is the predominant component of the plant call wall. – It is composed of D-glucose units. – Cellulose is not digested by human enzymes. It is a major constituent of dietary fiber.	

So the liver is the first filter of carbohydrates and has a major role in storage and distribution. Glucose is the body's most readily available source of energy. There are numerous metabolic pathways from beginning to the end **(Fig. 4.6)**.

Carbohydrates are not only obtained from food but are also produced in the body. Amino acids, glycerol, etc. are the different components from which the synthesis of carbohydrates takes place.

The chemical reactions which occur in the body are mainly divided into three pathways:
a. **Catabolic pathways:** Catabolic pathways are those which result in breaking down of compounds:
  - Glycolysis
  - Glycogenolysis

Fig. 4.6: Overview of carbohydrate metabolism.

b. **Anabolic pathways:** Anabolic pathways are those which build compounds or synthesize substances for the body:
   - Gluconeogenesis
   - Glycogenesis
c. **Amphibolic pathway:** It has a dual role: both catabolic and anabolic:
   - TCA cycle

GLYCOLYSIS

Glycolysis means the breakdown of glucose or sugar. Glycolysis occurs, at least in part, in almost every living cell. This series of reactions is believed to be among the oldest of all the biochemical pathways. It is a set of reactions in which one glucose molecule produces two pyruvic acid molecules, 2 molecules of ATP, 2 molecules of NADH, and 2 molecules of water. In the glycolysis pathway, the breakdown of six-carbon glucose ($C_6H_{12}O_6$) into two molecules of three-carbon compound pyruvate ($C_3H_6O_3$) takes place.

Site

It occurs in the cytoplasm of the cells in almost all the tissues.

Importance

- It provides fuel in the form of ATP and intermediates for metabolic pathways.
- It can operate both in aerobic and anaerobic conditions forming different end products.
- It is the fastest pathway for supplying energy.
- Glycolysis is the only source of energy in erythrocytes.

Steps of Aerobic Glycolysis Pathway

Following are the steps of glycolysis cycle (**Figure 4.7**).
- **Step 1:** The enzyme hexokinase or glucokinase phosphorylates adds a phosphate group to glucose in the cell's cytoplasm. In the process, a phosphate group from ATP is transferred to glucose, producing glucose 6-phosphate.
  - Glucose ($C_6H_{12}O_6$) + Hexokinase + ATP → ADP + Glucose 6-phosphate ($C_6H_{11}O_6P_1$)
- **Step 2:** The enzyme phosphoglucoisomerase converts glucose 6-phosphate into its isomer fructose 6-phosphate. Isomers have the same molecular formula, but the atoms of each molecule are arranged differently.
  - Glucose 6-phosphate ($C_6H_{11}O_6P_1$) + Phosphohexose isomerase → Fructose 6-phosphate ($C_6H_{11}O_6P_1$)

Fig. 4.7: Steps of glycolysis pathway.

- **Step 3:** The enzyme phosphofructokinase uses another ATP molecule to transfer a phosphate group to fructose 6-phosphate to form fructose 1, 6-bisphosphate.
  - Fructose 6-phosphate ($C_6H_{11}O_6P_1$)+ phosphofructokinase + ATP → ADP + Fructose 1, 6-bisphosphate ($C_6H_{10}O_6P_2$)

- **Step 4:** The enzyme aldolase splits fructose 1, 6-bisphosphate into two sugars that are isomers of each other. These two sugars are dihydroxyacetone phosphate and glyceraldehyde phosphate.
  - Fructose 1, 6-bisphosphate ($C_6H_{10}O_6P_2$) + Aldolase → Dihydroxyacetone phosphate ($C_3H_5O_3P_1$) + Glyceraldehyde phosphate ($C_3H_5O_3P_1$)
- **Step 5:** The enzyme triose phosphate isomerase rapidly inter-converts the molecules dihydroxyacetone phosphate and glyceraldehyde phosphate. Glyceraldehyde phosphate is removed as soon as it is formed to be used in the next step of glycolysis.
  - Dihydroxyacetone phosphate ($C_3H_5O_3P_1$) → Glyceraldehyde phosphate ($C_3H_5O_3P_1$)
  - The net result for steps 4 and 5: Fructose 1, 6-bisphosphate ($C_6H_{10}O_6P_2$) ↔ 2 molecules of Glyceraldehyde phosphate ($C_3H_5O_3P_1$)
- **Step 6:** The enzyme glyceraldehyde 3-P dehydrogenase serves two functions in this step. First the enzyme transfers hydrogen (H^-) from glyceraldehyde phosphate to the oxidizing agent nicotinamide adenine dinucleotide (NAD^+) to form NADH. Next triose phosphate dehydrogenase adds a phosphate (P) from the cytosol to the oxidized glyceraldehyde phosphate to form 1, 3-bisphosphoglycerate. This occurs for both molecules of glyceraldehyde phosphate produced in step 5.
  a. Glyceraldehydes 3-dehydrogenase + 2 H^- + 2 NAD^+ → 2 NADH + 2 H^+
  b. Glyceraldehydes 3-phosphate dehydrogenase + 2P + 2 glyceraldehyde phosphate ($C_3H_5O_3P_1$) → 2 molecules of 1, 3-bisphosphoglycerate ($C_3H_4O_4P_2$)
- **Step 7:** The enzyme phosphoglycerokinase transfers a P from 1, 3-bisphosphoglycerate to a molecule of ADP to form ATP. This happens for each molecule of 1, 3-bisphosphoglycerate. The process yields two 3-phosphoglycerate molecules and two ATP molecules.
  - 2 molecules of 1, 3-bisphoshoglycerate ($C_3H_4O_4P_2$) + phosphoglycerokinase + 2 ADP → 2 molecules of 3-phosphoglycerate ($C_3H_5O_4P_1$) + 2 ATP
- **Step 8:** The enzyme phosphoglyceromutase relocates the P from 3-phosphoglycerate from the third carbon to the second carbon to form 2-phosphoglycerate.
  - 2 molecules of 3-phosphoglycerate ($C_3H_5O_4P_1$) + phosphoglyceromutase → 2 molecules of 2-phosphoglycerate ($C_3H_5O_4P_1$)
- **Step 9:** The enzyme enolase removes a molecule of water from 2-phosphoglycerate to form phosphoenolpyruvic acid (PEP). This happens for each molecule of 2-phosphoglycerate.
  - 2 molecules of 2-phosphoglycerate ($C_3H_5O_4P_1$) + Enolase → 2 molecules of phosphoenolpyruvic acid (PEP) ($C_3H_3O_3P_1$)
- **Step 10:** The enzyme pyruvate kinase transfers a P from PEP to ADP to form pyruvic acid and ATP. This happens for each molecule of PEP. This reaction yields 2 molecules of pyruvic acid and 2 ATP molecules.
  - 2 molecules of PEP ($C_3H_3O_3P_1$) + pyruvate kinase + 2 ADP → 2 molecules of pyruvic acid ($C_3H_4O_3$) + 2 ATP

Anaerobic Glycolysis Pathway

Anaerobic glycolysis serves as a means of energy production in cells that cannot produce adequate energy through oxidative phosphorylation. In poorly oxygenated tissue, glycolysis produces 2 ATP by shunting pyruvate away from mitochondria and through the lactate dehydrogenase reaction. In rapidly contracting skeletal muscle cells with energy demand exceeding what can be produced by oxidative phosphorylation alone, anaerobic glycolysis allows for the more rapid production of ATP. (**Glycolysis is approximately 100 times faster** than oxidative phosphorylation). In cells lacking mitochondria altogether, pyruvate cannot undergo oxidative phosphorylation regardless of oxygen levels.

Two major fermentation processes exist:

(i) **Lactic acid fermentation:** In lactic acid fermentation, the pyruvic acid from glycolysis is reduced to lactic acid by NADH, which is oxidized to NAD⁺. Lactic acid fermentation allows glycolysis to continue by ensuring that NADH is returned to its oxidized state (NAD⁺).
- This pathway is common for animal cells and lactic acid bacteria. Red blood cells take most of the energy from anaerobic metabolism. The lactate produced utilizes through diffusion from the tissues to the bloodstream and then to aerobic tissues, such as the liver and heart **(Fig. 4.8)**.
  Site: This commonly occurs in muscle cells.

(ii) **Alcoholic fermentation:** In alcoholic fermentation, the pyruvic acid from glycolysis loses one carbon in the form of carbon dioxide to form acetaldehyde, which is reduced to ethyl alcohol by NADH. When acetaldehyde is reduced to ethyl alcohol, NADH⁺ becomes NAD⁺ (is oxidized). This is the fermentation that commonly occurs in yeast. Like lactic acid fermentation, alcoholic fermentation allows glycolysis to continue by ensuring that NADH is returned to its oxidized state (NAD⁺) **(Fig. 4.9)**

Fig. 4.8: Anaerobic glycolysis pathway: Lactic acid fermentation.

Fig. 4.9: Anaerobic glycolysis pathway: Alcoholic fermentation.

Energetics of Glycolysis

Anaerobic glycolysis

Energy spent/molecule of glucose =	
• Hexokinase	1 ATP
• Phosphofructokinase (PFK)	1 ATP
Total	2 ATP
Energy generated/molecule of glucose =	
• Phosphoglycerate kinase 1 ATP × 2	= 2 ATP
• Pyruvate kinase 1 ATP × 2	= 2 ATP
Total	= 4 ATP
Net gain of ATP	= 2 ATP

■ GLYCOGENOLYSIS

Glycogenolysis is the biochemical pathway in which glycogen breaks down into glucose-1-phosphate and glucose. The reaction takes place in the hepatocytes and the myocytes. The process is under the regulation of two key enzymes: phosphorylase kinase and glycogen phosphorylase. Blood glucose is a source of energy for the entire human body. During the fasting state, to maintain normal blood glucose levels, the liver plays a central role in producing glucose via glycogenolysis and gluconeogenesis. Glycogen is a branched polysaccharide consisting of glucose units. In humans, it is the principal storage form of glucose. During times of need, the body breaks down glycogen to produce glucose.

The process is caused by the hormones glucagon and epinephrine which stimulate glycogenolysis.

The free glucose so formed is metabolized in two ways:
a. It is completely oxidized to carbon dioxide and water with the release of considerable energy as ATP molecules.
b. It is converted to other sugars, e.g., pentoses.

Site

It occurs in the liver when blood glucose falls below normal. Glycogenolysis occurs within the cytoplasm of cells.

Significance

❖ It occurs when glucose level in blood decreases.
❖ It also occurs during muscle contraction.

Steps of Glycogenolysis Pathway

Figure 4.10 presents the steps of glycogenolysis.
❖ At first step of glycogenolysis, glycogen phosphorylase cleaves α (1→ 4) linkage of glycogen to form glucose 1-phosphate. From the outermost chains of the glycogen molecule, the terminal glucosyl residues are detached sequentially until approximately four glucose residues remain on either side of an α (1→ 6) branch. Branches of glycogen are removed by two debranching enzymes such as α (1→ 4) → α (1→ 4)-glucan transferase and amylo- α (1→ 6)--glucosidase.
❖ Secondly, glucose 1-phosphate is converted to glucose 6-phosphate by phosphoglucomutase.
❖ Finally, in liver, but not in skeletal muscle, glucose 6-phosphatase enzyme hydrolyzes glucose

Fig. 4.10: Steps of glycogenolysis pathway.

Fig. 4.11: Steps of gluconeogenesis pathway.

6-phosphate, forming glucose that is exported to circulation, and leading to increased blood glucose.

GLUCONEOGENESIS

Gluconeogenesis is the process by which glucose is made, primarily in the liver, from non-carbohydrate sources. The body is able to make glucose from amino acids (protein), glycerol (the backbone of triglycerides, the primary fat storage molecule), and glucose metabolism intermediaries like lactate and pyruvate. Liver and kidneys are the major organs that carryout the gluconeogenesis. The steps of gluconeogenesis is depicted in **Figure 4.11**.

Site of Gluconeogenesis

It occurs mainly in the liver, and to a lesser extent in the renal cortex. The pathway is partly mitochondrial and partly cytoplasmic.

The major substrates for gluconeogenesis are:
a. Lactic acid
b. Glycerol
c. Some amino acid

Significance

- It meets the energy needs of the body when dietary carbohydrates are insufficient (as a continuous supply of glucose is vital for a delicate organ such as brain).
- Glucose is also required as a source of glycerol for the synthesis of triglycerol (fats) in the adipose tissues.
- Glucose is the only fuel that supplies energy to the skeletal muscles under anaerobic conditions.
- For the synthesis of lactose in the mammary gland, glucose is essential.
- The pathway uses lactic acid and glycerol and thus removes these metabolic products from the blood preventing their accumulation.
- It is the source of synthesis of other carbohydrates as well as provides oxaloacetate for the TCA cycle.

■GLYCOGENESIS

Glycogenesis is the formation of glycogen from glucose. Glycogen is synthesized depending on the demand for glucose and ATP (energy). If both are present in relatively high amounts, then the excess of insulin promotes the glucose conversion into glycogen for storage in liver and muscle cells. Glycogen, the principal storage form of glucose and primary source of non-oxidative glucose for skeletal muscle and liver, confers significant contributions via its degradation by maintaining normal blood glucose levels and providing fuel for muscle contraction.

Significance

It stores the excess glucose, thus maintaining the glucose level in blood within normal limits.

Steps of Glycogenesis

- Glucose is converted into glucose-6-phosphate by the action of glucokinase or hexokinase.
- Glucose-6-phosphate is converted into glucose-1-phosphate by the action of phosphoglucomutase, passing through an obligatory intermediate step of glucose-1, 6-bisphosphate.
- Glucose-1-phosphate is converted into UDP-glucose by the action of uridyl transferase (also called UDP-glucose pyrophosphorylase) and pyrophosphate is formed, which is hydrolyzed by pyrophosphatase into 2 molecules of Pi.
- Glucose molecules are assembled in a chain by glycogen synthase, which must act on a pre-existing glycogen primer or glycogenin (small protein that forms the primer). The mechanism for joining glucose units is that glycogen synthase binds to uridine diphosphate glucose (UDP-Glucose), causing it to breakdown into an oxonium ion, also formed in glycogenolysis. This oxonium ion can readily add to the 4-hydroxyl group of a glucosyl residue on the 4 end of the glycogen chain.
- Branches are made by branching enzyme (also known as amylo-α (1:4) → α(1:6) transglycosylase), which transfers the end of the chain onto an earlier part via α 1:6 glycosidic bond, forming branches, which further grow by addition of more α 1:4 glycosidic units.

TRICARBOXYLIC ACID (TCA) CYCLE

Following glycolysis, the mechanism of cellular respiration involves another multistep process—TCA cycle which is also known as ***Krebs cycle or citric acid cycle as it was proposed by Sir Hans Krebs in 1937.*** It is a series of reactions through which the final oxidation of acetyl CoA to carbon dioxide occurs. The Krebs cycle uses the two molecules of pyruvic acid formed in glycolysis and yields high-energy molecules of NADH and flavin adenine dinucleotide (FADH), as well as some ATP.

Site
It occurs in mitochondria of the cell.

Significance
* The importance of Krebs cycle lies in the efficiency with which it captures energy released from nutrient molecules and stores it in a usable form.
* It also produces the raw material for the biosynthesis of certain amino acids and of purines and pyrimidines.
* It is the final common oxidative pathway that oxidizes acetyl-CoA to CO_2.
* It is the source of reduced coenzymes that provide the substrate for the respiratory chain.
* It acts as a link between the catabolic and anabolic pathways.

Steps of TCA Cycle
Following are the steps of TCA cycles (**Fig. 4.12**).

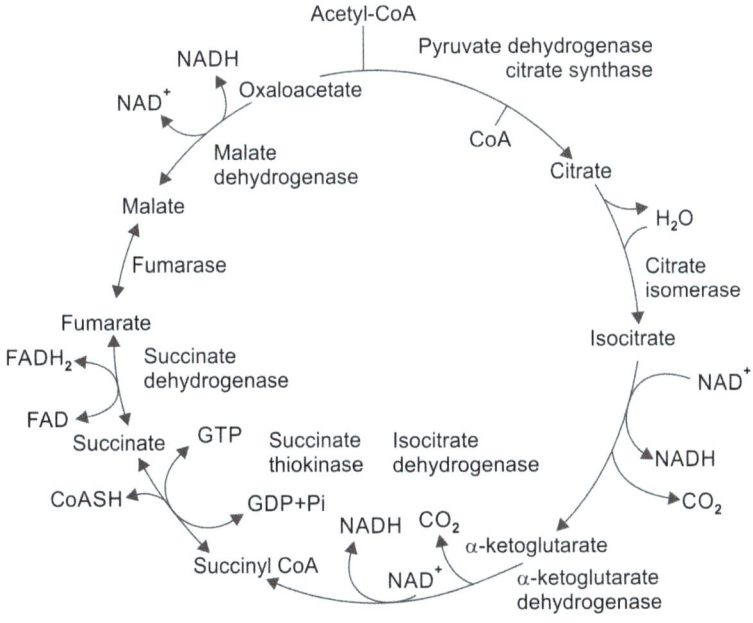

Fig. 4.12: Steps of TCA cycle pathway.

Preparatory Steps

Acetyl CoA enters the cycle, and completely oxidized. Pyruvate derived from glycolysis is oxidatively decarboxylated to acetyl CoA by the pyruvate dehydrogenase. All the enzymes of citric acid cycle are located inside the mitochondria.

Step 1: Formation of citric acid

The 4-carbon oxaloacetate condensed with 2-carbon acetyl CoA to form 6-carbon compound, the citrate. The enzyme is citrate synthase.

Step 2: Formation of isocitrate

Citrate is isomerized to isocitrate by aconitase. This reaction is a two-step process. At first, one water molecule is removed from citrate forming cis-aconitate. Immediately, one water molecule is added to aconitate to form isocitrate.

Step 3: Formation of α-ketoglutarate

- This reaction is a two-step process, both catalyzed by the same enzyme, isocitrate dehydrogenase. In the first part of the reaction, isocitrate is dehydrogenated to form oxalosuccinate. It is an unstable compound that undergoes spontaneous decarboxylation to form alpha ketoglutarate.
- The NADH generated in this step is later oxidized in the electron transport chain (ETC) to generate 3ATPs.
- Isocitrate (6 carbons) undergoes oxidative decarboxylation to form alpha ketoglutarate (5 carbons). In this reaction, one molecule of CO_2 is liberated.

Step 4: Formation of succinyl CoA

Next, alpha ketoglutarate is oxidatively decarboxylated to form succinyl CoA by the enzyme alpha ketoglutarate dehydrogenase. The NADH thus generated enters into ETC to generate 3 ATPs. Another molecule of CO_2 is removed in this step. This is the only irreversible step in the whole reaction cycle.

Step 5: Generation of succinate

- The next reaction involves a substrate-level phosphorylation, whereby a high energy phosphate is generated from the energy trapped in the thioester bond of succinyl CoA. The enzyme is succinate thiokinase. A molecule of GDP is phosphorylated to GTP and succinate is formed.
- The GTP can be converted to ATP by reacting with an ADP molecule.

$$GTP + ADP \longrightarrow GDP + ATP$$

Step 6: Formation of fumarate

Succinate is dehydrogenated to fumarate, an unsaturated dicarboxylic acid, by succinate dehydrogenase. The hydrogen atoms are accepted by FAD. $FADH_2$ then enters into ETC to generate 2 ATPs.

Step 7: Formation of malate

The formation of malate from fumarate is catalyzed by fumarase.

Step 8: Regeneration of oxaloacetate

Finally malate is oxidized to oxaloacetate by malate dehydrogenase. The coenzyme is NAD. The NADH is generated in this step, which enters the electron transport chain, when 3 ATPs

CHAPTER 4: Carbohydrates

are produced. The oxaloacetate can further condense with another acetyl CoA molecule and the cycle continues.

■ BLOOD GLUCOSE AND ITS REGULATION

Blood sugar regulation is the process by which the levels of blood sugar, primarily glucose, are maintained by the body. The maintenance of glucose levels in the blood within narrow limits is a finely and efficiently regulated system. This is important because it is essential to have a continuous supply of glucose to the brain. Even though it can utilize ketone bodies, the brain has an obligatory requirement for glucose. RBCs and renal medulla are dependent on glucose for meeting their fuel needs.

Mechanisms of Blood Sugar Regulation

The overview of the blood sugar regulation mechanism may also be seen in **Figures 4.13A** and **4.13B**.

Blood sugar levels are regulated by negative feedback in order to keep the body in homeostasis. The levels of glucose in the blood are monitored by the cells in the pancreas's Islets of Langerhans. If the blood glucose level falls to dangerous levels (as in very heavy exercise or lack of food for extended periods), the alpha cells of the pancreas release glucagon, a hormone whose effects on liver cells act to increase blood glucose levels. They convert glycogen into glucose (this process is called glycogenolysis). The glucose is released into the bloodstream, increasing blood sugar levels.

Fig. 4.13A: Mechanisms of blood sugar regulation.

Fig. 4.13B: Mechanisms of blood sugar regulation.

When levels of blood sugar rise, whether as a result of glycogen conversion or from the digestion of a meal, a different hormone is released from beta cells found in the Islets of Langerhans in the pancreas. This hormone, insulin, causes the liver to convert more glucose into glycogen (this process is called glycogenesis), and to force about 2/3rd of body cells (primarily muscle and fat tissue cells) to take up glucose from the blood through the GLUT4 transporter, thus decreasing blood sugar. When insulin binds to the receptors on the cell surface, vesicles containing the GLUT4 transporters come to the plasma membrane and fuse together by the process of exocytosis, thus enabling a facilitated diffusion of glucose into the cell. As soon as the glucose enters the cell, it is phosphorylated into glucose-6-phosphate in order to preserve the concentration gradient so glucose will continue to enter the cell. Insulin also provides signals to several other body systems and is the chief regulatory metabolic control in humans.

There are also several other causes for an increase in blood sugar levels. Among them are the 'stress' hormones such as epinephrine (also known as adrenaline), several of the steroids, infections, trauma, and of course, the ingestion of food.

Factors maintaining blood glucose are:
- The plasma glucose level at any instant depends on the balance between glucose entering and leaving the extracellular fluid.
- Hormones will make this balance possible.
- The major factors which cause entry of glucose into blood are:
  - Absorption from intestine
  - Glycogenolysis
  - Gluconeogenesis
  - Hyperglycemic hormones (glucagon, steroids)
- Factors leading to depletion of glucose in blood are:
  - Utilization by tissues for energy
  - Glycogen synthesis
  - Conversion of glucose into fat
  - Hypoglycemic hormone (insulin)

GLYCEMIA

- Glycemia is the concentration of glucose in the blood. It is usually expressed in milligrams per deciliter (mg/dL). Glycemia is controlled by several physiological processes.
- **Factors that may increase the blood glucose level:** Following are some of the essential factors that may increase the blood glucose levels.
  - After meals, due to the gastric and intestinal absorption of carbohydrates of low molecular weight present in the diet or broken down from other kinds of foodstuffs, such as starches (polysaccharides).
  - Another input to glycemia levels is gluconeogenesis, where amino acids and lipids are converted to glucose via several metabolic chains. Excess glucose is converted to glycogen or to triglycerides for energy storage.
  - Glycogenolysis, whereby glycogen stored in the liver breaks down to form glucose
  - Not being physically active
  - Side effects from some medications, such as steroids or antipsychotic medications
  - Illness—body release hormones to fight the illness, and those hormones raise blood glucose levels
  - Stress, which can produce hormones that raise blood glucose levels

- Short- or long-term pain, such as pain from a sunburn—your body releases hormones that raise blood glucose levels
- Menstrual periods, which cause changes in hormone levels
- Dehydration
❖ **Factors that may decrease the blood glucose level:** Following are some of the essential factors that may decrease the blood glucose levels:
  - With usage by catabolism or not enough food, such as a meal or snack with fewer carbohydrates than usual or a missed meal or snack. Stress can also decrease the level of glucose.
  - Temperature regulation
  - Physical exertion makes your body more sensitive to insulin and can lower blood glucose
  - Alcohol, especially on an empty stomach
  - Too much insulin or oral diabetes medications
  - Side effects from other medications
    - Glucose is the most important source of metabolic energy for the majority of cells, particularly for some cells (e.g., neurons and erythrocytes) which are almost totally dependent on it. The brain requires a fairly stable glycemia in order to function normally. Concentrations of less than about 30 mg/dl or greater than about 300 mg/dl can produce confusion, unconsciousness, and convulsions.
    - Several hormones are involved in the regulation of glucose metabolism, such as insulin, glucagon (secreted by the pancreas), epinephrine (adrenaline secreted by the adrenal glands), glucocorticoids, and steroid hormones (secreted by the gonads and adrenal glands).

Effects of Abnormal Values of Glycemia

❖ Many forms of severe stress and trauma, stroke, heart attack, and surgery can temporarily increase glucose levels.
❖ Glycemia can also be increased by certain drugs such as antidepressants, corticosteroids, diuretics, estrogens, lithium, phenothiazine, phenytoin and salicylic acids, or decreased by others, such as acetaminophen, alcohol, steroids, clofibrate, gemfibrozil.
❖ However, the disease most directly associated to chronic increase of glycemia is diabetes mellitus, due to a decrease in the secretion of insulin, excess of its breakdown or decreased capacity of cells to transport it across its membranes (insulin resistance).

GLUCOSE TOLERANCE TEST

The glucose tolerance test (GTT) is a laboratory method to check how the body breaks down (metabolizes) sugar. The glucose tolerance test is an aid to diagnosis in diabetes mellitus. If the glucose level peaks at a higher than normal level at 1 and 2 hours after injection or ingestion of glucose and are slower than normal to return to fasting levels, then diabetes mellitus is confirmed. The most common glucose tolerance test is:

❖ **The oral glucose tolerance test (OGTT):** A person cannot eat or drink anything for at least 8 hours before the test. For the test, after taking a fasting blood sample of the patient, he/she is asked to drink a liquid containing a certain amount of glucose (usually 75 grams). Then blood samples are taken every 30-60 minutes after drinking the glucose solution. The test takes up to 3 hours.
❖ **The intravenous glucose tolerance test (IGTT)** is rarely used, and is never used to diagnose diabetes. In this test, glucose is injected into vein. Blood glucone levels are measured before the injection, and again at 1, 2 and 3 hours after the injection. However, the timing may vary.

Indications of GTT
- Glucose tolerance tests are one of the tools used to diagnose diabetes. If a patient has symptoms of diabetes mellitus, but fasting blood glucose value is inconclusive.
- The oral glucose tolerance test is used to screen pregnant women for gestational diabetes between 24 and 28 weeks of pregnancy.
- To rule out benign renal glycosuria.

Preparation for the Test
- Make sure that patient eats normally for several days before the test.
- Ensure that patient has not consumed anything for 8 hours before the test and patient does not eat during test also.
- Certain medicines also may be discontinued which may affect the test results such as steroids, morning dose of insulin or oral hypoglycemic medicines, etc.
- Patients are advised to remain in the hospital during the waiting time of 2 hours without any active exercise.

Interpretations of GTT Results
Normal blood values for a 75-gram oral glucose tolerance test used to check for type 2 diabetes:
Fasting: 60–100 mg/dL
1. **Hour:** Less than 200 mg/dL
2. **Hours:** Less than 140 mg/dL.

Impaired Results for Type 1 Diabetes or Type 2 Diabetes
- **Fasting glucose level:** 100–125 mg/dL
- **Two-hour glucose level:** 140–200 mg/dL

Abnormal (Diagnostic) Results for Type 1 Diabetes or Type 2 Diabetes
- Fasting glucose level greater than 126 mg/dL
- Two-hour glucose level greater than 200 mg/dL

Normal Results for Gestational Diabetes
- Fasting glucose level less than 90 mg/dL
- One-hour glucose level less than 130–140 mg/dL
- Two-hour glucose level less than 120 mg/dL

Abnormal Results for Gestational Diabetes
- Fasting glucose level greater than 95 mg/dL
- One-hour glucose level greater than 140 mg/dL
- Two-hour glucose level greater than 120 mg/dL

Nursing Considerations
- Instruct the patient to eat a high-carbohydrate (200–300 g) diet for 3 days before the test.
- Instruct the patient to avoid alcohol, coffee and smoking for 36 hours before test.
- Instruct the patient to fast for 8–10 hours before test.
- Instruct the patient to avoid strenuous exercise for 8 hours before test and after the test.
- Instruct the patient with diabetes mellitus to withhold morning insulin or oral hypoglycemic medications.
- Instruct the patient that the test may take 3–5 hours that requires IV or oral administration of glucose and multiple blood samples.

HYPERGLYCEMIA AND DIABETES

Hyperglycemia, or high blood glucose (sugar), is a serious health problem for those with diabetes. Hyperglycemia develops when there is too much sugar in the blood. In people with diabetes, there are two specific types of hyperglycemia that occur:

- Fasting hyperglycemia is defined as a blood sugar greater than 90–130 mg/dL after fasting for at least 8 hours.
- Postprandial or after-meal hyperglycemia is defined as a blood sugar usually greater than 180 mg/dL. In people without diabetes postprandial or post-meal sugars rarely go over 140 mg/dL but occasionally, after a large meal, a 1–2 hour post-meal glucose level can reach 180 mg/dL. Consistently elevated high post-meal glucose levels can be an indicator that a person is at high-risk for developing type 2 diabetes.
  - It is important to treat the symptoms of hyperglycemia promptly to prevent complications from diabetes.

Factors contributing to hyperglycemia: Include reduced insulin secretion, decreased glucose utilization, and increased glucose production. Glucose homeostasis is a balance between hepatic glucose production and peripheral glucose uptake and utilization. Insulin is the most important regulator of glucose homeostasis.

Hyperglycemia in diabetes may be caused by:
- Skipping or forgetting insulin or oral glucose-lowering medicine
- Eating too many grams of carbohydrates for the amount of insulin administered or just eating too many grams of carbohydrates in general
- Eating too much food and having too many calories
- Infection
- Illness
- Increased stress
- Decreased activity or exercising less than usual
- Strenuous physical activity.

Secondary Cause of Hyperglycemia

The secondary causes of hyperglycemia include the following:
- Destruction of the pancreas from chronic pancreatitis, hemochromatosis, pancreatic cancer, and cystic fibrosis
- Endocrine disorders that cause peripheral insulin resistance like Cushing syndrome, acromegaly, and pheochromocytoma
- Use of medications like glucocorticoids, phenytoin, and estrogens
- Gestational diabetes is known to occur in 4% of all pregnancies and is primarily due to decreased insulin sensitivity
- Total parental nutrition and dextrose infusion
- Reactive as seen postoperatively or in critically ill patients

Major Risk Factors for Hyperglycemia

- Weight more than 120% of the desired body weight
- Family history of type 2 diabetes
- Presence of hyperlipidemia or hypertension
- History of gestational diabetes
- Presence of polycystic ovarian syndrome

Symptoms of Hyperglycemia

It is important to know the early signs of hyperglycemia. If hyperglycemia is left untreated, it may develop into an emergency condition called ketoacidosis (if type 1 diabetes) or HHNS (if type 2 diabetes).

Early signs of hyperglycemia in diabetes include:
- Increased thirst
- Headaches
- Difficulty concentrating
- Blurred vision
- Frequent urination
- Fatigue, weak and tired feeling
- Weight loss
- Blood glucose more than 180 mg/dL

Prolonged hyperglycemia in diabetes may result in:
- Vaginal and skin infections
- Slow-healing cuts and sores
- Decreased vision
- Nerve damage causing painful cold or insensitive feet, loss of hair on the lower extremities, and/or erectile dysfunction
- Stomach and intestinal problems such as chronic constipation or diarrhea.

Treatment of Hyperglycemia

If a person has diabetes and has any of the early signs of hyperglycemia, be sure to test blood glucose several times. Person will need to have a record of several blood glucose readings before contacting healthcare provider. They may recommend the following changes:
- **Drink more water:** Water helps remove the excess glucose from urine and helps avoid dehydration.
- **Exercise more:** Exercise will help to lower blood glucose. Caution: If type 1 diabetes and blood glucose is over 240 mg/dL, need to check urine for ketones. If ketones are positive, do NOT exercise. If type 2-diabetes and blood glucose is over 300 mg/dL, even without ketones, do NOT exercise.
- **Change eating habits:** Person may need to meet with the dietitian to change the amount and types of foods.
- **Change medications:** Healthcare provider may change the amount, timing, or type of diabetes medications take. Do not make adjustments in diabetes medications without talking to healthcare provider.

Complications of untreated or uncontrolled hyperglycemia over a prolonged period of time include:

Microvascular Complications
- Retinopathy
- Nephropathy
- Neuropathy

Macrovascular Complications
- Coronary artery disease

- Cerebrovascular disease
- Peripheral vascular diseases.

Prevention of Hyperglycemia

Make sure to following meal plan, exercise program and medicine schedule are instructed to patient.
- Know diet, count the total amounts of carbohydrate that are consuming.
- Test blood glucose regularly.
- Know when to contact healthcare provider if repeated abnormal blood glucose readings.
- Make sure always wear medical identification that states diabetes so you can receive proper treatment in the event of an emergency.

HYPOGLYCEMIA

Hypoglycemia is a condition that occurs when blood sugar (glucose) is too low. Blood sugar below 70 mg/dl is considered low and termed as hypoglycemia. **Hypoglycemia** is most often seen in patients who have diabetes that undergoing pharmacologic intervention. Among this group, patients with type 1 diabetes are three times as likely to experience **hypoglycemia** than patients with type 2 diabetes when receiving treatment.

Causes and Risk Factors of Hypoglycemia

The most common causes of low blood sugar in people with diabetes are:
- Taking insulin or diabetes medicine at the wrong time
- Taking too much insulin or diabetes medicine by mistake
- Not eating enough during meals or snacks after taken insulin or diabetes medicine
- Skipping meals
- Waiting to eat meals after insulin
- Exercising more or at a different time than usual
- Drinking alcohol
- Diabetes medications: Such as sulfonamides, metformin, insulin.
- In patients who do not have diabetes, **hypoglycemia** is uncommon, but when it occurs, there are a few major causes of **hypoglycemia**: pharmacologic, alcohol, critical illness, counter-regulatory hormone deficiencies, and non-islet cell tumors

Symptoms of Hypoglycemia

- Double vision or blurry vision
- Fast or pounding heartbeat
- Feeling cranky or acting aggressively
- Feeling nervous
- Headache
- Hunger
- Shaking
- Sleeping trouble
- Sweating
- Tingling or numbness of the skin
- Tiredness or weakness
- Unclear thinking.

Sometimes blood sugar may be too low, even without having symptoms. If blood sugar gets too low, a patient may:
- Faint
- Have a seizure
- Go into a coma.

Diagnosis of Hypoglycemia

Random blood sugar: Show readings lower than 70 mg/dL.

Treatment of Hypoglycemia

Treatment primarily depends on the cause.

Severe **hypoglycemia** can be treated with intravenous (IV) dextrose followed by infusion of glucose. For conscious patients able to take oral (PO) medications, readily absorbable carbohydrate sources (such as fruit juice) should be given. For patients unable to take oral agents, glucagon should be administered. Glucagon can be given intramuscularly. Once the patient is more awake, a complex carbohydrate food source should be given to achieve sustained euglycemia.

Give about 15 grams of carbohydrates. Examples are:
- 3 glucose tablets
- A 1/2 cup (4 ounces) of fruit juice or regular, non-diet soda
- 5 or 6 hard candies
- 1 tablespoon sugar, plain or dissolved in water
- 1 tablespoon honey or syrup
  - Wait about 15 minutes before giving anything else. Be careful not to over-treat by eating too much. This can cause high blood sugar and weight gain.
- **Check blood sugar again:** If person does not feel better in 15 minutes and blood sugar is still low (less than 70 mg/dL), eat something that has 15 grams of carbohydrates again.
- Person may need to eat a snack that has carbohydrates and protein if blood sugar is in a safer range (over 70 mg/dL) and next meal is more than an hour away.
  - If these steps for raising your blood sugar do not work, plan to administer 5% dextrose intravenously.

Prevention of Hypoglycemia

- Instruct the patient to follow advice about diet, medicine, and exercise.
- Preventing low blood sugar is better than having to treat it. So instruct the patient that when he/she exercises, check blood sugar levels.
- Make sure that patient eats food after administration of insulin or hypoglycemic treatment.
- Protein snacks may be advised for bedtime to prevent late night or early morning hypoglycemic episodes.
- Instruct the patient to avoid the alcohol drinks without eating food.
- Instruct the patient to have small, frequent meals that contain complex carbohydrates, fiber, and fat, and to avoid simple sugars, alcohol, and fruit juice.
- Instruct the patient to eat meals at regular times and eat extra food when carrying out more exercise.
- Instruct to keep sugar-containing snacks or drinks, which can be taken in the event of hypoglycemic symptoms.

CHAPTER 4: Carbohydrates

QUESTIONS

Q.1: What are the carbohydrates? How are they classified on the basis of number of saccharide units and number of carbon atoms; give an example of each class as well as their properties.

Q.2: What are the carbohydrates? Explain the classification and properties of carbohydrates. Describe the functions of carbohydrates in living cells.

Q.3: What is metabolism? Describe briefly the metabolism of carbohydrates.

Q.4: Describe TCA cycle. Give its bioenergetics.

Q.5: What is metabolism? Explain glycolysis and TCA cycle.

Q.6: Explain metabolism and biochemical basis of hypoglycemia.

BIBLIOGRAPHY

1. Bakker BM, Mensonides FIC, Teusink BS, et al. Compartmentation protects trypanosomes from the dangerous design of glycolysis. Proc Nat Acad Sci, USA 2000; 97(5):2087-92.
2. Fothergill-Gilmore LA, Michels PA. Evolution of glycolysis. Prog Biophys Mol Biol, 1993; 59:105-35.
3. Frommer WB, Schulze, WX, LaLonde S. Hexokinase, Jack-of-All-Trades. Science, 2003; 300:261, 263.
4. Grisham CM, Garrett R. Biochemistry. Philadelphia: Saunders College Pub, 1999: 426-7.
5. Malik VS, Schulze MB, Hu, FB. Intake of Sugar-sweetened beverages and weight gain: A systematic review. Am J Clin Nutr, 2006; 84:274-88.
6. Payne VA, Arden C, Wu C, et al. Dual role of phosphofructokinase-2/fructose bisphosphatase-2 in Regulating the compartmentation and expression of glucokinase in hepatocytes. Diabetes, 2005; 54:1949-57.
7. Piskur J, Rozpedowska E, Polakova S, et al. How Did Saccharomyces cerevisiae evolve to become a good brewer? Trends Genet, 2006: 22(4):183-6.
8. Smith AL (Ed). Oxford dictionary of biochemistry and molecular biology. Oxford: Oxford University Press, 1997.
9. Teusink B, Walsh MC, van Dam K, et al. The danger of metabolic pathways with turbo design. Trends Biochem Sci, 1998; 23(5):162-9.
10. Erica A. Melkonian; Mark P. Schury. Biochemistry, Anaerobic Glycolysis. Available on https://www.ncbi.nlm.nih.gov/books/NBK546695/. Cited on 03-02-2022
11. Manuel A. Paredes-Flores; Shamim S. Mohiuddin. Biochemistry, Glycogenolysis Available on https://www.ncbi.nlm.nih.gov/books/NBK554417/. Cited on 03-02-2022
12. Good to Know: Factors affecting blood glucose. Clin Diabetes, 2018 Apr; 36(2):202. Avaialble on https://www.ncbi.nlm.nih.gov/pmc/articles/PMC5898168/. Cited on 03-02-2022
13. Philip Mathew, Deepu Thoppil. Hypoglycemia. Available on https://www.ncbi.nlm.nih.gov/books/NBK534841/ Cited on 03-02-2022
14. Emily Eyth, Hajira Basit, Carrie J. Smith. Glucose Tolerance Test. Available on https://www.ncbi.nlm.nih.gov/books/NBK532915/ cited on 04-03-2022
15. MIchelle Mouri, Madhu Badireddy. Hyperglycemia. Available on https://www.ncbi.nlm.nih.gov/books/NBK430900/ cited on 04-02-2022
16. Vasudevan DM, S Sreekumari, Vaidyanathan Kannan. Textbook of Biochemistry for Medical Students. 9th edn. New Delhi:Jaypee Brothers Medical Publishers;2019.

CHAPTER 5

Proteins

Suresh K Sharma, Navjot Kaur

Chapter Outline
- Amino Acids
- Proteins
- Catabolism of Amino Acids
- Urea Cycle
- Gout
- Nitrogenous Constituents of Urine and Blood
- Plasma Proteins

■ AMINO ACIDS

Amino acids are the basic structural unit of proteins. They are also known as building blocks of proteins. Fundamentally, amino acids are organic compounds that are joined together by peptide bonds to form the basic structure of proteins. However, owing to the many 'side groups' that are part of the amino acids other sorts of bonds may form between the amino acid units. These additional bonds twist and turn the protein into convoluted shapes that are unique to the protein and essential to its ability to perform certain functions within the human body.

More than 300 amino acids are found in nature. There are twenty amino acids that are used to form proteins in the human body; these are called the proteinogenic amino acids.

All amino acids found in proteins have above basic structure, differing only in the structure of the R-group or the side chain. The simplest, and smallest amino acid found in proteins is glycine for which the R-group is hydrogen (H) (**Fig. 5.1**).

L-isomer: In proteins, only the L-isomer is found normally. Amino acids contain two functional groups:
1. An amino group (NH_2)
2. A carboxylic acid (COOH)

Amino group is basic in nature, while carboxylic group is acidic in nature. At physiological pH, free amino acids are ionized, that is, the carboxyl group loses its H^+ and amino group

Fig. 5.1: Basic structure of an amino acid.

gains H⁺ although the molecules net charge is zero. The main role of amino acids is in the synthesis of structural and functional proteins. In addition, a number of nitrogen-containing compounds are also synthesized using amino acids. Unlike carbohydrates and fats, there is no storage form of proteins in the body.

■ CLASSIFICATION OF AMINO ACIDS

There are many classification systems, four of which are presented here:

Based on the Nutritional Importance

Essential amino acids	Non-essential amino acids
These are not synthesized in our body and must be provided in the diet.	These are synthesized in the body. Hence they are not an essential component of diet.
• Histidine	• Alanine
• Isoleucine	• Arginine
• Leucine	• Aspartic acid
• Lysine	• Cysteine
• Methionine	• Cystine
• Phenylalanine	• Glutamic acid
• Threonine	• Glutamine
• Tryptophan	• Glycine
• Valine	• Proline
	• Serine
	• Tyrosine

Based on Polarity

Non-polar	Polar
Amino acids having hydrophobic side chain are known as non-polar amino acids, e.g.,	Amino acids having hydrophilic side chain are known as polar amino acids, e.g.,
Glycine	Phenylalanine
Alanine	Tryptophan
Valine	Serine
Leucine	Threonine
Isoleucine	Asparagine
Proline	Glutamine
Methionine	Cysteine
	Tyrosine

Based on the Number of —NH_2 and –COOH Group

Superstructure	Amino Acid
Monoamine, monocarboxylic	Glycine
	L-alanine
	L-valine
	L-leucine
	L-isoleucine
	L-proline
	L-phenylalanine
	L-tyrosine
	L-tryptophan
	L-methionine
	L-serine
	L-threonine
	L-cysteine
	L-asparagine
	L-glutamine
Monoamine, dicarboxylic	L-aspartate
	L-glutamate
Diamino, monocarboxylic	L-lysine
	L-arginine
	L-histidine

Based on the Structure

Classification	Amino acid	Structure
Aliphatic (do not contain N,O,S in side chain)	Glycine	H_2N-CH_2-COOH
	Alanine	$H_2N-CH(CH_3)-COOH$
	Valine	$H_3N-CH(CH(CH_3)_2)-COOH$
	Leucine	$H_3N-CH(CH_2CH(CH_3)_2)-COOH$
	Isoleucine	$H_2N-CH(CH(CH_3)CH_2CH_3)-COOH$
Sulfur-containing	Cysteine	$H_3N-CH(CH_2SH)-COOH$
	Methionine	$H_2N-CH(CH_2CH_2SCH_3)-COOH$

SECTION 1: Biochemistry

Aromatic (benzene ring in side chain)	Phenylalanine	(structure of phenylalanine)
	Tyrosine	(structure of tyrosine)
	Tryptophan	(structure of tryptophan)
	Serine	(structure of serine)
	Threonine	(structure of threonine)

Neutral (Hydroxyl or amide groups in side chain)	Asparagine	$H_2N-\underset{\underset{\underset{O=C-NH_2}{\mid}}{CH_2}}{\overset{H}{\underset{\mid}{C}}}-COOH$
	Glutamine	$H_3N^+-\underset{\underset{CH_2\ CH_2\ \overset{\parallel}{C}-NH_2}{\mid}}{\overset{H}{\underset{\mid}{C}}}-\overset{O}{\underset{\parallel}{C}}-O^-$
Acidic (carboxylate groups in side chain)	Aspartic acid	$H_2N-\underset{\underset{H}{\mid}}{\overset{\underset{\mid}{CH_2}}{\underset{\mid}{C}}}-COOH$ with $\overset{O}{\underset{\parallel}{C}}\!\!\diagup\!\!OH$ on side chain
	Glutamic acid	$H_3N^+-\underset{\underset{CH_2\ CH_2\ \overset{\parallel}{C}-OH}{\mid}}{\overset{H}{\underset{\mid}{C}}}-\overset{O}{\underset{\parallel}{C}}-O^-$
Basic	Lysine	$H_3N^+-\underset{\underset{CH_2\ (CH_2)_3-NH_2}{\mid}}{\overset{H}{\underset{\mid}{C}}}-\overset{O}{\underset{\parallel}{C}}-O^-$
	Arginine	$H_3N^+-\underset{\underset{(CH_2)_3-N-\overset{\parallel}{C}-NH_2}{\mid}}{\overset{H}{\underset{\mid}{C}}}-\overset{O}{\underset{\parallel}{C}}-O^-\ NH_2$
Imino acid (special case)	Proline	(cyclic structure) H_2N^+ — ring — $HC-\overset{O}{\underset{\parallel}{C}}-O$

Properties of Amino Acids

Physical Properties

- Amino acids are colorless and crystalline in nature.
- Amino acids are soluble in water, alcohol and insoluble in organic solvents.
- Amino acids melt at higher temperature.
- Amino acids can be sweet (glycine, alanine, and valine), tasteless (leucine), or bitter (arginine).

Standard Amino Acids are Optically Active Except Glycine

Chemical Properties

- **Reactions due to carboxylic (COOH) group:**
  - *Decarboxylation:* Decarboxylation produces biologically important amines, e.g.,

  $$\text{Histidine} \xrightarrow{\text{Decarboxylase}} \text{Histamine}$$

  - *Esterification:* Amino acids form esters with alcohols.
  - *Formation of amides:* Amino acids can form amides, when allowed to react with ammonia such as aspartic acid after reacting with ammonia, form asparagine, e.g.,

  $$\text{Aspartic acid} + NH_3 \longrightarrow \text{Asparagine}$$

  - *Salt formation:* Amino acids form salts when they react with bases.
- **Reactions due to amino group:**
  - *Transamination:* It is the transfer of α-amino group of an α-amino acid to form an α-keto acid.
  - *Deamination:* It is the removal of α-amino group of α-amino acid to form an α-keto acid.
  - *Oxidation:* Potassium permanganate or H_2O_2 oxidizes the $-NH_2$ group and converts the amino acids into imino acid which reacts with water to form ammonia and keto acid.
  - *Reaction with formaldehyde:* Formaldehyde reacts with $-NH_2$ group to form methylene compounds.
  - *Carbamino reaction:* In an alkaline solution, the $-NH_2$ group of an amino acid anion binds CO_2 to form a carbamino-acid anion.
  - *Ninhydrin reaction:* In this test α-amino group of an α-amino acid is mixed with ninhydrin and heated which causes the appearance of a purple/blue colored compound. This test is used to detect α-amino acids except for proline which gives yellow color as it contains amino acid.
- **Reactions due to side chain:**
  - *Transmethylation:* It is the transfer of the methyl group from the active form of methionine to noradrenaline to form adrenaline.
  - *Formation of disulfide bond:* It is the formation of disulphide bond between two cysteine molecules.
  - Cys – SH + HS – Cys   (–S –S) Disulphide bond of cysteine.
- **Peptide bond formation:**
  - α-carboxyl group of one amino acid and α-amino group of another amino acid reacts to form a peptide bond **(Fig. 5.2)**.

Functions of Amino Acids

- Phenylalanine helps in boosting the memory power.
- Valine acts as an important component in promoting muscle growth.
- Threonine helps in promoting the functions of the immune system.

Fig. 5.2: Chemical properties and structure of protein.

- Tryptophan is involved in the production of vitamin B3 and serotonin hormone. This serotonin hormone plays a vital role in maintaining our appetite, regulating sleep and boosting our moods.
- Isoleucine plays a vital role in the formation of hemoglobin, stimulating the pancreas to synthesize insulin, and in transporting oxygen from the lungs to the various parts.
- Methionine is utilized for the treatment of kidney stones, maintaining healthy skin and also useful in controlling the invasion of pathogenic bacteria.
- Leucine is involved in promoting protein synthesis, and growth hormones.
- Lysine is necessary for promoting the formation of antibodies, hormones, enzymes and in the development and fixation of calcium in bones.
- Histidine is involved in many enzymatic processes and in the synthesizing of both red blood cells (erythrocyte) and white blood cells (leukocytes).

■ PROTEINS

The name protein is derived from the Greek word *Proteios* which means primary or first. The name is so given because they are first among natural polymers essential for the growth and maintenance of life. Proteins are complex nitrogenous polymers containing C, H, O, N as major components and S, P as minor components. Proteins have high molecular weight.

In simple words, proteins are nitrogenous macromolecules made-up of many amino acids. Proteins are polymers of amino acids linked together by peptide bonds, commonly known as polypeptides.

Classification of Proteins

Proteins form the fundamental basis of the structure and function of life. Proteins are classified in several ways. There are three different types that are of major importance.

Protein Classification Based on Chemical Nature and Solubility

a. **Simple proteins:** They are composed of only amino acid residues. So these yield only amino acids on hydrolysis. The different kinds of simple proteins with description and examples are presented in **Table 5.1**.
b. **Conjugated proteins:** Besides amino acids, they contain a nonprotein moiety known as prosthetic group. So these yield amino acids and nonprotein products upon hydrolysis. Description and examples of different conjugated protein are depicted in **Table 5.2**.
c. **Derived proteins:** These are the denatured or degraded products of simple and conjugated proteins. Description of different derived proteins is depicted in **Table 5.3**.

Table 5.1: Different kinds of simple proteins.

S. No.	Kinds of protein	Description	Example
1.	Albumins	Soluble in water and are found in plant and animal tissues.	Blood (serumalbumin); milk (lactalbumin); egg white (ovoalbumin)
2.	Globulins	Sparingly soluble in water; soluble in neutral solutions; and by heat; distributed in both plant and animal tissues.	Blood (serum globulins); muscle (myosin)
3.	Glutelins	Insoluble in water; soluble in dilute acids; found in grains and cereals	Wheat (glutenin); rice (oryzenin)
4.	Prolamins	Insoluble in water and absolute alcohol; soluble in 70% alcohol; occurs in grain seeds	Wheat and rye (gliadin); corn (zein)
5.	Protamines	Soluble in water; occurs in sperm cells	sturgeon (sturine); mackerel
6.	Histones	Soluble in water, salt solutions, and dilute acids; combined with nucleic acids within cells.	Thymus gland; pancreas; nucleoproteins (nucleohistone)
7.	Scleroproteins	Connective tissues and hard tissues. Fibrous protein; insoluble in all solvents and resistant to digestion.	**Collagen:** Connective tissues, bones, cartilage, and gelatin. **Elastin:** Ligaments, tendons, and arteries **Keratin:** Hair, nails.

Table 5.2: Different kinds of conjugated proteins

S. No.	Kinds of protein	Description	Example
1.	Nucleoproteins	Contains nucleic acids, nitrogen, and phosphorus. Present in all living forms as a combination of protein with either RNA or DNA.	Cytoplasm of cells (ribonucleoprotein); nuclease of chromosomes (deoxyribonucleoprotein)
2.	Mucoprotein	Proteins combined with amino sugars, sugar acids, and sulfates.	Saliva (mucin); egg white (ovomucoid)
3.	Glycoprotein	Containing more than 4% hexosamine, mucoproteins; if less than 4%, then glycoproteins.	Bone (osseomucoid); tendons (tendomucoid); cartilage (chondromucoid)
4.	Phosphoproteins	Phosphoric acid joined in ester linkage to protein.	Milk (casein); egg yolk (ovovitellin)
5.	Chromoproteins	Protein compounds with such non-protein pigments as heme; colored proteins.	Hemoglobin; Myoglobin
6.	Lipoproteins	Water-soluble protein conjugated with lipids; found dispersed widely in all cells and all living forms.	Serum lipoprotein; brain, nerve tissues, milk, and eggs
7.	Metalloproteins	Proteins combined with metallic atoms that are not parts of a nonprotein prosthetic group	Ferritin; Carbonic anhydrase

Table 5.3: Description of different derived proteins.

S. No.	Kinds of protein	Description
1.	Proteins	Results from short action of acids or enzymes; insolvent in water.
2.	Peptones	Intermediate products of protein digestion. Same properties as proteases except that they cannot be salted out; of smaller molecular weight.
3.	Peptides	Intermediate products of protein digestion. Two or more amino acids joined by a peptide linkage; hydrolyzed to individual amino acids.

Classification of Proteins According to Shape and Solubility

Proteins can be broadly classified into three groups, based on their shape and solubility as depicted in **Table 5.4**.

Classification of Proteins Based on the Functions

Based on the functions they perform, proteins are classified into different groups as presented in **Table 5.5**.

Table 5.4: Comparative description of different proteins based on shape and solubility.

Fibrous proteins	Globular proteins	Membrane proteins
1. Long thread-like molecules whose helical strands often form fibers or sheets.	1. Spheroid or ovoid shape. These proteins are more or less spherical in nature.	1. These are proteins that are in association with lipid membranes.
2. These proteins have a rod like structure.	2. Due to their distribution of amino acids (hydrophobic inside, hydrophilic outside), they are very soluble in aqueous solution.	2. Those membrane proteins that are embedded in the lipid bilayer have extensive hydrophobic amino acids that interact with the non-polar environment of the bilayer interior.
3. They are not soluble in water.	3. Myoglobin is an example of a globular protein.	3. Membrane proteins are not soluble in aqueous solution.
4. Collagen, elastin, keratin are the examples of a fibrous protein.		4. Rhodopsin is an example of a membrane protein.

Table 5.5: Classification of proteins based on functions.

S. No.	Type	Example
1.	Structural proteins	Keratin of hair and nails, collagen of bone
2.	Enzymes or catalytic proteins	Hexokinase, pepsin, etc.
3.	Transport proteins	Hemoglobin, serum albumin
4.	Hormonal proteins	Insulin, growth hormone, etc.
5.	Contractile proteins	Actin and myosin
6.	Storage proteins	Glutelin
7.	Genetic proteins	Nucleoproteins
8.	Defense proteins	Immunoglobulins

Structure of Protein

- Each protein has a very unique folding pattern to perform its specific function in the cell. The linear sequence of amino acid residues in a polypeptide chain determines the three-dimensional configuration of a protein, and the structure of a protein determines its function. All proteins contain the elements carbon, hydrogen, oxygen, nitrogen, and sulfur some of these may also contain phosphorus, iodine, and traces of metals like ions, copper, zinc, and manganese.
- A protein may contain 20 different kinds of amino acids. Each amino acid has an amine group at one end and an acid group at the other and a distinctive side chain.
- The backbone is the same for all amino acids while the side chain differs from one amino acid to the next.

There are four levels of structural organization:

Primary Structure of Proteins

Primary structure is the sequence of chain of amino acids. Each amino acid is linked to another amino acid with the help of peptide bond and locations of disulfide bonds. The arranging sequence is very specific and is decided by genes and thus imparts specificity to function **(Fig. 5.3)**.

Proteins organize themselves into stable three dimensional structures shortly after synthesis due to close interaction between the adjacent amino acid and the side chains of amino acids forming polypeptide.

Secondary Structure of Proteins

- Secondary structure occurs when the sequence of amino acids are linked by hydrogen bonds making it more stable.
- The two most stable types of secondary structure include α-helix and β-pleated sheet **(Fig. 5.4)**:
- **α-helix:** It was predicted by Linus Pauling in 1951. The right handed α-helix formation is assisted by hydrogen bond between the –NH of peptide bond (at n position) and C=O of peptide bond (at n + 4 position) stabilizing the structure. A protein may have many α-helix at many locations. The α-helix has 3.6 amino acids per turn of helix. Hemoglobin and myoglobin have many α-helical regions.
- **β-pleated sheet:** It is a zigzag structure of proteins. In contrast to continuous sequence of α-helix, β-pleated sheet involves 5–10 amino acids and amino acids are fully stretched. The β-strands are aligned adjacent and close to each other and the C=O in one β-sheet forms hydrogen bond with the N-H of another β-sheet and the β-sheets so formed are pleated.

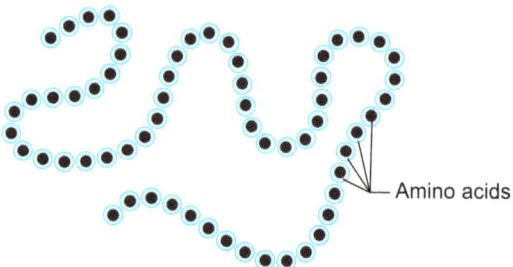

Fig. 5.3: Primary structure of protein.

α-helix   β-pleated sheet

Fig. 5.4: Secondary structure of protein.

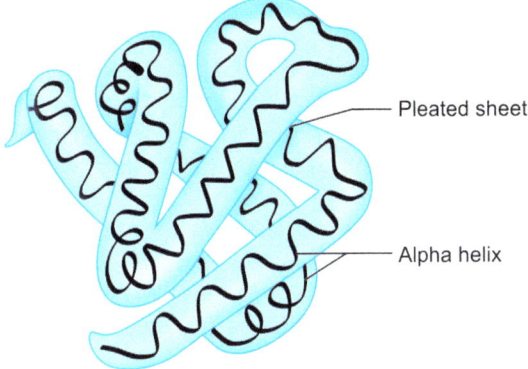

Fig. 5.5: Tertiary structure of protein.

Tertiary Structure of Proteins

The tertiary structure of a protein refers to its overall three-dimensional conformation. The tertiary structure of proteins is the result of further bonding between side chains within the protein and with any water that may be present around the protein. Polar amino acids move outwards and non-polar amino acids move inwards when placed in a polar solution. Bonds that are considered part of the tertiary structure include (**Fig. 5.5**):

- Bonds formed between non-polar side chains.
- Disulfide bonds formed between sulfur atoms in cysteine side chains.
- Ionic bonds formed between acidic and basic side chains.
- Hydrogen bonds formed between carbonyl groups and hydroxyl or amino groups.

Quaternary Structure of Proteins

Quaternary structure refers to the interaction of one or more subunits to form a functional protein. The quaternary structure of proteins is the result of the bonding between two or more polypeptides. The bonds formed are the same as those found in the tertiary structure of

Fig. 5.6: Quaternary structure of protein.

proteins. Hemoglobin, the oxygen-carrying component of blood, is an example of a protein in a quarternary structure **(Fig. 5.6)**.

Functions of Protein

Proteins are vital for growth and repair, and their functions are endless. They also have an enormous diversity of biological functions. Protein is the fundamental life force. Proteins are necessary in initiating every biochemical process in the body as well as in providing us an invaluable source of energy. In the absence of protein, the body would have deviation in many normal functions.

- **Protein as enzymes:** Proteins acts as enzymes, i.e., they facilitate biochemical reactions in which protein acts as a catalyst that increases the rate of reaction without themselves being changed in the process. Examples include enzymes like lactase and pepsin. Lactase breaks down the sugar lactose found in milk. Pepsin is a digestive enzyme that works in the stomach to break down proteins in food.
- **Transportation and storage:** Proteins have a unique ability to transport substances across cell membranes that other molecules cannot penetrate. Examples include hemoglobin and cytochromes. Hemoglobin transports oxygen through the blood. Cytochromes operate in the electron transport chain as electron carrier proteins.
- **Cell and tissue growth:** Continuous supply of amino acids is needed by the body in order to build the proteins that create tissue. Throughout our everyday lives, we constantly manufacture new tissues such as hair, teeth, skin and nails. The blood cells and skin cells last about a month while the cells situated in our digestive system lining last only two weeks. When the cells die and slough off, our bodies need new healthy tissue to replace them. It is only through the regeneration of new tissue that we can become healthy again. Collagens and elastin provide support for connective tissues such as tendons and ligaments.
- **Mechanical support:** Proteins are responsible for movement. Examples include actin and myosin. These proteins are involved in muscle contraction and movement.
- **Immune protection:** Antibodies are highly specialized proteins involved in defending the body from antigens (foreign invaders). The body produces a specific antibody to respond to an antigen and inactivate it.
- **Nerve generation and impulses:** The nervous system is responsible for keeping the body in balance. When a certain stimulus triggers the nervous system, it responds with an appropriate

reaction. This cannot occur without a receptor site awaiting the stimulus. These receptor sites are made of protein complexes and are responsible for transmitting nerve messages from cell to cell.
* **Fluid balance:** Proteins have the unique ability to regulate the amount of fluid within a cell. The amount of protein within a cell will determine the cell's water content, as water is attracted to protein. When protein levels are low, fluid imbalance results. This type of system is important to prevent dehydration, as well as to enhance muscle and nerve cell function.
* **Hormonal proteins:** These are messenger proteins which help to coordinate certain bodily activities. Examples include insulin, oxytocin, and somatotropin. Insulin regulates glucose metabolism by controlling the blood-sugar concentration. Oxytocin stimulates uterine contractions in females during childbirth. Somatotropin is a growth hormone that stimulates protein production in muscle cells.

Protein Synthesis

Protein synthesis is the process of creating protein molecules. In biological systems, it involves amino acid synthesis, transcription, translation, and posttranslational events. The process of protein synthesis is known as translation in which information present in the mRNA sequence is converted into an amino acid sequence of a protein. Firstly, the genetic information from the DNA is copied to mRNA. Then ribosome reads this genetic code and translates it into the structure of protein **(Fig. 5.7)**.

All the three types of RNAs, the tRNA, the rRNA and mRNA are involved in protein synthesis. Their functions and usefulness are as follows:
* tRNA (t for transfer RNA) serves as the carrier of amino acids.
* rRNA (r for ribosomal RNA) is a part of ribosomes which are workbenches for manufacturing proteins in the cell. Ribosomes are made-up of rRNA and ribosomal proteins.
* mRNA (m for messenger RNA) has the message responsible for directing the sequence of amino acids in a protein.

Process of Translation

The synthesis of protein is condensation reaction in which two amino acids form a peptide bond. Before initiation of translation, the amino acids should be added to tRNA and amino acids have to be activated. Activation is done by aminoacyl tRNA synthetases in the presence of Mg^{++}. In this activation process, each participating amino acid reacts with ATP to form amino acid AMP complex and pyrophosphate 20 aminoacyl tRNA synthetases are present. These enzymes are highly specific for the amino acid and the corresponding tRNA.

Activation

In this activation process, each participating amino acid reacts with ATP and takes up AMP from ATP to become adenylated amino acid and then recognized by an enzyme to form amino acid AMP complex and pyrophosphate.

$$\text{Amino Acid} + \text{tRNA} + \text{ATP} + H_2O \rightarrow \text{Aminoacyl - tRNA} + \text{AMP} + 2\text{PPi}$$

$$\text{DNA} \xrightarrow{\text{Translation}} \text{mRNA} \xrightarrow{\text{Transcription}} \text{Polypeptide}$$

Fig. 5.7: Protein synthesis pathway.

The process of protein synthesis can be summarized in the following four steps:
1. Initiation
2. Elongation
3. Translocation
4. Termination

Initiation

The protein synthesis is initiated when a ribosome has assembled on the mRNA and P site is occupied by the initiator codon. This complex is formed by the action of proteins known as initiation factors. There are above twelve different initiator factors which help in promoting the association of the small ribosomal subunit with the mRNA and a charged initiator tRNA.

Four steps are required for the specific initiation of translation:
a. Dissociation of ribosome into its 40S and 60S subunits.
b. Formation of a 43S pre-initiation complex with the initiator tRNA, GTP, eIF2, and the 40S subunit.
c. The mRNA is bound to the pre-initiation complex forming the 40S initiation complex.
d. Joining of the 60S ribosomal subunit to form 80S initiation complex.

Elongation

Elongation process involves sequential addition of amino acids to the carboxyl end of the growing polypeptide chain by formation of peptide bonds. Elongation factors are termed eEF1 and eEF2, the former consists of two subunits bringing the charged tRNA molecule to ribosome. The eEF2 moves the ribosome one codon down the mRNA. eEF2 is the specific target for inactivation by diphtheria toxin.

A charged tRNA molecule carrying its amino acid, enters the ribosome at the A site. The anticodon present on the arm of the tRNA locates and binds with the complementary codon of the mRNA chain by hydrogen bonds at A site in the ribosomes. The P-site tRNA is now empty and the A-site tRNA is covalently linked to the growing polypeptide chain. This step is somewhat of a mystery but is believed to be catalyzed by a region of the 50S subunit, called the peptidyl transferase complex. The complex utilizes both proteins and 23S rRNA. There is growing evidence that 23S rRNA actively catalyzes the peptidyl transfer step but the mode of action is yet unknown.

Translocation

The A-site tRNA with the growing polypeptide chain is then moved within the ribosome to the P-site while the uncharged tRNA is moved to the E-site. Simultaneously, the mRNA is shifted by exactly 3 ribonucleotides or 1 codon.

Termination

The mRNA Signal STOP Codons: UAA, UAG, or UGA. There are no tRNAs that recognize the STOP codons UAA, UAG, or UGA.

Soluble Protein Release Factors

RF1 responds to UAA or UAG RF2 responds to UAA or UGA
RF3, a GTPase (like EF-Tu and binds in a similar A-site location)

RF1/RF2 interacts with RF3-GTP, has a similar shape as EF-Tu-GTP-aa-tRNA or EF-G, and bind in a similar ribosomal site (A-site). In a manner similar to EF-G, GTP hydrolysis drives the movement of the terminal mRNA codon into the P-site, moving the last tRNA into the E-site and off. At the same time, the polypeptide chain is released after hydrolysis of the tRNA-peptide bond.

In eukaryotes, only a single release factor, eRF, is necessary. It recognizes all three STOP codons and interacts with GTP.

Role of Nucleic Acids in Protein Synthesis

The central dogma of protein synthesis is that DNA makes RNA, which in turn makes protein. This can be expressed as follows:

$$\text{DNA} \xrightarrow{\text{Replication}} \text{DNA} \xrightarrow{\text{Transcription}} \text{RNA} \xrightarrow{\text{Translation}} \text{PROTEIN}$$

Protein synthesis consists of two main events:
I. Transcription
II. Translation

I. **Transcription** is the copying of a complementary messenger RNA strand on a DNA strand. The DNA strand unwinds and one of the two strands forms mRNA strand. This strand is called antisense strand or template strand. The nucleotides of mRNA are complementary to those of the DNA strand. However, in mRNA uracil (U) replaces thymine (T) of DNA. As a result the complementary pairing is A-U and G-C. The mRNA thus formed makes its way through the pores in the nuclear membrane to the cytoplasm. Here it forms a complex with a group of ribosomes.
   - Transcription requires along with a template strand, ribonucleotide triphosphate (ATP, GTP, UTP, CTP), the enzyme RNA polymerase and divalent metal ions. RNA polymerase consists of a core enzyme (with subunits α, α, β, β and ω) and a sigma (σ) factor. The sigma factor initiates transcription of mRNA on the DNA template and the core enzyme continues transcription. All the RNA chains start with either pppG or pppA and are synthesized in the 5' - 3' direction. Chain termination is brought about by a rho factor.

II. **Translation:** During translation, the genetic information present in mRNA directs the order of specific amino acids to form a polypeptide or protein. The mRNA has a series of triplet bases, each triplet forming a codon. The codons pair with anticodons of the tRNA molecule. Each anticodon consists of three free bases. This pairing follows the A-U and G-C combination. Thus the codon GUC pairs with the anticodon CAG to tRNA. Thus the series of codons on mRNA determines the series of anticodons of the different tRNA molecules, and hence of the amino acids. Since the triplets of mRNA in turn depend upon the series of bases in DNA, it follows that the DNA molecule determines the sequence of amino acids, and thus the structure of the protein molecule. The translation process consists of activation of amino acids, transfer of the activated amino acid to tRNA, initiation of polypeptide chain synthesis, chain elongation, and chain termination.
   - **Activation of amino acids:** The 20 amino acids (aa) used in protein synthesis are activated by ATP in the present of specific activating enzymes (E) called amino acyl synthetases to form amino acyl adenylates (aaa), also called amino acyl AMP. Pyrophosphates (PPi) are released.

$$\text{aa} + \text{ATP} + \text{E} \longrightarrow \text{E-aa-AMP} + \text{PPi}$$

   - **Transfer of activated amino acids to tRNA:** The activated amino acid is transferred to a specific tRNA with the release of AMP and activating enzyme.

$$\text{E.aa.AMP} + \text{E} + \text{tRNA} \longrightarrow \text{aa-tRNA} + \text{AMP} + \text{E}$$

- **Initiation of chain synthesis:** This requires the ribosome subunits, mRNA, an energy source (GTP), activated amino acids attached to tRNA (aa-tRNA) and initiation factors (IF). These factors are called IF-1, IF-2, IF-3 in prokaryotes and eIF-2, e-IF2', eIF-2a1 eIF-2a2, eIF-2a3 and eIF-3 in eukaryotes.
    - The 30S ribosomal subunit attaches to mRNA to form an mRNA-30S complex. The process requires IF-3 and Mg^{++}.
    - The starting amino acid is methionine (Met) in eukaryotes and N-formyl methionine in prokaryotes. The amino acid-tRNA complex (fMEt-tRNA) attaches to the initiation codon, AUG, on mRNA through its anticodon UAC to form the 30S initiation complex. The process requires initiation factors IF-2 and IF-1 as well as GTP.
    - The larger ribosomal subunit (50S in prokaryotes) joins to the 30S initiation complex to form the complete initiation complex (70S).
    - The larger ribosomal subunit has two binding sites for tRNA, an A or acceptor site and a P or peptidyl site. fMet-tRNA binds to the P site.
- **Chain elongation:** Elongation of the polypeptide chain requires elongation factors (EF). These are EF-Tu. EF=Ts and EF-G in prokaryotes and EF-1 and EF-2 in eukaryotes:
    - The second amino acid-tRNA complex (aa2-tRNA) now occupies the A site. There is enzymatic recognition of internal codons. The process requires EF-Tu, GTP and Mg^{++}.
    - Formation of a peptide bond takes place by transfer of fMet to the second amino acid (aa2). Mg^{++} and K^+ are required. The catalyzing enzyme is peptidyl transferase.
    - **Translocation:** The aa2-tRNA complex moves from the A site to the P-site. This process is called translocation and requires EF-G, GTP and Mg^{++}. Translocation involves movement of ribosome relative to mRNA in the 5'—3' direction. The third amino acid-tRNA (aa3- tRNA) complex now occupies the vacant A-site.
- **Chain termination:** Chain elongation continues until a termination codon (UAA, UAG, UGA) reaches the ribosome. The chain is then terminated and released from the ribosome. This process requires release factors RF-1, RF-2 and RF-3 in prokaryotes and RF in eukaryotes:
    - The termination codon provides signals to the ribosome for the attachment of release factors.
    - The release factors interact with peptidyl transferase causing hydrolysis of the bond between tRNA and the polypeptide chain, and the chain is released from the ribosome.
    - Hydrolysis of GTP results in the dissociation of the release factors from the ribosome. The tRNA is also unloaded. The ribosomal subunits dissociate and mRNA is released, for breakdown to nucleotides.
    - Processing of the polypeptide chain, e.g., cleavage of the formyl residue or of methionine, takes place after release.

Metabolism of Proteins

The amino acids from the "pool" are utilized for two purposes:
- **Anabolic pathway:** It includes the synthesis of proteins like protein biosynthesis, tissue proteins, blood proteins, enzymes, hormones. This also includes the synthesis of non-protein nitrogen substances like creatinine, purines, pyrimidines, glutathione and choline.

Catabolic pathway: It includes:
- Transamination
- Deamination:
- Oxidative deamination

- Non-oxidative deamination
- Transdeamination
- Utilization of nitrogen residue
- Glutamine synthesis
- Urea cycle.

Catabolism of Amino Acids

Nitrogen catabolism consists of removal of alpha amino groups from amino acids as ammonia by transamination and deamination, conversion to NH_3 and then to urea and uric acid and finally excretion in the urine.

Metabolism of amino acids can be discussed under the following headings:
- Transamination
- Deamination
  - Oxidative deamination
  - Non-oxidative deamination
- Trans deamination
- NH_3 transport
- Formation of urea

Transamination

It is a reversible reaction in which there is transfer of alpha amino group from an amino acid to a keto acid forming a new amino acid and a keto acid **(Fig. 5.8)**.
  e.g., Alanine + Ketoglutarate $\xrightarrow{ALT}$ Pyruvate + Glutamate
  ALT = Alanine transaminase

Deamination

It is a process in which there is removal of amino group from an acid to form NH_3. It is of two types:
- **Minor oxidative of deamination:** Oxidative deamination is the mechanism by which amino group is removed from the alpha carbon to form a keto acid and free NH_3. *Oxidative deamination takes place in two steps* **(Fig. 5.9)**:
  - The amino acid is first dehydrogenated by the flavoprotein of enzyme, L-amino acid oxidase, forming an alpha amino acid.
  - The water molecule is added spontaneously and decomposes to the corresponding alpha-keto acid and NH_3.
- **Major oxidative deamination:** It is the deamination of L-glutamine acid. It involves transamination coupled with oxidative deamination, hence the process called transdeamination **(Figure 5.10)**.

Fig. 5.8: Transamination.

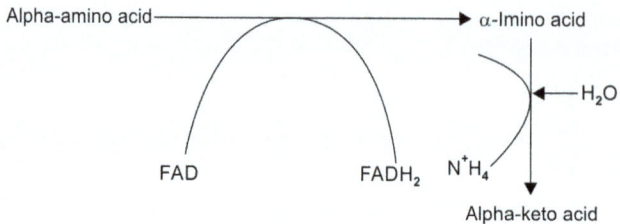

Fig. 5.9: Minor oxidative deamination pathway.

Fig. 5.10: Major oxidative deamination pathway.

* **Non-oxidative deamination:** There are certain amino acids, which can be non oxidatively deaminated to form NH_3 by specific enzymes:
  - Histidine $\xrightarrow{\text{Histidase}}$ Urocanic acid + NH_3
  - Serine $\xrightarrow{H_2O}$ Pyruvate + NH_3

Ammonia Transport

NH_3 is removed or metabolic fate of NH_3 in the body is by three ways. As discussed in previous steps, NH_3 is released from α-amino group of amino acids. Even in minute concentration, ammonia can be neurotoxic. Hence, it needs to be converted to harmless substances by which it can be transported to liver and finally converted to urea. Three forms in which ammonia is transported to liver are:
1. **Glutamine:** Major participant in interogen transport of urea, even from brain.
2. **Asparagine:** The minimal urea is also tranported in this form from cells to liver.
3. **Alanine:** Serves as transport form of ammonia from muscles.

FORMATION OF UREA

The final step of the amino acid is formation of urea as discussed in underneath as urea cycle.

Urea Cycle

Urea formation takes place mainly in the liver. The liver catabolizes toxic ammonia into urea. Urea is the major excretory product in humans, accounting for an average of 86% of nitrogen eliminated. The enzymes involved in urea formation are located in mitochondria of hypatocytes and cytoplasm. When this process is not working efficiently, toxic ammonia (NH_3) accumulates

Fig. 5.11: Steps of urea cycle.

within the body and may elicit clinical manifestations such as lethargy, slurred speech, cerebral edema, and asterixis.

Steps of Urea Cycle
The steps of urea cycle are presented in **Figure 5.11**.

1. **Formation or Synthesis of Carbamoyl Phosphate**
    - CO_2 is first activated and the first active CO_2 combines with NH_3 to form carbamoyl phosphate.
    $CO_2 + NH_3 + 2ATP \xrightarrow{\text{N-acetyl glutamate}} $ Carbamoyl phosphate + 2ADP + Pi

2. **Formation of Citrulline**
    Ornithine reacts with carbamoyl phosphate to form citrulline.

3. **Synthesis of Arginosuccinate**
    Citrulline combines with aspartate to form arginosuccinate catalyzed by arginosuccinate synthetase. The reaction requires ATP.

4. Cleavage of Arginosuccinate

Cleavage of arginosuccinate to arginine and fumarate is catalyzed by arginosuccinase or arginosuccinate lyase.

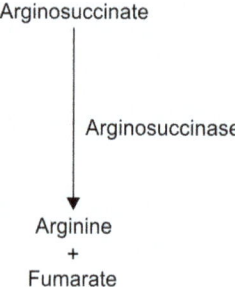

5. Hydrolysis of Arginine

Cleavage of arginine to ornithine and urea is catalyzed by arginine.

The overall process in each turn of cycle requires three molecules of ATP.
* **Glutamine Formation**
  Increased NH_3 concentration also increases glutamine synthesis from glutamic acid. It is catalyzed by glutamine synthetase and requires ATP. The reaction is irreversible.

$$\text{Glutamate} \xrightarrow[\text{ATP} \quad \text{NH}_4^+ \quad \text{ADP} \quad \text{Pi}]{} \text{Glutamine}$$

Glutamate (CH₂–COO⁻, CH₂, CH-NH₃⁺, COO⁻) + ATP + NH₄⁺ → Glutamate/Glutamine (CH₂–CONH₂, CH₂, CH-NH₃⁺, COO⁻) + ADP + Pi

- **Amination of Alpha-keto Acids**
  NH_3 is also used to aminate certain alpha-keto acids to form corresponding alpha-amino acids, e.g.,

  $$\text{Pyruvic acid} + NH_3 \longrightarrow \text{Alanine}$$

GOUT

Gout is a disease characterized by abnormal metabolism of uric acid, resulting in an excess of uric acid in the tissues and blood. People with gout either produce too much uric acid, or more commonly, their bodies have a problem in removing it. Gout is one of the most common causes of chronic inflammatory arthritis, characterized by monosodium urate (MSU) monohydrate crystals deposition in the tissues.

The prevalence of gout appears to be increasing.

Causes of Gout

Uric acid is generated as we metabolize the food we eat and as the body's tissues are broken down during normal cell turnover.
- Hereditary 20% possibility.
- British people are five times more likely to develop gout.
- American Blacks, but not African Blacks, are more likely to have gout than other populations.
- Intake of alcoholic beverages, especially beer, increases the risk for gout.
- Diets rich in red meats, internal organs, yeast, and oily fish increase the risk for gout.
- Uric acid levels increase at puberty in men and at menopause in women, so men first develop gout at an earlier age (after puberty) than do women (after menopause). Gout in premenopausal women is distinctly unusual.

Attacks of gouty arthritis can be precipitated when there is a sudden change in uric acid levels, which may be caused by:
- Overindulgence in alcohol and red meats
- Trauma
- Starvation and dehydration
- IV contrast dyes
- Chemotherapy
- Medications
- Diuretics and some other antihypertensive medications
- Nicotinic acid (B-3-50, B3-500-Gr, Niacin SR, Niacor, Niaspan ER, Slo-Niacin)
- Cyclosporine A.

Fig. 5.12: Signs and symptoms of gout.

Symptoms and Signs of Gout
- Sudden onset of a hot, red, swollen joint with severe tenderness **(Fig. 5.12)**.
- Kidney stones are more frequent in people with gout.
- Uric acid crystals can form outside joints. Collections of these crystals, known as tophi, can be found in the earlobe, elbow, and Achilles tendon (back of the ankle), or in other tissues. Typically, these tophi are not painful but can be a valuable clue for the diagnosis as the crystals that form them can be removed with a small needle for microscopic examination. Microscopic evaluation of a tophus reveals a nest-like accumulation of uric acid crystals embedded with white blood cells of inflammation.

Laboratory Study
The examination usually reveals elevations in the white blood cell count, erythrocyte sedimentation rate (ESR), and C-reactive protein (CRP) during a gout flare-up. Still, these features are non-specific and do not confirm the diagnosis.

Treatment of Gout
- Drugs like corticosteroids may be given to manage the acute attack of gout.
- Ibuprofen or nonsteroid anti-inflammatory drugs may be given to manage the pain.
- Allopurinol decreases uric acid level by decreasing its production, usually prescribed as a long-term treatment for gout. Anti-inflammatory drugs like colchicine may be prescribed by the physician for acute attack of gout.

Prognosis
The prognosis of gout depends on the comorbidity of each individual. Mortality is higher in individuals with cardiovascular comorbidity. When gout receives proper treatment, most patients will live a normal life with mild sequelae. Patients whose symptoms appear earlier in life will usually have a more severe disease at presentation. For those who do not modify their lifestyle, recurrent flare-ups are common.

Lifestyle modification and strategies to reduce the risk of gout flares and progression of gout:
- Lifestyle changes are encouraged in gout patients, including weight loss, limiting alcohol intake, and avoiding certain foods. These changes will complement medical therapy but often are not enough by themselves to combat or reverse gout.
- Weight gain and increased adiposity are risk factors for gout, while in overweight patients with established gout, weight loss likely benefits in reducing serum urate and gout symptoms.
- The diet composition optimum for gout is likely to be one with adequate protein intake, especially from plant sources and low-fat dairy sources, with reduced intake from animal sources of purine such as shellfish or red meat; decreased saturated fat; and replacement of simple sugars with complex carbohydrates.
- Avoid or minimize the frequency of sugar-sweetened juices and alcohol-containing beverages or beverages containing highfructose.

Prevention of Gout
The disorder itself may not be preventable, but one can avoid things that trigger such symptoms. Limit alcohol consumption and follow a low-purine diet.

■ NITROGENOUS CONSTITUENTS OF URINE AND BLOOD
In a healthy individual, urine has following nitrogenous constituents as given below:
- Water 96%
- Urea 2%
- Uric acid
- Creatinine
- Ammonia
- Sodium
- Potassium   2 %
- Chlorides
- Phosphates
- Sulfates
- Oxalates.

Constituents of Blood
Blood consists of 55% plasma and 45% formed elements.

Plasma
- Plasma is a clear, slightly yellow liquid, containing a large number of organic and inorganic substances dissolved in water.
- Plasma contains approximately 91% water and 9% solids. Of the solids, about 7% are the plasma proteins which consist of serum albumin, serum globulin, and fibrinogen.
- Other organic substances present are glucose, amino acids, fatty acid, phospholipids, cholesterol, hormones, enzymes, antibodies, etc.
- Inorganic substances are sodium, potassium, calcium, magnesium, iron, copper, zinc, chloride, bicarbonate, etc.

Formed Elements
The formated elements of the blood which form 45% portion are:
- The red blood corpuscles (RBC)
- The white blood corpuscles (WBC)
- The platelets.

Plasma Proteins

Plasma proteins are proteins found in the blood plasma. These proteins play a number of important roles in the human body. Plasma proteins make-up around 7% of the total blood volume.

Levels of plasma proteins are sometimes evaluated in a laboratory analysis to gather information about a patient's general health and specific health issues which a patient may be experiencing.

Some common plasma proteins include albumin, which is by far the most common, along with fibrinogen and globulin, which is subclassified into globulin alpha, globulin beta, and globulin gamma. Trace amounts of other proteins can also be found in the blood plasma, usually in concentrations of less than one percent of the total plasma, which can make them difficult to identify, especially with only basic blood screening tools available.

Functions of Plasma Proteins
Following are the main functions of the plasma proteins:
- **Transport:** Plasma proteins are responsible for the following things:
  - Transferrin transports iron.
  - Ceruloplasmin transports copper.
  - Albumin transports fatty acids, bilirubin calcium, many drugs, etc.
  - Transcortin transports cortisol and corticosterone.
  - Retinol-binding protein transports retinol.
  - Lipoproteins transports lipids.
  - Haptoglobin transports free hemoglobin.
  - Thyroxine binding globulin transports thyroxine.
- **Osmotic regulation:** Plasma proteins are colloidal and non-diffusible and exert a colloidal osmotic pressure which helps to maintain a normal blood volume and a normal water content in the interstitial fluid and the tissues. Albumin content is most important in regulation of colloidal osmotic or oncotic pressure. Decrease in albumin level results in loss of water from blood and its entry into interstitial fluids causing edema.
- **Catalytic function (enzymes),** e.g., lipases for removal of lipids from the blood.
- **Protective function:** Immunoglobulin combines with foreign antigens and removes them. Complement system removes cellular antigens. Enzyme inhibitors remove enzymes by forming complexes with them, e.g., α_1 antitrypsin combines with elastase, trypsin and protects the hydrolytic damage of tissues such as lungs. Some proteins increase during acute phase and protect the body. For example, CRP (C-reactive protein), α_1 antitrypsin, α_2 macroglobulins.
- **Blood clotting:** Many factors are involved in clotting mechanism and prevent loss of excessive amount of blood. For example, clotting factors IX, VIII, thrombin, fibrinogen, etc. An excess or deficiency can lead to diseases. For example, hemophilia, thrombus formation.
- **Anticoagulant activity (thrombolysis):** Plasmin breaks down thrombin and dissolves the clot.
- **Buffering capacity:** Proteins in plasma help to maintain acid–base balance.

QUESTIONS

Q.1: Write a short note on the classification of proteins.
Q.2: Write a short note on proteins.
Q.3: Discuss transamination and oxidative deamination of amino acids.
Q.4: Classify proteins on the basis of nutrition.
Q.5: What is isoelectric points of alpha-amino acids? Describe with examples.
Q.6: What is protein? Describe its various levels of structure and its classification on a structure basis.
Q.7: Write a short note on oxidative deamination.
Q.8: What is meant by denaturation of proteins? Write names of some agents (chemical or actions) by which protein can be denatured? Explain transamination and deamination.
Q.9: Write a short note on functions of protein.
Q.10: Briefly discuss gout.

BIBLIOGRAPHY

1. Ahlborg G, Felig P, Hagenfeldt L, et al. Substrate turnover during prolonged exercise in man. J Clin Invest, 1974;53:1080-90.
2. Anthony JC, Anthony TG, Layman DK. Leucine supplementation enhances skeletal muscle recovery in rats following exercise. J Nutr, 1999;129:1102-6.
3. Attaix D, Taillandier D, Temparis S, et al. Regulation of ATP- ubiquitin-dependent proteolysis in muscle wasting. Reprod Nutr Dev, 1914;34:583-97.
4. Baar K, Esser K. Phosphorylation of p70(S6k) correlates with increased skeletal muscle mass following resistance exercise. Am J Physiol, 1999;276:C120-7.
5. Balon TW. Role of nitric oxide in contraction induced glucose transport. Adv Exp Med Biol, 1998;441:87-95.
6. Bennet WM, Rennie MJ. Protein anabolic actions of insulin in the human body. Diabetic Med, 1991;8:199-207.
7. Bergstrom J, Furst P, Vinnars E. Effect of a test meal, without and with protein, on muscle and plasma free amino acids. Clin Sci, 1990;79:331-7.
8. Biolo G, Chinkes D, Zhang XJ, et al. A new model to determine in vivo the relationship between amino acid transmembrane transport and protein kinetics in muscle. J Parenter Enter Nutr, 1992.16:305-15.
9. Biolo G, Tipton KD, Klein S, et al. An abundant supply of amino acids enhances the metabolic effect of exercise on muscle protein. Am J Physiol Endocrinol Metab, 1997;273:E122-9.
10. Blomstrand E, Saltin B. Effect of muscle glycogen on glucose, lactate and amino acid metabolism during exercise and recovery in human subjects. London, 1999;514:293-302.
11. Booth J, Physiol FW, Tseng BS, et al. Molecular and cellular adaptation of muscle in response to physical training. Acta Physiol Scand, 1998 162:343-50.
12. Brahm H, Piehl-Aulin K, Ljunghall S. Biochemical markers of bone metabolism during distance running in healthy, regularly exercising men and women. Scand J Med Sci Sports, 1996;6:26-30.
13. Brouns F, Saris WH, Stroecken J, et al. Eating, drinking, and cycling. A controlled Tour de France simulation study. II. Effect of diet manipulation. Int J Sports Med, 1989;10 (Suppl.1): S41-8.
14. Matthews DE, Marano MA, Campbell RG. Splanchnic bed utilization of leucine and phenylalanine in humans. Am J Physiol, 1993;264:E109-18.
15. Nair KS, Halliday D, Griggs RC. Leucine incorporation into mixed skeletal protein muscle in humans. Am J Physiol, 1988;254:E208-13.
16. Nelson AG, Arnall DA, Loy SF, et al. Consequences of combining strength and endurance training regimens. Phys. Ther, 1990;70:287-94
17. Phillips SM, Tipton KD, Ferrando AA, et al. Resistance training reduces the acute exercise-induced increase in muscle protein turnover. Am J Physiol, 1999;276:E118-24.

18. Radha E, Bessman SP. Effect of exercise on protein degradation: 3-methylhistidine and creatinine excretion. Biochem. Med, 1983;29:96-100.
19. Sartorelli V, Kurabayashi M, Kedes L. Muscle-specific gene expression: a comparison of cardiac and skeletal muscle transcription strategies. Circ. Res, 1993;72:925-31.
20. Smith K, Rennie MJ. Protein turnover and amino acid metabolism in human skeletal muscle. Baillieres Clin Endocrinol Metab. 1990;4:461-98.
21. Smith K, Reynolds N, Downie S, et al. Effects of flooding amino acids on incorporation of labeled amino acids into human muscle protein. Am J Physiol. 1998;275:E73-8.
22. Tipton KD, Ferrando AA, Phillips SM, et al. Postexercise net protein synthesis in human muscle from orally administered amino acids. Am J Physiol, 1999;276:E628-34.
23. Wong TS, Booth FW. Protein metabolism in rat gastrocnemius muscle after stimulated chronic concentric exercise. J Appl Physiol, 1990;69:1709-17.
24. Barmore W, Azad F, Stone WL. Physiology, Urea Cycle. [Updated 2021 May 19]. In: StatPearls [Internet]. Treasure Island (FL): StatPearls Publishing;2022 Jan-. Available from: https://www.ncbi.nlm.nih.gov/books/NBK513323/
25. Hoerter JE, Ellis SR. Biochemistry, Protein Synthesis. [Updated 2021 Jul 22]. In: StatPearls [Internet]. Treasure Island (FL): StatPearls Publishing;2022 Jan-. Available from: https://www.ncbi.nlm.nih.gov/books/NBK545161/
26. Fenando A, Rednam M, Gujarathi R, et al. Gout. [Updated 2021 Dec 7]. In: StatPearls [Internet]. Treasure Island (FL): StatPearls Publishing;2022 Jan-. Available from: https://www.ncbi.nlm.nih.gov/books/NBK546606/
27. Rambabu K, Ravikiran, PB Kameswari. Fundamentals of Biochemistry. 2nd edition. India;ATBS publishers: 2019

CHAPTER 6

Lipids

Navjot Kaur, Suresh K Sharma

Chapter Outline

- Function of Lipids
- Classification of Lipids
- Role of Liver in Fat Metabolism
- Biological Importance of Important Lipids and their Functions
- Alcohols Present in Lipids
- Cholesterol and Lipoproteins
- Phospholipids
- Glycolipids
- Lipoproteins and their Functions
- Metabolism of Fatty Acids

INTRODUCTION

Fat (lipids) are organic substances insoluble in water and soluble in organic solvents such as ether, alcohol, acetone, etc. There are heterogeneous group of compounds. These are made-up of fatty acids. Lipids-include fats, oils, waxes, and related compounds. Fats act as a stored form of energy in many organisms. Lipids form about 3.5% of cell content and generally, they do not polymerize to form macromolecules. However, they may combine with carbohydrates and proteins to form macromolecules. Fats and lipids are an essential component of the homeostatic function of the human body.

Biomedical importance: Lipids are important dietary constituents because of

- Their high energy value (9 Kcal/gm).
- The fat-soluble vitamins and the essential fatty acids contained in the fat of natural foods.
- Lipids are found primarily in three compartments in the body: plasma, adipose tissue, and biological membranes.

FUNCTIONS OF LIPIDS

- **Energy source:** Lipids are the storage form of energy. One gram of lipid provides 9.1 Kcal of energy.
- **Structural component:** Lipoproteins, phospholipid, and cholesterol form an important cellular constituent of cell membranes and cell organelles.
- **Insulating material:** They insulate against changes in the external temperature, e.g., in subcutaneous tissues and around organs like kidneys.

- **Emulsifying agent:** Bile salts act as emulsifying agents during the digestion and absorption of lipid.
- **Electrical insulator:** The fat content of nerve tissue is particularly high and is essential for proper function.
- **Surfactant:** Dipalmitoyl lecithin acts as a surfactant and maintains surface tension in the alveoli, without which they will collapse.
- They are also sources of vitamins A, D, E, and K and carriers of triglycerides, cholesterol and phospholipid in the body.

CLASSIFICATION OF LIPIDS

Bloor (1925) classified lipids based on their chemical nature. They are classified as simple, compound and derived lipids. They are discussed in details as below:

1. **Simple lipids:** Simple lipids are esters of fatty acids with alcohol. Simple lipids are further classified into, neutral fats and waxes as depicted in **Table 6.1**.
2. **Compound lipids:** These are having two components lipid plus nonlipid part. They are further classified into, phospholipid and glycolipids as presented in **Table 6.2**.
3. **Derived lipids:** These are derived from simple and compound lipids after hydrolysis. Example, fatty acids, steroids and sterols, glycerol, prostaglandins, leukotrienes, terpenes, monoacylglycerol (MAG), diacylglycerol (DAG), fat soluble vitamins and ketone bodies.

Table 6.1: Description of simple lipids.

Type	Description	Occurrence
Neutral fats	Neutral fats are fatty acid esters of glycerol and are commonly called triglycerides.	These are mainly present in adipose tissues, butter fat, fish oils, olive oil, corn oil, etc.
Waxes	Waxes are esters of fatty acids with alcohol other than glycerol.	These mainly occur in beeswax, head oil of sperm whale, cerumen, carnauba oil and lanolin.

Table 6.2: Description of compound lipids.

Type	Description	Occurrence
Phospholipid	These contain phosphate groups, in addition to the lipid part, e.g., lecithin, sphingomyelins	These occur in animal tissues, brain, egg yolk, organ meats, nervous tissue and red blood cells.
Glycolipid	These contain carbohydrate group along with lipid part, e.g., gangliosides, cerebrosides.	These occur in myelin sheaths of nerves, brain and other tissues.
Lipoproteins	These contain protein groups in addition to lipid, e.g., chylomicrons, high-density lipoproteins (HDL)	These are found in the white matter of brain and nerve tissue.
Sulfolipid	These contain sulfated carbohydrates with lipid part, e.g., sulfatides	These are found in the white matter of brain, liver and testicle, also found in plant chloroplast.

CHAPTER 6: Lipids

ROLE OF LIVER IN FAT METABOLISM

Liver plays a significant role in fat metabolism. It is involved in the synthesis as well as the oxidation of fatty acids. It also produces bile salts and bile acids which are primarily responsible for fat emulsification, digestion, and metabolism. In fat metabolism, the liver cells break down fats and produce energy. They also produce about 800 to 1,000 mL of bile per day. In addition, some other essential functions are:

- Fatty acids are breakdown by hepatocytes to generate ATPs.
- Liver synthesizes lipoproteins, which transport fatty acids, triglycerides, and cholesterol to and from body cells.
- Ketone bodies such as acetoacetate, β-hydroxybutyrate, and acetone are produced in the liver from acetyl-CoA, which is metabolized outside the liver to produce liver energy except acetone, which is exhaled unmetabolized.
- Liver synthesizes cholesterol and uses cholesterol to make bile salts.
- The major metabolic activities that happen in the liver are lipolysis (catabolism of lipid) and lipogenesis (anabolism of lipid). During lipolysis, triglycerides are split into glycerol and fatty acids and utilized to produce the ATPs. In lipogenesis extra consumed glucose and amino acids are converted into lipids and stored in the body.

BIOLOGICAL IMPORTANCE OF IMPORTANT LIPIDS AND THEIR FUNCTIONS

I. FATTY ACIDS

Fatty acids are the building blocks of fat in our bodies and in the food we eat. Fatty acid is a carboxylic acid consisting of hydrocarbons and a terminal carboxyl group. Fatty acids exist in free form and ester form.

Classification of Fatty Acids

Fatty acids can be saturated fatty acids and unsaturated fatty acids.

1. Saturated Fatty Acids

Saturated fatty acids having 10 or less than 10 carbon atoms are called "short-chain fatty acids". Examples, acetic acid, butyric acid, etc.

Saturated fatty acids having more than 10 carbon atoms are called "long-chain fatty acids", e.g., palmitic acid, stearic acid, etc. **(Table 6.3)**.

Table 6.3: Saturated fatty acids.

S. No	Fatty acid	Source
1.	Acetic acid (CH_3COOH)	It is the major end product of carbohydrate fermentation by rumen organisms.
2.	Propionic acid (CH_3CH_2COOH)	It is the end product of carbohydrate fermentation by rumen organisms.
3.	Butyric acid ($CH_3(CH_2)_2COOH$)	Butter. An end product of carbohydrate fermentation by rumen organisms.
4.	Caproic acid ($CH_3(CH_2)_4COOH$)	Butter. An end product of carbohydrate fermentation by rumen organisms.
5.	Caprylic acid ($CH_3(CH_2)_6COOH$)	Butter, fats of plant origin.
6.	Palmitic acid ($CH_3(CH_2)_{14}COOH$)	Common in all animal and plant fats.
7.	Stearic acid ($CH_3(CH_2)_{16}COOH$)	Common in all animal and plant fats.

Table 6.4: Unsaturated fatty acids.

S. No.	Fatty acid	Source
1.	Oleic acid $CH_3(CH_2)_7CH=CH(CH_2)_7COOH$	Found in nearly all fats.
2.	Linoleic acid $CH_3(CH_2)_4CH=CHCH_2CH=CH(CH_2)_7COOH$	Peanut oil, corn oil, cotton seed oil, soybean oil, egg yolk, etc.
3.	Linolenic acid $CH_3(CH_2)_4CH=CHCH_2CH=CH(CH_2)_7COOH$	Linseed oil, rapeseed oil, soybean oil, fish visceras, cod liver oil.
4.	Arachidonic acid $CH_3(CH_2)_4CH=CHCH_2CH=CHCH_2CH=CHCH_2CH=CH(CH_2)_3COOHNIST$	Peanut oil, animal fats, e.g., silver fats. Also found with linoleic acid and linolenic acid

2. Unsaturated Fatty Acids

- Unsaturated fatty acids contain one or more double bonds. They are classified according to the degree of saturation.
- **Monounsaturated fatty acids:** Monounsaturated fatty acids are the ones that contain one double bond, e.g., oleic acid.
- **Polyunsaturated fatty acids:** Polyunsaturated fatty acids contain two or more double bonds, e.g., linoleic acid, linolenic acid and arachidonic acid.

Refer to **Table 6.4** for the description of the chemical structure and source of unsaturated fatty acids.

Essential Fatty Acids

Essential fatty acids are those which cannot be synthesized in the body. They have to be provided in the diet.

Traditionally, linoleic acid, linolenic acid, and arachidonic acid are collectively known as "essential fatty acid". The term essential fatty acids (EFA) refers to those polyunsaturated fatty acids (PUFA) that must be provided by foods. There are two families of EFA, omega-3 (ω-3) and omega-6 (ω-6)

Functions of Essential Fatty Acid

- *Structural elements:* These are the structural components of the cell membranes, membranes of mitochondria, and the gonads, which suggests their reproductive function.
- *Regulation of blood clotting:* Omega-6 FAs encourage blood clot formation, whereas Omega-3 oil reduces clotting. The ideal is to achieve a balance between omega-6 and omega-3 FAs
- *Hypocholesterolemic agent:* EFAs are hypocholesterolemic, e.g., PUFA tend to lower serum level of cholesterol. This provides an anti-atherogenic effect.
- *Precursor:* Arachidonic acid functions as a precursor of hormone-like substances such as prostaglandins, leukotrienes, and thromboxane.
- *Biomedical importance:* These help in the prevention of many diseases like fatty liver, artherosclerosis, eczema, etc.
- Proper development and functioning of the brain and nervous system
- Proper thyroid and adrenal activity
- Support healthy skin and hair

II. PROSTAGLANDINS

Prostaglandins are 20 carbon-containing derivatives of unsaturated fatty acids. They contain a cyclopentane ring. These are derived from arachidonic acid **(Fig. 6.1)**.

They usually act as local hormones and have a short half-life.

Fig. 6.1: Chemical structure of prostaglandins.

Classification of Prostaglandins
Classification is based on the presence of number of a double bonds and the presence of substituent group.
1. Based on the presence of number of double bonds:
   a. If one double bond—PG_1
   b. If two double bonds—PG_2
   c. If three double bonds—PG_3
2. Based on the substituent groups such as CH_3, OH, and keto groups on the linear part, they are denoted as PGD, PGE, PGG, and PGH.

Occurrence of Prostaglandins
PGs are named because of their origin from the prostate gland. PGs occur in animal tissues, body fluids, seminal vesicles, synovial fluid, menstrual fluid, renal medulla, thymus and blood plasma. Prostaglandins are naturally occurring compounds that are easily separable from other biologically active substances because of their acidic lipid nature. They are divided into 4 series, the A, B, E, and F-alpha series, which differ in the structure of the characteristic 5-membered ring.

Functions of Prostaglandins
- Act as a vasodilator, hence lower blood pressure.
- Increase capillary permeability.
- Inhibit platelet aggregation.
- Inhibit gastric secretions.
- Increase intestinal mucus secretions.
- Are used for the treatment of status asthmaticus.
- Prostaglandins play a role in various reproductive functions: 1. conception; 2. luteolysis; 3. menstruation; and 4. parturition. Are purgative in action.
- Cause hypercalcemia by affecting the bones.

III. THROMBOXANES
These are 20 carbon containing derivatives of unsaturated fatty acids and contain oxane ring. Thromboxane A2 (TxA2) is in the family of lipids known as eicosanoids, which are metabolites of arachidonic acid **(Fig. 6.2)**.

Classification of Thromboxanes
1. Based on the presence of the number of double bonds present:
   a. If one double bonds are present—TX_1
   b. If two double bonds are present—TX_2
   c. If three double bonds are present—TX_3
2. Based on the presence of substituent groups in the linear part such as CH_3, OH, C=O and based on the position of these groups, thromboxanes are designated as TXA, TXB.

Fig. 6.2: Chemical structure of thromboxanes.

Occurrence of Thromboxanes
* These are mainly formed in platelets, neutrophils, lungs, brain, kidney, spleen, etc.
* They also occur in animal tissues, body fluids and smooth muscles.

Functions of Thromboxanes
* It acts principally by decreasing cAMP levels in target cells. It can also use Ca^{++} as a second messenger, e.g., in muscle fibers. Its main functions are: It increases platelet aggregation and promotes thrombosis.
* It produces contraction of smooth muscles.

IV. LEUKOTRIENES

These are 20 carbon containing derivatives of unsaturated fatty acids and possess no ring structure.

These are derived from arachidonic acid. These contain 3 conjugated double bonds **(Figure 6.3)**.

Occurrence of Leukotrienes

Leukotrienes first found in leukocytes and are formed from eicosanoid acids in leukocytes, mast cells and macrophages by the lipoxygenase pathway in response to both immunologic and noninflammatory stimuli.

Functions of Leukotrienes

Following are the main functions of leukotrienes:
* Contraction of smooth muscles.
* Capillary dilation and increases vascular permeability.
* Constriction of bronchioles.
* Chemotaxis and chemokinesis of neutrophils and eosinophils at the site of inflammation.

Fig. 6.3: Chemical structure of leukotrienes.

CHAPTER 6: Lipids

ALCOHOLS PRESENT IN LIPIDS

Lipids molecules contain alcohols like glycerol, sphingosine, cholesterol, etc.

Glycerol

- This is trihydroxy alcohols, capable of forming 3 esters bond with three molecules of fatty acids to form triglycerides.

$$\begin{array}{c} CH_2\text{-}OH \\ | \\ CH\text{-}OH \\ | \\ CH_2\text{-}OH \end{array}$$

- Glycerol is colorless, oily fluid with a sweetish taste.
- Glycerol is miscible with water and alcohol, but insoluble in ether.
- When exposed to moist air, it absorbs water (hydroscopic) as well as gasses such as hydrogen sulfide and sulfur dioxide.

Source of Glycerol

It is mainly derived from diet. It is also obtained endogenously from lipolysis of fat in adipose tissue.

Uses of Glycerol

- It is an important component of fats, oils and phosphoglycerides.
- It is a component of many pharmaceutical and cosmetic preparations, it is used as a laxative given orally, as an enema and given as a suppositories
- Intravenous glycerol has been given to reduce cerebral edema and hence reduce intracranial pressure and have many other uses in pharmaceuticals.
- It is having a definitive nutritive value, as it can be converted to glucose and glycogen.

Sphingosine

It is 18 carbon containing derivative of unsaturated amino acid and is present as a constituent of phospholipid, sphingomyelin and various glycolipid **(Fig. 6.4)**.

It is the precursor of important cell signaling molecules, such as ceramides, through amide binding of a fatty acid to the C2 amino group.

Sphingosine is a "bioactive lipid". It has been found to inhibit protein kinase C in human platelets.

Steroids and Sterols

- Steroids are normally found in association with fats and can be separated after the process of "saponification" of fat in the form of "unsaponifiable residue".
- All steroids have "phenanthrene" like cyclic nucleus of a complex ring system, known as "cyclopentano phenanthrene nucleus" **(Fig. 6.5)**.

$$H_3\text{-}C\text{-}(CH_2)_{12}\text{—}CH=CH\text{—}\underset{OH}{CH}\text{—}\underset{NH_2}{CH}\text{—}\underset{OH}{CH_2}\text{—}$$

Fig. 6.4: Chemical structure of sphingosine.

Fig. 6.5: Cyclopentano phenanthrene ring.

Table 6.5: Types of steroids.	
Types	Examples
Sterols	Cholesterol, ergosterol
Bile acids	Glycocholic acid, taurocholic acid
Sex hormones	Testosterone, estradiol
Vitamin D	Vitamin D_2 and D_3
Adrenocortical hormone	Corticosterone
Cardiac glycosides	Digoxin
Saponins	Digitonin

Sterol

If is the steroid compound having one or more –OH groups and no carbonyl or carboxyl groups, it is called sterol. The most important sterol in the human body is known as cholesterol. The term sterol means solid alcohol. Different types of steroids may be perused from **Table 6.5**.

CHOLESTEROL AND LIPOPROTEINS

Cholesterol

- Cholesterol is a lipophilic molecule that is essential for human life. It has many roles that contribute to normally functioning cells.
- It is 27 carbon compound and its molecular formula is $C_{27}H_{44}OH$.
- It possesses OH group at C_3 position, a double bond between C_5 and an eight-carbon side chain at C_{17} position **(Fig. 6.6)**.

Source of Cholesterol

It is derived from diet such as in butter, milk, cream, egg yolk, meats, hen's egg. It can be endogenously synthesized from acetyl-CoA approximately 1 gm/day.

Occurrence of Cholesterol

Cholesterol is widely present in the body tissue, such as the brain, nervous tissue, liver, skin, intestinal mucosa, adrenal cortex and corpus luteum. The relatively high content of cholesterol

Fig. 6.6: Chemical structure of cholesterol.

in the skin may be related to vitamin D formation by UV rays and that in the adrenal gland and gonads to steroid hormone synthesis. Cholesterol is present in the blood and bile and is usually a major constituent of gallstones.

Features of Cholesterol
- Cholesterol occurs both in free form and in ester form, in which it is esterified with a fatty acid at –OH group at C_3 position. Various fatty acids such as linoleic acid, oleic acid, palmitic acid, arachidonic acid, etc. can form cholesterol esters.
- Free cholesterol is equally distributed between plasma and RBC, but cholesterol esters are found in plasma and absent in RBC.
- Cholesterol occurs as a white or faint yellow color, almost odorless and pearly leaflets or granular form.
- It is insoluble in water, sparingly soluble in alcohol, and soluble in ether, chloroform, ethyl acetate, and vegetable oil.
- Cholesterol is the precursor of all other steroids in the body such as corticosteroids, sex hormones, bile acid, vitamin D, etc.

Blood Level of Cholesterol

• Cholesterol	• < 200 mg/dL
• Triglycerides	• 50–190 mg/dL
• LDL	• <130 mg/dL
• HDL	• >40 mg/dL

Functions of Cholesterol
- Normal total serum cholesterol level in young adults is 150 to 240 mg.
- It is the structural component of cell membrane.
- It is a poor conductor of electricity and function, probably as an insulating mechanism for nerve impulses.
- The genetic deficiency of LCAT causes Norum's disease.
- Cholesterol functions as a precursor molecule in the synthesis of vitamin D, steroid hormones (e.g., cortisol and aldosterone and adrenal androgens), and sex hormones (e.g., testosterone, estrogens, and progesterone).
- Cholesterol is also a constituent of bile salt used in digestion to facilitate absorption of fat soluble vitamins A, D, E, and K

While cholesterol is central to many healthy cell functions, it also can harm the body if it is allowed to reach abnormal blood concentrations. When LDL-cholesterol levels are too high, the condition referred to as hypercholesterolemia, the risk for premature atherosclerotic cardiovascular diseases (ASCVD) increases.

Bile Acids and Bile Salts

Bile is a complex fluid containing water, electrolytes and organic molecules including bile acids, cholesterol, phospholipids and bilirubin that flow through the biliary tract into the small intestine. Adult humans produce 400 to 800 mL of bile daily.

There are two fundamentally important functions of bile:
- Bile contains bile acids, which are critical for digestion and absorption of fats and fat-soluble vitamins in the small intestine.
- Many waste products, including bilirubin, are eliminated from the body by secretion into bile and elimination in feces.

Bile Acids

Bile acids are derivatives of cholesterol synthesized in the hepatocyte. Cholesterol, ingested as part of the diet or derived from hepatic synthesis is converted into the bile acids cholic and chenodeoxycholic acids, which are then conjugated to an amino acid (glycine or taurine) to yield the conjugated form that is actively secreted into canaliculi.

Bile acids carry out two important functions:

- **Emulsification of lipid aggregates:** Bile acids have detergent action on particles of dietary fat which causes fat globules to break down or be emulsified into minute, microscopic droplets. Emulsification is not digestion per se, but is of importance because it greatly increases the surface area of fat, making it available for digestion by lipases, which cannot access the inside of lipid droplets.
- **Solubilization and transport of lipids in an aqueous environment:** Bile acids are lipid carriers and are able to solubilize many lipids by forming **micelles**—aggregates of lipids such as fatty acids, cholesterol and monoglycerides—that remain suspended in water. Bile acids are also critical for transport and absorption of the fat-soluble vitamins.

Bile Salts

Bile salts are a component of bile, a fluid secreted from the gallbladder during the digestion of lipids. The presence of bile salts gives bile the ability to emulsify, or mix, lipids in the aqueous environment of the intestine. Bile salts play a crucial role in hepatobiliary and intestinal homeostasis and digestion. The liver synthesizes primary bile salts from cholesterol. Enzymatic modifications during their enterohepatic circulation lead to the formation of secondary and tertiary bile salts.

The common primary bile salts are:
- Glycocholic acid
- Taurocholic acid
- Glycochenodeoxycholic acid
- Taurochenodeoxycholic acid

Triacylglycerols (TAG)/Neutral Fats/ Triglycerides (TG)

Esters of fatty acids with glycerol are:
- **Monoacylglycerol:** When glycerol contains only one molecule of fatty acid.

- **Diacylglycerol:** When glycerol contains two molecules of fatty acids.
- **Triacylglycerol:** When glycerol contains three fatty acid residues.

A molecule of triacylglycerol may contain similar or dissimilar fatty acids (saturated or unsaturated).

Naturally occurring fats have apparently the D- structural configuration.

$$\begin{array}{c} CH_2-O-\overset{\displaystyle O}{\underset{\displaystyle \|}{C}}-R_1 \\ R_2-\overset{\displaystyle O}{\underset{\displaystyle \|}{C}}-O-CH \\ CH_2-O-\underset{\displaystyle O}{\overset{\displaystyle \|}{C}}-R_3 \end{array}$$

Fats are transported either in chylomicrons or VLDL and oxidized in mitochondria to give energy.

Physical Properties
- Neutral fats are colorless, odorless and tasteless.
- These are insoluble in water but soluble in organic solvents.
- Saturated fatty acids are generally hard, while unsaturated fatty acids are soft.

Chemical Properties
- **Hydrolysis:** Fats can be hydrolyzed by heating at high temperature, by acids or alkalies as well as by enzymes like lipases. They give glycerol and fatty acids after hydrolysis.
- **Hydrogenation:** Unsaturated fatty acids become saturated fatty acids after hydrogenation, e.g., vegetable oil.
- **Oxidation:** Fats are very rich in double bonds in their fatty acids and undergo spontaneous oxidation to form aldehyde, ketones and resins forming a transparent coating on the surfaces to which the oil is applied. These so-called drying oils are used in the manufacture of paints and varnishes.
- **Rancidity:** It is the process of the formation of a complex product known as rancid fat. It is formed because of exposure of fats and oils to warm, moist air for long time. This exposure results in the auto-oxidation, splitting and aldehyde formation of fats and oils resulting in unpleasant taste, e.g., moisture in butter fat and enzymes of airborne bacteria produces a variety of volatile fatty acids.

Characterization of Fats and Oils
- **Saponification number:** The number of mgs of KOH required to saponify the free and the combined fatty acids in one gram of a given fat is called its saponification number.
  - The saponification number depends on the number of –COOH groups, which is higher in short-chain fatty acids.

Human fat	194–198
Butter	210–230
Coconut oil	253–262
Castor oil	175–180

- **Iodine number:** It is defined as number of grams of iodine absorbed by 100 gm of fat. It is an index of degree of saturation.

Coconut oil	7–10
Butter	25–28
Palm oil	45–55
Olive oil	80–85

- **Acid number:** It is the number of mgs of KOH required to neutralize the fatty acids in a gm of fat. The acid number indicates the degree of rancidity of the given fat.
- **Acetyl number:** It is the number of mgs of required to neutralize the acetic acid obtained by saponification of 1 gm of fat after it has been acetylated by means of acetic anhydride.

PHOSPHOLIPIDS

- Phospholipids are a heterogeneous group of compounds that contain a phosphate group and a nitrogenous or non-nitrogenous group. In addition, they also contain long-chain fatty acids.
- **Classification of phospholipids:** Phospholipids are classified into three main groups, on the basis of type of alcohol present in them **(Fig. 6.7 and Table 6.6)**.

Properties of Phospholipids
- They are signal mediators.
- They are amphipathic molecules.
- They anchor proteins within the cell membranes.
- They are the major constituents of cell membranes.
- They are the components of bile and lipoproteins.

Functions of Phospholipids
- Phospholipids constitute the matrix of cell walls and membranes, the myelin sheath, mitochondria and microsomes.
- Certain enzymes require tightly bound phospholipids for their action, e.g., mitochondrial enzyme system.
- Phospholipids help in the coagulation of blood by activating certain coagulation factors.
- Choline acts as a lipotropic agent to prevent fatty liver formation.
- Lecithin also helps in the emulsification of lipids in water.

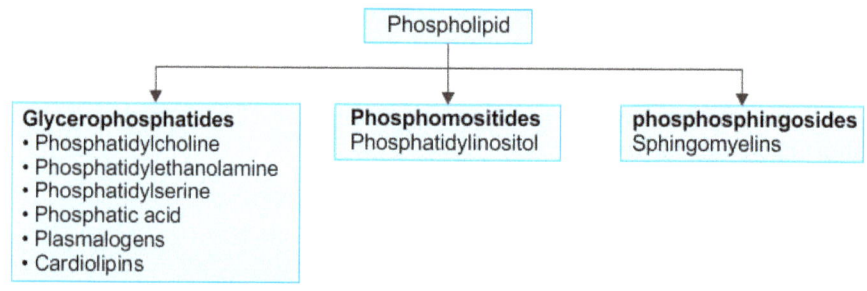

Fig. 6.7: Types of phospholipids.

Table 6.6: Classification of phospholipids.

Sr. No.	Name of phospholipid	Description	Occurrence
1	Phosphatidylcholine (Lecithin)	Lecithin contains two fatty acids, glycerol, phosphoric acid and a nitrogen base "choline". Lecithin emulsify the lipid-water mixture and is required for the digestion and absorption of the lipids from intestine.	In liver, brain, nerve tissue, egg yolk, sperm and plasma. Along with the lecithin in brain liver, cardiac muscles, erythrocytes and nervous tissue.
2	Phosphatidyletha-nolamine (Cephalins)	These are structurally identical with lecithins with the exception that the base ethanolamine replaces choline.	
3	Phosphatidylserine	It contains the amino acid serine in place of ethanolamine	In brain and nervous tissue as well as in small amount in other tissues and blood.
4	Phosphatidic acid	It contains a molecule of glycerol, two fatty acids and a phosphate group.	
5	Plasmalogens	These compounds on hydrolysis yield one molecule each of long-chain aliphatic aldehyde, a fatty acid, glycerol, phosphate and a nitrogenous base which is usually ethanolamine, but may sometimes choline.	About 10% of total phospholipid of brain, nervous tissue, muscles, and mitochondria.
6	Cardiolipin	These are two molecules of phosphatidic acid combined with glycerol.	In mitochondria and bacterial cell wall.
7	Phosphatidylinositol	It replaces the base choline of lecithin.	Firstly found in acid-fast bacilli. Later, in brain and nervous tissue as well as in other plants phospholipids.
8	Sphingomyelins	It contains a molecule of fatty acid, phosphoric acid, nitrogenous base choline and sphingol in place of glycerol	In the brain and nervous tissues and in very small amounts in other tissues.

- They also play an active part in the transport of lipids such as chylomicrons, lipoproteins from the intestine.
- They act as a carrier of inorganic ions across the membranes.
- Phospholipids of myelin sheaths provide insulation around the nerve fibers.
- Phospholipids act as a source of arachidonic acid, which is utilized for the synthesis of prostaglandins and leukotrienes.

GLYCOLIPIDS

Glycolipids are compound lipids that contain carbohydrates in the form of galactose, and sphingol. They do not contain glycerol, phosphatidic acid and a nitrogenous base. They are of two types, i.e., cerebrosides and gangliosides. The description of the classification of glycolipids is given in **Table 6.7**.

Table 6.7: Classification of glycolipids.

S. No.	Name of glycolipid	Description	Occurrence
1	Cerebrosides	Cerebrosides contain galactose, a high molecular weight fatty acid and sphingosine. On the basis of fatty acid content, they are classified into: Kerasin Cerebron Nervon Oxynervon	In white matter of the brain and in the myelin sheaths of nerves
2	Gangliosides	They contain N-acetylneuraminic acid (sialic acid), fatty acids, sphingosine and 3 molecules of hexose. Four important types are: GM-1 GM-2 GM-3 GM-4	Found in ganglion cells, neuronal bodies, dendrites, spleen and RBC stroma and in high amount in gray matter of brain.

Functions of Glycolipids

- It provides energy to the cells.
- It is an essential part of cell membranes.
- It helps in determining the blood group of an individual.
- It acts as receptors at the surface of the red blood cells.
- It also functions by assisting the immune system by destroying and eliminating the pathogen from the body
- Cerebrosides function in transmission of nerve impulses across the synapses.
- In Gaucher's disease, large amount of cerebrosides is accumulated in the liver and spleen.
- Gangliosides serve as a specific membrane binding site on a cell membrane for circulating hormones, thereby influence various metabolic processes.
- In Tay-Sachs disease, gangliosides accumulate in the brain due to genetic lack of the enzyme "Hexosaminidase-A" required for its degradation.

LIPOPROTEINS AND THEIR FUNCTIONS

Lipoproteins are the complexes of lipids with proteins to form lipoproteins. Since lipids are insoluble in water, they cannot be transported as such in plasma. Therefore, they are complexed with proteins to form lipoproteins. Protein part of lipoproteins is called apolipoprotein/apoprotein.

Type of Lipoproteins

There are five main types of lipoprotein depending on the density, all of which have slightly different functions.
1. **Chylomicrons:** Made in the small intestine; carry dietary fatty acids directly from the gut to the liver and peripheral tissues where it will be used or stored as fuel.
2. **Very-low-density lipoproteins (VLDLs):** Made in the liver; carry excess fatty acids from the liver to adipose tissue (fat tissue), where free fatty acids are released and taken up by fat cells for storage.

3. **Intermediate-density lipoproteins (IDLs):** Made from VLDLs after free fatty acids are released; taken up by the liver and converted into LDL particles.
4. **Low-density lipoproteins (LDLs):** The main carrier of cholesterol, taking it to peripheral tissues with excess returning to the liver.
5. **High-density lipoproteins (HDLs):** Made in the liver and intestines; collect cholesterol from cell membranes in peripheral tissues and transport it back to the liver for processing (reverse cholesterol transport).

Functions of Lipoproteins

The function of lipoprotein particles is to transport lipids (fats) (such as triacylglycerol) around the body in the blood.

METABOLISM OF FATTY ACIDS

Fatty Acid Oxidation

Fatty acids are an important source of energy for many cellular organisms. Oxidation of fatty acids occur in multiple regions of the cell within the human body; the mitochondria, in which only beta-oxidation occurs; the peroxisome, where alpha- and beta-oxidation occur; and omega-oxidation, which occurs in the endoplasmic reticulum. Fatty acids in the body are mainly oxidized by β-oxidation. Metabolism of fatty acids consists of catabolic processes that generate energy and primary metabolites from fatty acids, and anabolic processes that create biologically important molecules from fatty acids and other dietary carbon sources. Fatty acid oxidation provides an alternative mode of high-efficiency energy production while simultaneously sparing muscles from catabolic breakdown. The oxidation of fatty acid is the cyclic process. In each cycle, active fatty acid is degraded to give acetyl-CoA and acyl-CoA, two carbon less than original acyl-CoA.

The enzymes of fatty acid oxidation are mainly present in the mitochondria, and the sites of oxidation are most of the tissues except brain, RBC and adrenal medulla.

For oxidation to occur, fatty acids have to undergo the following steps:
- Activation of fatty acid
- Transport of fatty acid into mitochondria
- β-oxidation

I. Activation of Fatty Acid

Long-chain fatty acids are first activated to "active fatty acid" or " acyl-CoA" in the cytosol. The reaction follows **(Fig. 6.8)**:

Fig. 6.8: Fatty acid activation pathway.

Fig. 6.9: Mitochondrial transportation of fatty acid pathway.

II. Transport of Fatty Acid into Mitochondria

Active fatty acids penetrate the inner mitochondrial membrane in combination with carnitine and in the presence of enzyme carnitine acyl transferase-I, which converts acyl-CoA into "acyl-carnitine". Acyl carnitine is then transported across the membrane to mitochondrial matrix by another enzyme "carnitine-acylcarnitine translocase" **(Fig. 6.9)**.

III. β-Oxidation

It occurs in the mitochondrial matrix and involves four steps, i.e.,
a. FAD linked dehydrogenation
b. Hydration
c. NAD^+ dependent dehydrogenation
d. Thiolysis

The details of these steps are given below:

Steps of Fatty Acid Oxidation

- The first reaction after entering into the mitochondrial matrix is of dehydrogenation, in which Acyl-CoA is converted into α, β-unsaturated acyl CoA by the enzyme acyl CoA dehydrogenase, with the production of 2 ATP molecules.
- The next reaction is of hydration, where water is added to saturate the double bond to form β-hydroxyl acyl-CoA, catalyzed by enoyl-CoA hydratase.
- Further, it undergoes dehydrogenation, forming β-keto acyl-CoA, catalyzed by the enzyme β-hydroxyl acyl CoA dehydrogenase in the presence of NAD and production of 3 ATP molecules.
- Next, β-keto acyl CoA splits at the β position by thiolase, forming acyl CoA (2 carbon less) and acetyl CoA. Acyl CoA undergoes further oxidation, where acetyl CoA enters Krebs cycle and undergoes oxidation **(Fig. 6.10)**.

Energetics of β-Oxidation of Fatty Acid

- Palmitic acid oxidation (7 cycles)—7 × 5   = 35 ATP
- 8 Molecules of acetyl CoA oxidized by
  Krebs cycle 8 × 12   = 96 ATP
  Total   **= 131 ATP**
  Energy utilized for activation   = 2 ATP
  of fatty acid
  Net Yield   **= 129 ATP**

Fig. 6.10: Steps of fatty acid oxidation.

De Novo Synthesis of Fatty Acid

Fatty acid synthesis is the creation of fatty acids from acetyl-CoA and malonyl-CoA precursors through action of enzyme complex called fatty acid synthase. It is an important part of the lipogenesis process, which - together with glycolysis - stands behind creating fats from blood sugar in living organisms.

The cytoplasmic synthesis of fatty acids from acetyl-CoA is called *De Novo* synthesis, which mainly occurs in the cytosol of cells of liver, mammary glands, and adipose tissue.

Steps

1. The first reaction is conversion of acetyl-CoA to malonyl-CoA by acetyl-CoA carboxylase in the presence of ATP and active CO_2.
2. Then, there is transfer of an acetyl-CoA to the Cysteinyl-SH group of Ketoacyl synthase (I) by acetyl-CoA-transacetylase (I) subunit of fatty acid synthase complex (I) leading to the formation of acetyl-S-cys(I).
3. The next step is condensation of acetyl and malonyl groups by keto-acyl synthase (I) to form acetoacetyl-S-ACP(II). In this process, CO_2 is released and -Cys-SH becomes free.
4. Further, reduction of acetoacetyl-S-ACP to β-hydroxybutyryl-S-ACP (II) occurs with the help of enzyme ketoacyl reductase.
5. The next step is dehydration of β-OH-butyryl-S-ACP (II) by the enzyme dehydratase to form α, β-unsaturated butyryl-S-ACP(II).

6. Then, there is reduction of α, β-unsaturated butyryl-S-ACP (II) by enzyme enoyl-reductase to form butyryl-S-ACP.
7. New malonyl CoA combines with -SH of ACP and acyl group is transferred to -Cys-SH.
8. This sequence of reaction is repeated till a 16-carbon palmityl-S-ACP is formed.
9. Finally, palmityl-S-ACP is released as Palmitic acid by the enzyme thioesterase (deacylase) **(Fig. 6.11)**.

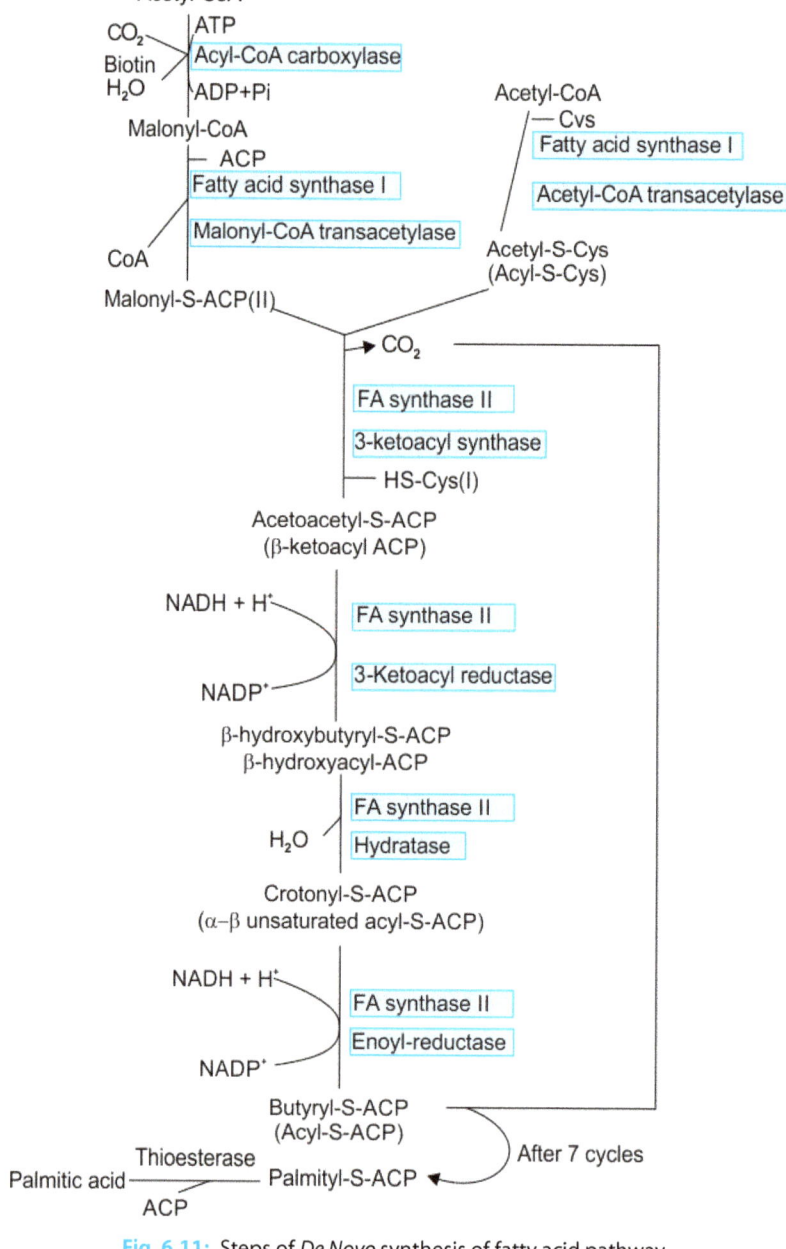

Fig. 6.11: Steps of *De Novo* synthesis of fatty acid pathway.

Energetic of Fatty Acid Synthesis

1. One high energy bond of ATP is spent in producing each acetyl-CoA from citrate by ATP-citrate lyase in the cytoplasm
   - Therefore, 7 high energy phosphate bonds are spent in providing 8 acetyl-CoA molecules for synthesizing one palmitate molecule.
2. Seven of the acetyl-CoA molecules have to be carboxylated to seven malonyl-CoA molecules by acetyl-CoA carboxylase, each involving the expenditure of one high energy bond of ATP.
   - Therefore, 7 high energy phosphate bonds are spent in providing seven malonyl-CoA molecules for one palmitate.

Interrelationship in Metabolism

- Glucose 6-phosphate
- Pyruvic acid
- Acetyl-CoA

These three molecules play a key role in metabolism.

1. **Glucose 6-phosphate:** There are four possible fates of glucose 6-phosphate:
   a. Synthesis of glycogen in liver and muscle cells.
   b. Release of glucose into bloodstream.
   c. Synthesis of nucleic acids from pentose phosphate pathway.
   d. Glycolysis through its conversion into pyruvic acid.
2. **Pyruvic acid:**
   a. Under aerobic condition, pyruvic acid is converted to acetyl-CoA.
   b. Under anaerobic condition, lactic acid is produced in skeletal tissues.
   c. Production of alanine through transamination of pyruvic acid.
   d. Gluconeogenesis by conversion of pyruvic acid to oxaloacetic acid. By glycolytic reversal again, it is converted into glucose 6-phosphate.
3. **Acetyl CoA:**
   a. Under aerobic condition, pyruvic acid is converted to acetyl CoA. It enters into Krebs cycle for ATP production.
   b. Synthesis of lipids including fatty acid, ketone bodies, and cholesterol.

■ KETONE BODIES

Ketone bodies are produced by the liver and used peripherally as an energy source when glucose is not readily available. The two main ketone bodies are acetoacetate (AcAc) and 3-beta-hydroxybutyrate (3HB), while acetone is the third, and least abundant, ketone body. Ketones are always present in the blood and their levels increase during fasting and prolonged exercise. They are also found in the blood of neonates and pregnant women.

Metabolism of Ketone Bodies

Ketogenesis: Ketogenesis is a metabolic pathway that produces ketone bodies, which provide an alternative form of energy for the body. Ketogenesis can be upregulated by hormones such as glucagon, cortisol, thyroid hormones, and catecholamines, by causing a more significant breakdown of free fatty acids, thus increasing the amount available to be used in the ketogenic pathway. However, insulin is the primary hormonal regulator of this process. Insulin regulates many key enzymes in the ketogenic pathway, and a state of low insulin triggers the process.
- It occurs in the liver
- Enzymes responsible for ketogenesis are found in mitochondria.
- Acetoacetate is the first substance produced.

Utilization

Acetoacetate and beta-hydroxybutyrate are the two ketone bodies used by the body for energy.

The brain uses them as a major source of energy during periods where glucose is not readily available.

■ INTERRELATIONSHIP IN METABOLISM

Carbohydrates, Lipid and Proteins

- Acetyl-CoA is the link between carbohydrate and lipid pathways
- Glucose, glycerol and fatty acids all degrade into acetly-CoA
- Bio-synthesis of fatty acids, ketone bodies and cholesterol all uses acetyl-CoA
- Glycerol is the only component of lipids that is involved in the synthesis of carbohydrates.
- On the other hand, lipase can be formed from carbohydrates (**Fig. 6.12**).

Fig. 6.12: Inter-relation between metabolism of carbohydrates, fats and proteins.

CHAPTER 6: Lipids

■ QUESTIONS

Q.1: Metabolism of fatty acids.
Q.2: What are lipids? Explain the classification of lipids.
Q.3: Describe in what way the lipids are useful for human body?
Q.4: Write the functions of lipids.
Q.5: Oxidation of fatty acids.
Q.6: What is auto-oxidation, hydrogenation and saponification of fatty acids?
Q.7: Classification of fats.

■ BIBLIOGRAPHY

1. Alley JT, Mohiuddin SS. Biochemistry, Fatty Acid Oxidation. [Updated 2021 Jan 30]. In: StatPearls [Internet]. Treasure Island (FL): StatPearls Publishing; 2022 Jan. Available from: https://www.ncbi.nlm.nih.gov/books/NBK556002/
2. Bach AC, Babayan VK. Medium-chain triglycerides: an update. American J Clin Nutr, 1982: 36: 950–62.
3. Berning JR. The role of medium-chain triglycerides in exercise. Int. J. Sport Nutr. 1996: 6: 121–33.
4. Beynen AC, Katan M/B. Why do polyunsaturated fatty acids lower serum cholesterol? American J Clin Nutr, 1985: 42: 560–3.
5. Essén-Gustavsson B, Blomstrand E, Karlström K, et al. Influence of diet on substrate metabolism during exercise. Proc 3rd Int Conf. Equine Exercise Physiology, 1991: 288–98.
6. Grisham, Charles M, Garrett HR. Biochemistry. Philadelphia: Saunders College Pub, 1999: 426–7.
7. Huff T, Boyd B, Jialal I. Physiology, Cholesterol. [Updated 2021 Mar 2]. In: StatPearls [Internet]. Treasure Island (FL): StatPearls Publishing; 2022 Jan. Available from: https://www.ncbi.nlm.nih.gov/books/NBK470561/
8. InformedHealth.org [Internet]. Cologne, Germany: Institute for Quality and Efficiency in Health Care (IQWiG); 2006-. How does the liver work? 2009 Sep 17 [Updated 2016 Aug 22]. Available from: https://www.ncbi.nlm.nih.gov/books/NBK279393/
9. Jones RL. Functions of prostaglandins. Pathobiol Annu. 1972;2:359-80. PMID: 4589748.
10. Kaur N, Chugh V, Gupta AK. Essential fatty acids as functional components of foods–a review. J Food Sci Technol. 2014;51(10):2289-2303. doi:10.1007/s13197-012-0677-0
11. Laffel L. Ketone bodies: a review of physiology, pathophysiology and application of monitoring to diabetes. Diabetes Metab Res Rev. 1999 Nov-Dec;15(6):412-26. doi: 10.1002/(sici)1520-7560(199911/12)15:6<412::aid-dmrr72>3.0.co;2-8. PMID: 10634967.
12. Marks DB, Marks AD, Smith CM. Basic Medical Biochemistry: A Clinical Approach, Williams & Wilkins, 1996.
13. Meisenberg G, Simmons WH. Principles of Medical Biochemistry, Mosby, 1998.
14. Murray RK, Granner DK, Mayes PA, et al. Harper's Biochemistry, Appleton and Lange, 1999.
15. Rambabu K, Ravikiran and PB Kameswari. Fundamentals of Biochemistry. 2nd edition. India; ATBS publishers: 2019
16. Vasudevan DM, S Sreekumari, Vaidyanathan Kannan. Textbook of Biochemistry for Medical students. 9th edition. New Delhi: Jaypee Brothers Medical Publishers; 2019.

Section 2

Biophysics

Section Outline

- Chapter 7: Introduction to Biophysics
- Chapter 8: Motion
- Chapter 9: Gravity
- Chapter 10: Force, Energy and Work
- Chapter 11: Heat
- Chapter 12: Light
- Chapter 13: Pressure and Fluid Mechanics
- Chapter 14: Sound Waves
- Chapter 15: Electricity and Electromagnetism
- Chapter 16: Nuclear Physics
- Chapter 17: Electronics in Nursing

CHAPTER 7

Introduction to Biophysics

Suresh K Sharma, Navjot Kaur

Chapter Outline
- Meaning of Biophysics
- Importance of Biophysics in Nursing
- Concept of Units
- Fundamental and Derived Units
- Systems of Units
- Fundamental Units in Various Systems

■ INTRODUCTION

Nature around us is colorful and full of phenomena of many varieties. The air, light, sands, water, planets, heating, electricity, functioning of the human body, there are a large number of objects and events happening around us. Physics is the study of all this. Events of nature take place according to some basic laws and knowing these basic laws from observed events is physics. Understanding physics leads to many applications in the bio and medical sciences. Biophysics is a branch of science that uses methods of physics to study biological systems.

Modern biophysics combines state-of-the-art physical measurements with computational models to understand the detailed physical mechanisms underlying the behavior of complex biological systems. Biophysics is a growing enterprise worldwide, driven primarily by the widespread realization of the major contribution that can be made to biological science by a combination of truly state-of-the-art physical measurements with modern molecular biology. The field occupies a unique and central position at the intersection of the biological, chemical, physical, and computational sciences.

Biophysics is intrinsically interdisciplinary. Biophysics takes a quantitative, physical, and non-phenomenological approach to biology that is firmly rooted in the principles of condensed phase of physics and physical chemistry. Biophysicists are driven primarily by their curiosity about how biological systems work at the molecular level. While they routinely employ the methods of molecular biology, their primary focus is on the development of novel structures and dynamical tools that enable uniquely incisive studies of systems ranging in complexity from single proteins *in vitro* to the complex interactions of biopolymers in live cells. Biophysicists as a group most often develop novel, sophisticated experimental methods that reveal molecular level details with unprecedented clarity. The state-of-the-art in X-ray crystallography, solution phase, and solid-state NMR, atomic force microscopy, single-molecule methods, EPR, and fluorescence microscopy continues to evolve in ways that better elucidate biological structure and function. In parallel, biophysicists are developing powerful new computational tools based on firmly established physical principles that are sufficiently accurate to greatly enhance insights from the experiment. Just as the tools of molecular biology gradually become useful to biophysicists, over time the new tools developed by biophysicists gradually find widespread use among all biological scientists.

■ MEANING OF BIOPHYSICS

The term biophysics was first used in 1892 by Karl Pearson in his book "The Grammar of Sciences".
- "Biophysics is defined as the science where there is the application of the laws of physics to life process".
- "Biophysics is the application of physical principles and methods to the study of the structure of living organisms and the mechanisms of the life process".
- "It is the science of living physics; the form of physics applies the knowledge of physics to explain biological questions, such as the transmission of nervous impulses or muscle control".
- "Biophysics is a branch of science that deals with the study of physical or biophysical principles and their application to health sciences".
- Biophysics is an interdisciplinary scientific discipline which uses physical techniques and methods to study the functions, structures, and energetics of biological objects.

■ IMPORTANCE OF BIOPHYSICS IN NURSING

The study of biophysics immensely benefits the nurses, because it helps them to acquire:
- Practical, functional knowledge of physical principles that underline nursing procedures and the operation of machinery that nurses use.
- Technical knowledge from the science of physics that applies specifically to nursing performance and understanding of certain biomedical phenomena, like how does a suction apparatus operate? What is the most efficient way to move a heavy object or a patient? How does air get in and out of the lungs? etc.

The study of biophysics help to understand movement, electrophysiology, membrane physics, the three-dimensional structure of proteins, protein-DNA interactions, glycoprotein structure and function, gene expression, and network theories applied to cellular metabolism and macromolecular interactions.

In addition study of biophysics helps a nurse to understand the following contents of nursing:

Measurement
- Accuracy in preparation of medications.
- Assessment of patients by measurement of vital signs

Motion
- Inertia in accidents
- The physiological reaction to high-velocity centrifuges

Gravity
- Circulation of blood
- Postural drainage

- Postoperative position
- ESR estimation
- Dependent position for edema patient

Center of Gravity

- Body mechanics
- Lifting and turning patients
- Crutch walking

Specific Gravity

- Underwater exercises
- Examination of the body fluids

Force

- Torques in traction
- Muscle action
- Vector addition and analysis in traction.

Pressure

- Suction
- Internal and external respiration
- Positive pressure ventilation
- Oxygen therapy
- Administration of irrigation and parental fluid.

Heat

- Thermometry
- Application of heat and cold application
- Steam inhalation
- Basal metabolism
- Thermography
- Autoclave and sterilization.

Light and Sound

- Actions of lenses
- Use of mirrors in apparatus
- Microscopy
- Ophthalmoscope
- Refraction
- Visual fields
- Audiometry
- Human audibility.

Electricity

- Patient monitors, ECG, EEG, EMG
- Diathermy
- Electrosurgical procedures
- Electric shock therapy

- Use of transistors in apparatus
- Cardiac pacemakers.

Work and Energy
- Circulation of blood
- Pulse formation
- Work done by heart and skeletal muscles.

Molecular Physics
- Artificial kidney
- Colloidal dispersions
- The surface tension of antiseptics
- The viscosity of blood.

Atomic Physics
- High energy radiation
- X-ray therapy
- Radioisotopes
- Tracer studies of metabolism
- Precautions in the use of radioactive material
- Half-life in radiotherapy.

■ CONCEPT OF UNITS

Nursing care demands several measurement tasks like measuring vital signs, patient's height, weight, body mass index, 24 hours fluid balance, and so many others. In this situation, a nurse takes a measurement of a physical quantity and compares the measured value of the physical quantity with a standard to determine its relationship with that standard. The standard of measurement is called a unit.

"The unit of any measurement is defined as a conventional quantity used as the reference or standard of measurement to which measurements with that unit can be compared".

■ FUNDAMENTAL AND DERIVED UNITS

Fundamental units are the units of the fundamental physical quantities in the SI system which are not formed from other units. There are a total of seven fundamental units such as meter, kilogram, ampere, and second. Derived units are those units that are used for derived quantities. Examples of derived units are meter per second (distance), mole per cubic meter (amount of substance concentration) and specific volume (cubic meter per kilogram). Total of 21 derived SI units are present. "Units of various physical quantities, which can be expressed in terms of the fundamental units of mass, length and time, are called derived units."

The unit of measurement is fixed by definition and is independent of such physical conditions as temperature, humidity, etc. The numerical value of a physical quantity, therefore, refers to the number of standard unit of measurement. For example, when we say that a patient's temperature is 38°C; it means that the patient's temperature is 38 times the unit of measurement, called degree Celsius (°C). Thus, measurement of any quantity has two characteristics—a numerical value and a unit. For example, you measure the birth weight of a baby as 3.5 Kg. Then 3.5 is the numerical value and Kg is the unit.

Although the number of physical quantities that we measure is very large, we do not need a very large number of standards to compare every measurement. It is so because all the physical quantities are not independent quantities in so far as their measurement is concerned. For example, the velocity of a body is measured in units of length (meter) and time (seconds). A few independent standards have been chosen to fix the units of certain physical quantities. The measurement of most of the other physical quantities can be expressed in terms of these independent current standards. These independent standards are length, mass and time. Such units fixed by independent standards are called fundamental units. For example, fundamental units of length, mass and time are:

- *One meter:* the unit of length
- *One kilogram:* the unit of mass
- *One second:* the unit of time

Units of measurement of many physical quantities such as density, speed, volume, pressure, and force can be derived from these fundamental or basic units using physical equations. These units are called derived units. For example, the unit of volume is a cubic meter, which is derived from the unit of length. Speed is defined as the distance covered per unit of time and its unit is m/s. The unit of speed is derived from units of length and time.

SYSTEMS OF UNITS

A system of units is a set of related units that are used for calculations. The system includes base units, which represent base dimensions, and derived units. There are several systems of units that have been used for measuring physical quantities. The commonly used systems are the centimeter-gram-second (CGS), the foot-pound-second (FPS), the metre-kilogram-second (MKS), and the International System of Units (SI). They differ from each other because different standards of measurement are used for fundamental quantities. **Table 7.1** contains the standards of measurement for fundamental quantities in these systems.

The two systems of measurement most frequently used in nursing practice are the MKS (also called metric) and the FPS (also called English). You may note from **Table 7.1** that the units for these physical quantities are the same in the metric and SI systems. The International System of Units (abbreviated SI) is the metric system used in science, industry, and medicine.

Table 7.1: Systems of units with their standards of measurement.

Physical quantity	CGS system	FPS system	MKS system	SI system
Length	Centimeter (cm)	Foot (f)	Meter (m)	Meter (m)
Mass	Gram (gm)	Pound (d)	Kilogram (kg)	Kilogram (kg)
Time	Second (s)	Second (s)	Second (s)	Second (s)
Temperature	–	Fahrenheit (F)	Celsius (°C)	Kelvin (K)
Electric current	–	–	–	Ampere (A)
Light intensity	–	–	–	Candela (Cd)
Amount of substance	–	–	–	Mole (mol)

SECTION 2: Biophysics

Table 7.2: Multiples of units of length in English and metric systems.

English system	Metric system
12 inches = 1 foot	10 millimeters (mm) = 1 centimeter (cm)
3 feet = 1 yard	10 centimeters (cm) = 1 decimeter
5 ½ yards = 1 rod	10 decimeters = 1 meter (m)
1,760 yards = 1 mile	10 meters = 1 decameter
5,280 feet = 1 mile	10 decameters = 1 hectometer
	10 hectometers = 1 kilometer (km)
	10 kilometers = 1 myriameter

Note: 1 feet = 12 inches = 30 cm (1 inch = 2.5 cm)

■ FUNDAMENTAL UNITS IN VARIOUS SYSTEMS

Units of Length

Length is defined as the distance between two points in space. The unit of length in the English system is the foot. The unit of length in the metric system is the meter. The bigger unit of measuring length is kilometer. Smaller measurement units are decimeter, centimeter and millimeter. The standard unit of length is 'Meter' which is written in short as 'm'.

In the health care system, one can observe the use of different systems like patient's height recorded in feet, whereas small size papule on the skin is measured in millimeters. Similarly, in microscopic work, a very small unit—a micron is used. The micron is 1/1,000 mm.

The various multiples of units of length are listed in **Table 7.2** for both metric and English systems.

The instruments used to measure length are an infantometer, measuring tape, stadiometer (measuring height)

Unit of Mass and Weight

The mass of a body refers to the quantity of matter contained in it. The unit of mass in the metric system and SI system is the kilogram (kg). A physical balance ordinarily measures the mass of a body. **Table 7.3** shows the unit of mass in the English system and metric system. Some of these units are used in measuring food items for special diets, amount of drugs, weights of patients, etc.

Although commonly we use the terms mass and weight in the same sense, the two terms have different meanings in physics. In physics, concepts of mass and weight are different. The mass of a body is the quantity of matter contained in it. On the other hand, weight is defined as the gravitational force with which a body is pulled towards the center of the earth. Mathematically, we write:

$$W = mg$$

Where 'W' denotes the weight of the body, 'm' is its mass and 'g' is the acceleration due to gravity.

The kilogram is the SI unit of mass and it is the almost universally used standard mass unit. In the SI system, the unit of weight is Newton. 1 kilogram weighing 9.8 Newtons.

Since the value of the acceleration due to gravity varies with the distance of an object from the center of the earth, the weight of the object changes with its position on the earth.

CHAPTER 7: Introduction to Biophysics

Table 7.3: Multiples of units of mass in the metric and English systems.

English system	Metric system
Troy units	10 milligrams = 1 centigram
24 grains = 1 pennyweight	
20 pennyweights = 1 ounce	10 centigrams = 1 decigram
12 ounces = 1 pound	
Avoirdupois units	10 decigrams = 1 gram
27.34 grains = 1 dram	
16 drams = 1 ounce	10 grams = 1 decagram
16 ounces = 1 pound	
25 pounds = 1 quarter	
4 quarters = 1 hundredweight	
20 hundredweights = 1 shorts ton	10 decagrams = 1 hectogram
2,240 pounds = 1 long ton	10 hectograms = 1 kilogram
Apothecaries unit	1,000 kilograms = 1 metric ton
20 grains = 1 scruple	
3 scruples = 1 dram	
8 drams = 1 ounce	
12 ounces = 1 pound	

For example, an object at sea level weighs more than it does on a high mountain because the value of the acceleration due to the gravity of the earth on the object is greater at sea level. The mass, however, remains the same everywhere. The mass of an object is measured by a physical balance, whereas its weight is measured by a spring balance.

Mass is a scalar quantity while weight is a vector quantity because it is directed toward the center of the earth. The mass of a person is the same on the earth as well as on the moon, but the weight of the person is different in these two places because their pulls on the person are different. A person weighs six times more on earth than on the moon.

Whereas mass and weight have the same numerical value, it is important in solving problems to indicate the unit specifically, as one of force (weight) or as one of mass. One gram (gm) is a unit of mass; one gram weight is a unit of weight **(Table 7.4)**.

Units of Time

Time is defined as the continued progress of existence in the past, present and future. The unit of time is the second and is based on the natural clock. The natural clock is governed by the time taken by the earth to complete one revolution around the moon. According to this clock, one second is defined as (1/86,400) part of a mean solar day; a solar day is a period between noon of two consecutive days, and a mean solar day is the average solar day over a year, which is 24 hours. Since one hour contains 60 minutes and one minute contains 60 seconds, a mean solar day of 24 hours would have $24 \times 60 \times 60 = 86,400$. Thus, one second is 1/86400th part of a mean solar day.

Table 7.4: Conversion of weight and measurements.

Weight	Fluid volume
1 ounce = 8 drams	60 minims = 1 fluid dram
12 ounces = 1 pound	8 fluid drams = 1 fluid ounce
1000 micrograms (mcg) = 1 milligram (mg)	20 fluid ounces = 1 pint
1000 milligrams (mg) = 1 gram (gm)	2 pints = 1 quart (1000 ml)
1000 grams (g) = 1 kilogram (kg)	8 pints = 1 gallon
1 kilogram (kg) = 2.2 pounds	1 milliliters (ml) = 15–16 minims (15–16 drops)
1 grain = 60 milligrams (mg)	1 liter = 35 fluid ounce
1 dram = 4 grams (g)	1 fluid ounce = 30 ml
	1 fluid dram = 4 ml
1 ounce = 30 grams	1 gallon = 4.5 liters
1 pound = 375 grams	1 minimus = 0.04 ml = 1 drop
1 milligram = 1/60 grains (gr)	1 pint = 500 ml
	Household measurements
	1 teaspoonful = 4 or 5 ml = 1 fluid dram = 60 drops

Table 7.5: Prefixes and symbols used with SI units and metric units.

Prefix	Symbol	Power	Value
Tera	T	10^{12}	1,000,000,000,000
Giga	G	10^{9}	1,000,000,000
Mega	M	10^{6}	1,000,000
Kilo	K	10^{3}	1,000
Hecto	H	10^{2}	100
Deca	Da	10	10
Meter	M	1	1
Deci	D	10^{-1}	.1
Centi	C	10^{-2}	.01
Milli	Mm	10^{-3}	.001
Micro	U	10^{-6}	.000001
Nano	N	10^{-9}	.000000001
Pico	P	10^{-12}	.000000000001
Femto	F	10^{-15}	.000000000000001
Atto	A	10^{-18}	.000000000000000001

Let us consider some of the measurements of time you make in the course of your work. You will see that the second's hand of your watch is sufficiently accurate for recording a patient's pulse rate (number of pulse beats per minute). However, for studying the heartbeat of a patient by electrocardiography, greater accuracy in the measurement of time is required. In this case, the beating of the heart must be accurately measured in tenths or hundredths of a second.

Table 7.5 lists some of the prefixes and symbols used with SI and metric units to express a very large or very small value:

Table 7.6: Conversion between metric and English systems.

Weight	Length	Volume
1 gram = 15 grains	2.54 centimeters = 1 inch	1 cubic centimeter = 15 minims
4 grams = 1 dram	1 meter = 39.37 inches	4 cubic centimeters = 1 fluid dram
30 grams = 1 ounce		30 cubic centimeters = 1 fluid ounce
454 grams = 1 pound		
1 kilogram = 2.2 pounds		

In nursing practice, one may come across situations when a measurement is taken in the metric unit must be changed to the corresponding English unit and vice versa. For this reason, approximate equivalents commonly used in the hospital are given in **Table 7.6**.

QUESTIONS

Q.1: Discuss the meaning and importance of biophysics in nursing.
Q.2: Discuss the concept of units and fundamental and derived units.
Q.3: Describe the different systems of the units.
Q.4: List out the basic units of length, weight, mass, and time.

BIBLIOGRAPHY

1. Cantor CR, Schimmel PR. Biophysical Chemistry, Volumes 1–3. WH Freeman, San Francisco, 1980.
2. Cantor CR, Schimmel PR. Biophysical Chemistry, Volumes 1–3. WH Freeman, San Francisco, 1980.
3. Cotterill RMJ. Biophysics: An Introduction, Wiley, 2002.
4. Cotterill RMJ. Biophysics: An Introduction, Wiley, 2002.
5. Dogonadze RR, Urushadze ZD. "Semi-Classical Method of Calculation of Rates of Chemical Reactions Proceeding in Polar Liquids". J Electroanal Chem, 1971; 32: 235–45.
6. Flitter HH, Rowe HR. An Introduction to Physics in Nursing. St Louis: The CV Mosby Company, 1995.
7. Glaser R. Biophysics, Springer, 2001.
8. Glaser R. Biophysics: An Introduction (Corrected Edition). Springer, 2004: 11-23.
9. Glaser R. Biophysics: An Introduction. Springer Verlag, Heidelberg, 2004.
10. 10 Gomber KL, Gogia KL. Fundamental Physics. Ambala: Publishers, 2004.
11. Goyal RP, Tripathi SP. Concise Physics. New Delhi: Selina Publishers, August 2007.
12. Hobbie RK, Roth BJ. Intermediate Physics for Medicine and Biology (4th Edition). Springer, 2006.
13. Hobbie RK, Roth BJ. International Physics for Medicine and Biology (4th Edition). Springer, 2006.
14. Jackson B. Molecular and cellular biophysics. New York: Cambridge Publication, 2006.
15. Lal S. Principles of Physics. Ambala: Paedeep Publishers, 2004.
16. Mielczarek VE, Greenbaum E, et al. Biological Physics. New York. American Institute of Physics, 1993.
17. Nelson PC. Biological Physics (Updated Edition). WH Freeman, 2007.
18. Perutz MF. "The haemoglobin molecule". Proceedings of the Royal Society of London. Series, 1969;B 173(31)113-40.
19. Perutz MF. Electrostatic Effects in Proteins, Science. 1978;201:1187-91.
20. Perutz MF. Proteins and Nucleic Acids, Elsevier, Amsterdam, 1962.
21. Perutz MF. Proteins and Nucleic Acids: Structure and Function. Amsterdam: Elsevier, 1962.
22. Phillips R, Kondev J, Theriot J. Physical Biology of the Cell. Garland Science, Oxford, 2008.
23. Rashevsky N. Mathematical biophysics. Rev. ed., University of Chicago Press, 1948.

24. Rashevsky N. Mathematical Biophysics: Physico- Mathematical Foundations of Biology - Vol.2, New York: Dover Publications, Third Revised Edition, 1960.
25. Ruch TC, Fulton JF. Medical Physiology and Biophysics. Saunders, 1974: 1232.
26. Sneppen K, Zocchi G. Physics in Molecular Biology, Cambridge University Press, 2005.
27. Sneppen K, Zocchi G. Physics in Molecular Biology, First edition. Cambridge University Press, 2005:10-7.
28. Volkenshtein MV, Dogonadze RR, Madumarov AK, et al. Theory of Enzyme Catalysis. Molekuliarnaya Biologia (Moscow)1972; 6: 431-9 (In Russian, English summary).
29. Biophysics in nursing education. AIP Conference Proceedings 2152, 030019 (2019); https://doi.org/10.1063/1.5124763
30. Miroslava Líšková, Ľubomíra Valovičová, and Ján Ondruška. Collection Development Guidelines of the National Library of Medicine [Internet]. Bethesda (MD): National Library of Medicine (US); 2019-. Biophysics. [Updated 2004 Jan 2]. Available from: https://www.ncbi.nlm.nih.gov/sites/books/NBK518712/

CHAPTER 8

Motion

Suresh K Sharma, Navjot Kaur

Chapter Outline
- Scalars and Vectors
- Rest and Motion
- Speed
- Velocity
- Acceleration
- Applications of Motion in Nursing

■ INTRODUCTION

Motion is such an important phenomenon that life cannot be imagined without it. In physics, motion is the phenomenon in which an object changes its position over time. Motion is mathematically described in terms of displacement, distance, velocity, acceleration, speed, and time. The motion of the earth around the Sun gives rise to different seasons and the earth's motion on its own axis results in the occurrence of day and night. Most of the human body functions cannot be accomplished without motion, as the motion of the heart helps in pumping the blood in the body. Breathing is also only possible with the motion of the lungs. Similarly, there are several other body functions or activities of human life, where motion is essential to accomplish them, like transfer of a patient from bed to chair or administration of blood or fluid is only possible with the existence of the phenomenon of motion.

To understand the concept of motion, it is important to be familiar with scalar and vector quantities:

■ SCALARS AND VECTORS

- **Scalar quantities:** The physical quantities, which have a magnitude (how much) but no direction, are called scalars. For example, mass, length, temperature, work, charge, specific heat, time, density, etc. It may be positive or negative.
- **Vector quantities:** The physical quantities, which possess both magnitude and direction (which way), are called vectors. For example, displacement, velocity, acceleration, force, weight, momentum, etc.

To appreciate the difference between a scalar quantity and a vector quantity **(Table 8.1)**, suppose that an ambulance picks up a patient from a point "X" and travels along a path shown by the dashed curve and arrives at the hospital at point "P". The distance traveled by

SECTION 2: Biophysics

Table 8.1: Difference between a vector and scalar quantity.

	Vector	Scalar
Definition	A physical quantity with both the magnitude and direction	A physical quantity with only magnitude.
Representation	A number (magnitude), direction using unit cap or arrow at the top and unit	A number (magnitude) and unit
Symbol	Quantity symbol in bold and an arrow sign above	Quantity symbol
Direction	Yes	No
Example	Velocity and acceleration	Mass and temperature

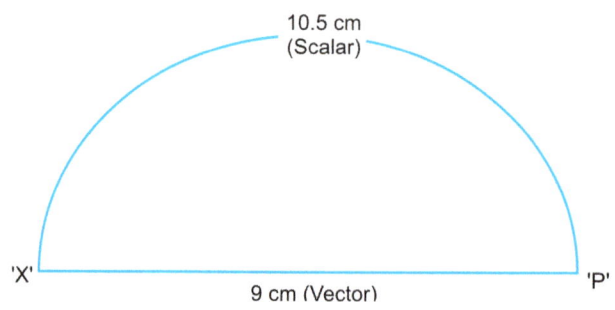

Fig. 8.1: Scalar and vector quantity.

the ambulance is the total length of the dashed line, irrespective of the direction in which it travels. The curved line "XP" is 10.5 cm long. This is the value of the distance covered by the ambulance. Note that, in this case, the direction along which the ambulance travels is not important. That is why we say that distance is a scalar quantity. It has magnitude but no direction. Further, as mentioned above displacement is the shortest distance between the initial and the final positions. Thus, in **Fig. 8.1**, the straight line "XP" (= 9 cm) represents the displacement and the direction of displacement is along "XP". Displacement, therefore, is a vector quantity and has magnitude as well as direction. From the knowledge of the distance covered by the vehicle, we may form an idea about the petrol consumed but we cannot locate the vehicle. For this we must know its displacement from a certain location.

Therefore, here total distance covered by ambulance is a scalar quantity and displacement of ambulance for 'X' place to 'P' is vector quantity.

▪ REST AND MOTION

There are two states of objects in physics i.e. Rest and motion. While traveling in a train, you find that your co-passenger is at rest but the viewer on ground tells that person is moving. The book in your hands is at rest if viewed from the room and is moving if viewed from moon. When we say an object is moving or is at rest… what exactly do we mean?

Motion is a combined property of the body under observation and observer. There is no meaning of rest and motion without a viewer. The viewer on ground is moving with respect to the train and train is moving with respect to that person. The moon is moving with respect to the book and the book is moving with respect to the moon.

From the above discussion, we can conclude if a body changes its position with respect to the viewer as time passes, it is said to be in motion and if it does not change its position, then it is at rest.

Motion is defined as "An act of change in position of an object with time with respect to some fixed position, which is taken as the reference point".

If an object or subject changes its position in reference to a fixed point with a time interval, it is said to be in motion. Basically, motion is a result of the force. One may experience several kinds of forces in day-to-day life to have motion. Such as muscular force causes blood circulation of the body or movement of lungs results in respiration. Gravitational forces contribute toward motion of fluids; therefore administration of nasogastric feed or intravenous fluids can be possible. Several other examples of motion like walking, exercise, lifting a load all the activities need some or other kind of force.

Types of Motion

In physics, motion is classified into various categories:
- **Translatory motion:** It is also called as linear motion. Motion in a straight path is named as translatory motion like walking.
- **Circular motion:** In a circular motion, the object just moves in a circle. The revolution of the earth around the sun, artificial satellites going around the Earth at a constant height. Movements of the magnetic fields around the body parts of the patient during Magnetic Resonance Imaging (MRI) or rotation of test tubes in a centrifuge are the another good examples for circular motion.
- **Rotational motion:** The object rotates about an axis, e.g., earth rotating on its own axis.
- **Oscillatory motion:** Something that oscillates moves back and forth. Anything that repeats the motion cycle after a certain period is considered to be oscillating. The pendulum of the clock oscillates about a point. In process of breathing, lungs move inside the chest in oscillatory manner. Similarly our intestines exhibit rhythmic motion as they move food towards its final destination.

Primarily the motion of objects can be studied under two separate headings:
- **Kinematics:** The study of the motion of the objects without taking into account the cause of their motion is called kinematics.
- **Dynamics:** The study of the motion of the objects by taking into account the cause(s) of their change of state is called dynamics. For example, gas molecules are always in causeless random motion, though their motion is not visible to the naked eye.

■ SPEED

Speed is a scalar quantity. Speed refers to the distance traveled by an object in a particular interval of time and is defined as a measure of distance covered in a time limit. In other words the time rate of covering the distance by a particle is called its speed. Consider the flow of blood inside our bodies. Its flowthrough capillaries is very slow, whereas, in larger vessels, it moves relatively rapidly. To quantify such observations, we define a physical parameter called speed as the rate of change of distance with time. Mathematically.

$$\text{Speed} = \frac{\text{Distance}}{\text{Time}}$$

The SI unit for speed is meter per second (ms^{-1}). The unit of speed is derived from the unit of length and unit of time. Speed indicates how fast a body is moving and does not specify the direction along which the body is moving.

VELOCITY

The physical parameter, which specifies how fast a body is moving and in which direction it is moving is called the velocity of the body. Thus, velocity is a vector quantity. The velocity of an object is the rate of change of its position with respect to a frame of reference, and is a function of time

Speed of the object in a particular direction. Mathematically, we write

$$\text{Velocity} = \frac{\text{Displament}}{\text{Time}}$$

The SI unit of velocity is the same as that of speed. But it is expressed with direction (because it is a vector quantity), for example, 50 ms^{-1} from A to B, or 50 ms^{-1} eastwards. Generally, in real-life situations, the direction is understood according to the situation and not expressed explicitly.

Types of Velocity

- **Uniform velocity:** An object is said to be moving with uniform velocity, if it undergoes equal displacements in equal intervals of time, however small these intervals of time may be.
- **Variable velocity:** An object is said to be moving with variable velocity, if either its speed or its direction of motion or both change with time.
- **Average velocity:** The ratio of total change in position or displacement to the total time taken is called average speed.
- **Instantaneous velocity:** The velocity of an object at a particular instant of time or at a particular point of its path is called the instantaneous velocity of the object.

ACCELERATION

Another useful physical parameter that specifies a change in velocity with time is called acceleration. It is defined as follows:

The rate of increase in speed is known as acceleration. In other words "the time rate of change of velocity of an object is called the acceleration of the object". The object is said to be moving with constant acceleration and such a motion is called uniformly accelerated motion.

The SI unit of acceleration is ms^{-2}. An example of accelerated motion is the flow of blood inside the human body, which circulates in different parts with different velocities. Acceleration, like velocity, is a vector quantity. Acceleration is regarded as positive if the velocity is increasing with time. A decreasing velocity refers to negative acceleration and it is usually called deceleration.

You can visualize the blood flow from arteries to the capillaries as deceleration and from capillaries to the heart as acceleration.

Types of Accelerations

Average acceleration: An object's average acceleration over a period of time is its change, divided by the duration of the period.

Instantaneous acceleration: Acceleration at a specific instant of time.

APPLICATIONS OF MOTION IN NURSING

With study of motion, nurses will be able to understand:

Motion during Walking

Walking is energy efficient. In a walking human, one leg swings forward while the other leg's foot stays planted on the ground. When walking at natural speed (defined below), the swinging leg uses muscle force to move forward and immediately relaxes, allowing the force of gravity to move it to the ground. Simultaneously, the planted leg moves forward with largely passive rotation at the hip. The plant leg only needs to stay straight and the swinging leg's knee only slightly bends to allow it to pass underneath the body. We have difficulty in walking on wet surface due to less friction and labored walking on sand which is having high friction.

So condition of floor and footwear of patient should be kept in mind while moving the patient and there should be enough friction for smooth walking and maintaining gait.

Motion Sickness

During the movement of body endolymph moves in inner ear and our balance is maintained by input from vision, nerves of the muscles and joints, and the vestibular system (inner ear) which is processed into meaningful information by the central vestibular system (brainstem). When movements are jerky and in rotational manner fluid moves in same direction due to inertia but the body is either stationary or moving in another direction so contradictory inputs from vision and vestibular system result in the sensations of dizziness, vertigo, or disequilibrium and this can be treated by medication or by Epley maneuver or Brandt-Daroff exercise.

Motion in Centrifuge Devices

A centrifuge is a metal rotor with holes to accommodate vessels of liquid, spun at selected speeds by a motor. Low-speed centrifuges generally operate at up to 10,000 revolutions per minute (rpm) and may be non-refrigerated or refrigerated. High-speed centrifuges generally operate at 10,000–30,000 rpm and some are refrigerated to cool the rotor chamber.

Centrifuges apply centrifugal (outward pushing) force to separate suspended particles from a liquid or to separate liquids of different densities. These liquids can include body fluids (e.g., blood, serum, urine), commercial reagents, or combinations of the two with other additives. By creating forces many times greater than gravity, centrifuges can greatly accelerate separations that occur naturally as a result of density differences. The applications includes study of viruses, proteins, nucleic acids, polymers and blood.

Motion and Orthostatic Hypotension

Normally, the gravitational stress of sudden standing causes 500 mL to 800 mL of blood to pool in the veins of the legs and trunk. That leads to a decrease in venous return which reduces cardiac output and thus BP. In the response to this fall in BP, baroreceptors in the aortic arch and carotid sinus activate autonomic reflexes to rapidly return the BP to normal. The sympathetic nervous system increases heart rate and contractility and increases the vasomotor tone of the capacitance vessels. Simultaneous parasympathetic (vagal) inhibition also increases heart rate. In most people, changes in BP and heart rate upon standing are minimal and transient, and symptoms do not occur. But nurses should be cautious in moving an old age person and the person who was on bed for long period, out of bed. Because they are prone to develop orthostatic hypotension. This should also be kept in mind while moving the patient through lifts.

Health implications of high velocity motion vehicles like airplanes and rockets where a person moving in a highly accelerated vehicle is known as acceleration stress.

Inertia in Accidents

According to law of inertia if a body is moving it remains in motion unless external force is applied, during accident body remains in speed even after vehicle stopped so due to this, a person remaining in vehicle without seat belt may have severe injuries hitting himself with body of the vehicle and due to jerk, there may be a fracture in the spine without external injury.

According to the definition, force is equal to the rate of change in momentum with time ($F = m \times v/t$) showing that if time is reduced then force will be increased. Using this principle karate player can break tiles with a high speed hand and if during accident, time of collision is less, then injury will be severe even with a light vehicle. So for assessment during road traffic accident special precaution should be given to spine and head.

QUESTIONS

Q.1: Discuss the types of motion.
Q.2: Explain the application of principles of the motion in nursing.
Q.3: A fast moving wheelchair on which a patient is sitting should not be stopped suddenly, discuss.

BIBLIOGRAPHY

1. Bowen R. Gastrointestinal Transit: How Long Does It Take? Colorado State University, 2006.
2. David H, George H, Keith B. "Velocity and Drag Forces on motor-protein-driven Vesicles in Cells". American Physical Society, the 69th Annual Meeting of the Southeastern, 2002.
3. Fischer M, Franzeck UK, Herrig I. "Flow velocity of single lymphatic capillaries in human skin". Am J Physiol Heart Circ Physiology, 1996; 270.
4. Hubble E. "A Relation between Distance and Radial Velocity among Extra-Galactic Nebulae" Proceedings of the National Academy of Sciences of the United States of America, 1929;15 (3), 1929: 168-73.
5. Kogut A, Lineweaver C, Smoot GF, et al. Dipole Anisotropy in the COBE Differential Microwave Radiometers First- Year Sky Maps. Astrophysical Journal, 1993; 419: 1.
6. Meschede M, Udo Barckhausen U. (November 20, 2000). "Plate Tectonic Evolution of the Cocos-Nazca Spreading Center". Proceedings of the Ocean Drilling Program. Texas A and M University. http://www-odp.tamu.edu/ publications/170_SR/chap_07/chap_07. htm Retrieved, 2007: 04-02.
7. Nave R. Motion HyperPhysics. Georgia State University, 2005.
8. Newton's . "Axioms or Laws of Motion" can be found in the "Principia" volume-1, 1729: 19.
9. Penny P. Hemodynamic: Blood Velocity, 2003.
10. Safkan Y. "The term 'absolute motion' has no meaning, then why do we say that the earth moves around the sun and not vice versa?" Ask the Experts. Physics Link, 2007.
11. Tyson DG, Liu NC, Irion R. One Universe: At home in the cosmos. Joseph Henry Press, 2000.
12. Wahlin L. "THE DEADBEAT UNIVERSE". Chapter 9. Colutron Research Corporation, 1997.
13. Kiseleva TA, Klochkov YV, Nikolaev AP. Comparison of scalar and vector FEM forms in the case of an elliptic cylinder. Comput. Math. and Math. Phys. 2015;55:422–31. https://doi.org/10.1134/S0965542515030094

CHAPTER 9

Gravity

Suresh K Sharma, Navjot Kaur

Chapter Outline
- Specific Gravity
- Center of Gravity
- Principles of Gravity
- Mass and Weight
- Effects of Gravitational Forces on Human Body and Applications of Principles of Gravity in Nursing

INTRODUCTION

Gravity is defined as the accelerating tendency of the bodies toward the center of the earth or towards the center of the other heavenly bodies, such as the moon. Gravity is very important to us. We could not live on Earth without it. The sun's gravity keeps Earth in orbit around it, keeping us at a comfortable distance to enjoy the sun's light and warmth. It holds down our atmosphere and the air we need to breathe. Gravity is what holds our world together. Gravitation is the force with which all bodies in the universe attract one another. According to Newton's law of universal gravitation, the gravitational force between any two bodies in the universe is proportional to the product of their masses and inversely proportional to the square of the distance between them.

$$F = \frac{G M_1 M_2}{d^2}$$

Where,
F = gravitational force
M_1 and M_2 = any two masses in the universe
d = distance between two masses
G = universal gravitational constant = 6.67×10^{-11} Nm^2/Kg^2

SPECIFIC GRAVITY

Specific gravity is the ratio of the density of any substance to that of water at a specified temperature. It is also known as relative density and clinically expressed as specific gravity. Specific gravity actually signifies how many times lighter or heavier a substance is than an equal volume of water.

$$\text{Specific density} = \frac{\text{Density of the object}}{\text{Density of the water}}$$

It is common to use the density of water at 4 °C as a reference point, as water at this point has the highest density of 1000 kg/m³. The specific gravity of a substance is expressed numerically by the values of its density in grams per cubic centimeter (gm/cm³), but with the unit omitted. For example, the specific gravity of a substance 'A' with a density of 5 gm/cm³ will be 5. It means the substance is five times heavier than water under the same circumstances.

It is clear that specific gravity depends on the density of the substance; for example, if urine is concentrated and has more salts dissolved, will likely have higher specific gravity and if urine is less concentrated then specific gravity will be likely to be lower (Normal specific gravity of urine is 1.010–1.030). Similarly, the specific gravity of blood ranges between 1.055 and 1.066; blood with higher plasma proportion in comparison to blood cells will have lower specific gravity.

As we have learned that specific gravity is the ratio of the density of any substance to that of water. So to determine the specific gravity of a solid substance when weight the substance in air and then water **(Table 9.1)**. The difference between the two weights gives the apparent loss of weight in water. The apparent loss of weight is equal to the weight of water displaced. Therefore, in physical properties, specific gravity can also be estimated by the following formula.

$$\text{Specific gravity} = \frac{\text{Weight of the object in air}}{\text{Weight of equal volume of water}}$$

■ CENTER OF GRAVITY

The center of gravity is considered to be the point at which all external forces are applied to an object. If an object is suspended from this point, it will remain in balance without turning whatever its position is.

In general, the center of gravity or center of mass of a body is the point at which all the mass is considered to be centered.

When a person is standing, her/his center of gravity is located in the pelvic cavity. A line drawn perpendicularly downwards from the center of gravity of a person passes through the

Table 9.1: Specific gravity of some substances.

Substance	Density (kg/m²)	Relative density/Specific gravity
Pure water	1000	1.00
Alcohol	790	0.79
Whole blood	1060	1.06
Blood plasma	1030	1.03
Aluminum	2700	2.70
Platinum	21400	21.40
Lead	11400	11.40
Gold	19300	19.30
Iron	7950	7.90
Mercury	13550	11.55

CHAPTER 9: Gravity

Center of gravity

Fig. 9.1: Center of gravity in a person standing.

Center of gravity

Fig. 9.2: Center of gravity in a person using crutches.

area bounded by her/his feet **(Fig. 9.1)**. It is for this reason that while carrying a heavy object, balance is obtained easily if the feet are placed farther apart.

In nursing practice, it is often necessary for a nurse to carry heavy objects close to the body, so that the center of gravity does not deviate and does not put extra strain on the body. For example, carrying a large water basin in hands away from the body will put extra strain on back muscles since a heavy object in the hands adds weight to the front of the body, the center of gravity shifts forward; in order to keep the normal position and maintain equilibrium, muscles of the back exert a backward pull. To minimize this strain, one should keep the object in hand as close to the body as possible, i.e. as close to the center of gravity as possible.

For Example

- In folding a blanket, the arms should be held relaxed at the side of the body and forearms should be flexed because outstretched extremities increase the distance through which the force act on the center of rotation at the shoulder.
- During the use of crutches, the area bounded by the crutches and the uninjured foot becomes the base through which the vertical line through its center of mass must pass. These supports must be kept far enough apart so that the vertical line always passes through the base area, otherwise, the patient may fall **(Fig. 9.2)**.

■ MASS AND WEIGHT

Although commonly we use the terms mass and weight in the same sense, the two terms have different meanings in physics. In physics concepts of mass and weight are different. The mass of a body is the quantity of matter contained in it. Everything we see around us has mass. For example, a table, a chair, your bed, a football, a glass, and even air has mass. That being said, all objects are light or heavy because of their mass.

The SI unit of mass is the kilogram (kg). The formula of mass can be written as:

$$\text{Mass} = \text{Density} \times \text{Volume}$$

On the other hand, weight is defined as the gravitational force with which a body is pulled towards the center of the earth.

Mathematically, we write

$$W = mg$$

where 'W' denotes the weight of the body, 'm' is its mass and 'g' is the acceleration due to gravity.

Since the value of the acceleration due to gravity varies with the distance of an object from the center of the earth, the weight of the object changes with its position on the earth. For example, an object at sea level weighs more than it does on a high mountain because the value of the acceleration due to the gravity of the earth on the object is greater at sea level. The mass, however, remains the same everywhere.

The mass of an object is measured by a physical balance, whereas its weight is measured by a spring balance.

Mass is a scalar quantity while weight is a vector quantity because it is directed toward the center of the earth.

The mass of a person is the same on the earth as well as on the moon, but the weight of the person is different in these two places because their pulls on the person are different. A person weighs six times more on earth than on the moon.

Whereas mass and weight have the same numerical value, it is important in solving problems to indicate the unit specifically, as one of force (weight) or as one of mass.

One gram (gm) is a unit of mass.

One gram weight is unit of weight.

	Mass	Weight
Definition	Mass is defined as the amount of matter in a substance	Weight is defined as the amount of force acting on the mass of an object because of acceleration due to gravity.
Denotation	Mass is represented by "M."	Weight is represented by "W."
Formula	• Mass is always constant for a body. • One way to calculate mass: Mass = density × volume.	• Weight is the measure of the gravitational force acting on a mass. • Formula of weight: Weight = mass × acceleration due to gravity
Unit of measurement	The SI unit of mass is "kilogram".	The SI unit of weight is Newton (N).
Quantity type	• Mass is a base quantity. • Mass only has magnitude and hence, it is a scalar quantity	• Weight is a derived quantity. • Weight has both magnitude and direction (toward the center of gravity) and hence, it is a vector quantity.
Measuring instrument	Mass can be easily measured using any ordinary balance. For example, beam balance, lever balance, pan balance, etc.	Weight can be measured by a spring balance or by using its formula given above.

■ PRINCIPLES OF GRAVITY

The most important principle of gravity is Archimedes' Principle. Archimedes, a Greek mathematician gave Archimedes' Principle.

It is a common experience for all of us that while standing in water, we feel as if we are being pushed upwards by force acting from below. Similarly, balloons filled with a gas, say hydrogen, rise in the atmosphere on their own. In fact, all bodies experience an upward force when held inside a fluid.

The force of thrust is opposite to the force of gravity. When pressure is put on any fluid, the body is submerged in it, and this force is thrust. The force reduces as it goes down because of gravity and thus the body feels light. Swimming is an example of this concept.

$$\text{Thrust} = \text{Pressure} \times \text{Area}$$

"The tendency of a fluid to exert an upward force on an object immersed in it is called buoyancy. The upward force acting on the object is known as the buoyancy force."

The upthrust due to buoyancy results in an apparent loss in the weight of the body **(Fig. 9.3)**.

You can see its manifestation if you draw water from a well using a bucket-rope arrangement. As soon as the bucket comes out of the water, it suddenly feels heavier.

We know that when a body is immersed in a fluid, it displaces some amount of fluid. If we imagine that the space occupied by the body is replaced by the fluid, then the center of gravity of this fluid is called the center of buoyancy. The upthrust on a body acts through the center of buoyancy. If a body of uniform density is submerged fully in a fluid, then its center of gravity coincides with the center of buoyancy. The quantitative measure of buoyant force is given by Archimedes' principle.

Archimedes' principle may be stated as follows:

"When a body is wholly or partially immersed in a fluid, it experiences an upward thrust, which is equal to the weight of the fluid displaced."

Fig. 9.3: Buoyant force.

Fig. 9.4: Archimedes' Principle.

This principle can also be stated as follows:
- When a body is wholly or partially immersed in a fluid, it experiences an apparent loss in its weight (due to upward thrust), which is equal to the weight of the fluid displaced by it **(Fig. 9.4)**.
- Sometimes this principle is also known as the principle of buoyancy. Archimedes' principle can be used to determine the specific gravity of a solid substance.

APPLICATIONS OF ARCHIMEDES' PRINCIPLE

- Submarine – Ballast tank inside the submarine makes the weight of the submarine greater than the buoyant force.
- Hot air balloon – The buoyant force of a balloon is less than the surrounding air by varying the quantity of hot air in the balloon
  - A hydrometer, used for measuring the specific gravity of liquids operates on this principle.
  - Urinometer also works on the same principle.
  - Underwater exercises, where patients with joint or muscular problems can be facilitated for exercise, where they feel easy to perform exercises in water due to buoyancy forces **(Fig. 9.5)**.

Fig. 9.5: Exercise in and out of water.

EFFECTS OF GRAVITATIONAL FORCES ON THE HUMAN BODY AND APPLICATION OF PRINCIPLES OF GRAVITY IN NURSING

Diagnosis using principles of gravity
- The erythrocyte sedimentation (ESR) is based on gravity only. In this test, the sedimentation rate is measured by the depth of surface between the clear plasma and the cells in a test tube for over an hour. The faster this happens, the higher the ESR and there may be more inflammation in the body because during inflammation there may be more protein in RBCs or they may clump together due to surface proteins and become heavier as a result more gravitational force is applied to make them settle fast.
- Haemoglobin screening is done during blood donation using an appropriately standardized $CuSO_4$ solution having a specific gravity of 1.053 based on gravitation force. If the drop of blood float on the surface it is assumed the person is having Hb level below 12 g/dl so he or she is not fit for blood donation. This is very useful during blood donation camps.
- A urine-specific gravity test compares the density of urine to the density of water by using principles of gravity. This quick test can help determine how well kidneys are diluting or concentrate the urine.

Position of the patient according to principles of gravity
- Brain surgery is frequently done with the patient in a sitting or semi-sitting position to lessen the danger of haemorrhage.
- After a rib resection, the patient is kept in a semi-sitting position to increase drainage from the thorax through the drainage tube by gravity.
- When a patient who is under the effect of anesthesia or an unconscious patient, his or her head is placed on one side, then tongue and oral secretions drop down due to gravity that makes a larger passageway for air to enter and respiration will improve.
- A dependent position with legs dragged on one side of beds, for a patient with congestive cardiac failure, it accumulate excess fluid in legs and facilitate breathing (also achieved through gravity).
- Oscillating beds are used to change the positions to facilitate the circulation of blood and lymph is achieved with gravity.
- Post radical mastectomy affected sidearm is kept in a high position, so that with gravity lymph can be drained effectively and swelling on the arm can be prevented.

Fluid movement due to gravity
- Infusion of intravenous fluid, blood transfusion, nasogastric tube feeding, irrigation of body cavities, urinary drainage, or drainages from other body cavities cannot be imagined without principles of gravity.
- Without gravity, there would be no pressure in the liquid. So we cannot give intravenous infusion or blood transfusion in the absence of gravity **(Fig. 9.6)**.
- Blood circulation in the body mainly depends on gravity. Changes in body position alter the pressure of blood in different parts of the body. If a person faints, his head should be lowered. This helps the blood to return to the head (by gravity).
- A person standing for a long period of time may have edema of the legs **(Fig. 9.7)**. Gravity exercises are sometimes prescribed for patients with circulatory disorders of the lower extremities.
- During thoracentesis, Paracentesis, the peritoneal dialysis fluid is drained with principles of gravity.
- Postural drainage after the chest physiotherapy is also based on gravity only.

Fig. 9.6: IV fluid administration with gravity.

Fig. 9.7: Edema due to gravity.

Stability and gravity

Body alignment is achieved by placing one body part in line with another body part in a vertical or horizontal line. Correct alignment contributes to body balance and decreases strain on muscle-skeletal structures. Without this balance, the risk of falls and injuries increases. In the language of body mechanics, the **center of gravity** is the center of the weight of an object or person. A lower center of gravity increases stability. This can be achieved by bending the knees and bringing the center of gravity closer to the base of support, keeping the back straight. A wide base of support is the foundation for stability. A wide **base of support** is achieved by placing feet a comfortable, shoulder-width distance apart. When a vertical line falls from the center of gravity through the wide base of support, **body balance** is achieved. If the vertical line moves outside the base of support, the body will lose balance.

- Persons with obesity may have a greater risk of falling while walking or running because some timeline of gravity may fall out base of support, so we should be careful while moving the obese patient.
- Chronic low back pain may be due to having the center of gravity located excessively towards the back caused by decreased low back strength and decreased amount of normal low back curve. If center of gravity is too far, a black person might have strength and balance challenges to overcome in order to re-establish postural control. So the right posture should be maintained during the working and shifting of patients.

Patient handling and gravity

Principles of body mechanics should be applied properly during all patient-handling activities.

- Assess the weight of the load before lifting and determine if assistance is required. Plan the move; gather all supplies and clear the area of obstacles. Avoid stretching, reaching, and twisting, which may place the line of gravity outside the base of support.

- Tighten abdominal, gluteal, and leg muscles in anticipation of the move.
- Stand up straight to protect the back and provide balance.
- Place the weight of the object being moved close to your center of gravity for balance. Equilibrium is maintained as long as the line of gravity passes through its base of support.
- Facing the direction prevents abnormal twisting of the spine. Turning, rolling, pivoting, and leveraging requires less work than lifting.
- Do not lift if possible; use mechanical lifts as required.
- Encourage the patient to help as much as possible.
- Keep all work at waist level to avoid stooping. Do not bend at the waist.
- Reduce friction between surfaces so that less force is required to move the patient. Bending the knees maintain your center of gravity and let the strong muscles of your legs do the lifting.
- It is easier to push an object than to pull it.
- Less energy is required to keep an object moving than it is to stop and start it.
- Use assistive devices (gait belt, slider boards, mechanical lifts) as required to position patients and transfer them from one surface to another.
- The person with the heaviest load should coordinate all the effort of the others involved in the handling technique.

A new horizon of gravity used in medical treatment:
Neural plasticity, the ability of the brain to learn from experience and to adapt to new environments is recognized to be profound and exposure to altered gravity has an effect on communication sites between the sensory cells and the nerve fibers ending on them. This could lead to the assumption that similar exposure to a force greater than 1G on a centrifuge on earth might one day prove useful in restoring a sense of balance to disabled people who have lost it. There are cases of children with medical disorders, such as autism, attention deficit disorders, fragile X etc.

A newborn baby whose brain is damaged at birth, like in the case of cerebral palsy, may require hypergravity, a higher intensity of gravity stimulus, before a child's brain becomes programed to respond to direction and acceleration and eventually learn to walk. Increasing gravity could modify or alter his perception of it prior to responding, by triggering gravity sensors and the brain blood flow. This would mean that rehabilitation exercises in children with cerebral palsy should be more effective if done in the upright position in a way that the body may experience some load, even if the child had to be supported by a harness. Alternately, the movement therapy could be done on a centrifuge.

■ QUESTIONS

Q.1: The point where the whole weight of the body may be supposed to act is called as.....................
Q.2: Hydrometer works on the principle of …………..
Q.3: Back should be kept upright while carrying a tray; why explain?
Q.4: What is the principle of lactometer in measuring specific gravity of milk?
Q.5: What do you understand by the terms specific gravity, density and center of gravity/mass? How does the presence of gravitational force affects the human body?
Q.6: Why should the principles of center of gravity be considered before undertaking any strenuous activity.
Q.7: What role does the center of gravity have to play in a normal upright person carrying a large basin of water and a person with crutches, explain?

BIBLIOGRAPHY

1. ASBC Methods of Analysis Preface to Table 1: Extract in Wort and Beer, American Society of Brewing Chemists, St Paul, 2009.
2. Dana ES. A Textbook of Mineralogy: With an Extended Treatise on Crystallography. New York, London (Chapman Hall): John Wiley and Sons, 1992.
3. Fox RW, McDonald AT. Introduction to Fluid Mechanics (4th edn). Wiley, 2003.
4. Hough JS, Briggs DE, Stevens R, et al. Malting and Brewing Science, Vol. II, Hopped Wort and Beer, Chapman and Hall, London, 1991.
5. Munson BR, Young DF, Okishi TH. Fundamentals of Fluid Mechanics (4th edn.). Wiley, 2001.
6. Schetz JA, Fuh E. Fundamentals of Fluid Mechanics. Wiley, John and Sons, Incorporated, 1999.
7. Atomi Y. Gravitational Effects on Human Physiology. Subcell Biochem. 2015;72:627-59. doi: 10.1007/978-94-017-9918-8_29. PMID: 26174402.

CHAPTER 10

Force, Energy and Work

Suresh K Sharma, Navjot Kaur

Chapter Outline

- Force
- Newton's Law of Motion
- Forces in the Circular Motion
- Work
- Energy
- Types and Transformation of Energy
- Energy in the Body
- Power
- Principles of Machines
- Efficiency and Mechanical Advantage of a Machine
- Principles of Friction
- Body Mechanics
- Simple Machine
- Lever
- Pulley
- Traction
- Inclined Plane
- Screw
- Application of Principles of gravity in Nursing

FORCE

We all have a basic understanding of force from everyday experience. An object (such as a drug trolley) at rest cannot change its position unless it is pushed or pulled. You exert a force on a ball when you throw or kick it. We have to push the drug into the syringe while giving the injection. Similarly, a car or a train moving at a constant speed cannot be stopped unless brakes are applied. In these examples, the word force is associated with muscular activity and some change in the velocity of an object. You should realize that a force is applied through the brakes in a direction opposite to the motion. These examples lead us to define force as:

"Force changes the state of rest or of uniform motion of a body".

There are three defining characteristics of force:
- It starts with an interaction between two or more physical objects (which could include the air)
- The interaction causes a push or pull to occur between the objects
- The resulting push or pull has a direction associated with it

Forces do not always cause motion, however. For example, as you sit reading this book, a gravitational force acts on your body, and yet you are stationary. As a second example, you can push (i.e., exert a force) on a large wall and not be able to move it.

A force produces acceleration in its direction. If several forces are acting on an object, the object accelerates only if the net force acting on it is not zero. Net force or resultant force is the vector sum of all the forces acting on the object. If the net force on a body is zero, then its acceleration will be zero, and it remains either at rest or moving at a constant velocity. A body is said to be in equilibrium when its velocity is constant (zero acceleration) or it is at rest.

So far we have considered only examples where one force was acting on the body, but often several forces act on the same body. Traction is an example of several forces on muscles. When a block is moving on a horizontal surface under the action of some external force, four forces are acting on it: External force (responsible for the motion of the block), the contact force of the surface, frictional, force, and gravitational force of the earth. Similarly, you can easily visualize various forces acting on a flying airplane:
- Force of gravity
- The force of air on the wings and body of the plane
- The force is associated with engine thrust.

■ UNITS OF MEASUREMENT

The SI unit of force is Newton (N). A force of 1N applied to a mass of 1 kilogram produces an acceleration of 1 m/s^2. Force is a vector quantity. To describe a force, we must specify three things its magnitude, its direction, and its point of application.

■ NEWTON'S LAW OF MOTION

Facts related to the motion were first enunciated by Sir Isaac Newton in the form of his famous laws of motion. In 1687, Newton introduced the three laws in his book "Philosophiae Naturalis Principia Mathematica" (Mathematical Principles of Natural Philosophy), which is generally referred to as the "Principia." This is where he also introduced his theory of universal gravitation, thus laying the entire foundation of classical mechanics in one volume.

Newton's First Law

Stated in Newton's words, the first law of motion is:

"*Everybody continues in its state of rest or of uniform motion in a straight line unless it is compelled to change that state by forces impressed upon it*." This is sometimes called the Law of Inertia, or just inertia. Essentially, it makes the following two points:
- An object that is not moving will not move until a force acts upon it.
- An object that is in motion will not change velocity (or stop) until a force acts upon it.

We come across numerous illustrations of the first law in our daily lives. Some such situations are discussed below:
- Sitting loosely or standing on a bus, we experience a backward jerk when the bus suddenly starts. This is because the lower part of the body moves forward with the bus, whereas the upper part tends to remain at rest.
- While handling the wheelchair, both starting and stopping should be gradual. If the wheelchair suddenly gets into motion, the patient's head may be thrown back, causing an injury. Likewise, if a moving wheelchair is suddenly stopped, the patient may fall forward to the ground.
- A bed at rest has a tendency to stay at rest. We need to apply a large force to move it and when it is set into motion, it continues to be in motion. Force of friction opposes the motion, and

so it requires some force (which is less than the force needed to start or stop the motion) to keep it moving. We thus conclude that, due to the inertia of motion, it is easier to keep the bed moving, then to start and stop suddenly.

❖ You may have seen a person fall on the road while getting down from a moving bus. This is because the lower part of the body comes to rest suddenly, while the upper part tends to continue in a state of motion. So to avoid falls, it is advisable to run for a while with the vehicle.

❖ Consider a stationary car that is struck from behind by another vehicle. The forces act through the seat, and move the trunk of the driver ahead. But, the inertia of the driver's head causes it to stay in place in the position of rest. Such accidents cause severe stretching of the neck. This can lead to injury of the neck in the cervical region of the spine. To reduce the impact of the collision, seat belts are provided in automobiles.
  • Apart from inertia, another aspect of the first law is force. Since a body cannot change its state of rest or of uniform motion unless an external force acts on it, we can define force with the help of this law as:
  • "Force is an external cause which changes or tends to change the state of rest or the state of uniform motion of a body".
  • A force can change the speed of the body, direction of motion of the body, or shape of the body. That is, force produces acceleration in the body on which it acts. When a force is applied to a stationary body, it starts moving. Its initial velocity was zero; the force produced acceleration in the body, making it move faster.

Newton's Second Law

Imagine performing an experiment in which you push a book across a frictionless table. When you exert some horizontal force 'F' on the book, it moves with some acceleration 'a'. If you apply a force twice as great, you find that the acceleration of the book doubles. If you increase the applied force to 3F, the acceleration triples, and so on.

From such observations, we conclude that the acceleration of an object is directly proportional to the force acting on it.

The acceleration of an object also depends on its mass, as stated in the preceding section. We can understand this from the previous thought experiment. If you apply a force 'F' to a book on a frictionless table, the book undergoes some acceleration 'a'. If the mass of the book is doubled, the same applied force produces acceleration $a/2$. If the mass is tripled, the same applied force produces acceleration $a/3$.

If you are struck by a fast-moving cricket ball, you get injured. However, a flower moving with same velocity as of cricket ball and hit you, it will not cause injury or pain. Similarly, if the ball is moving slowly, the injury will be less serious. This suggests that an impact made by an object depends on two things: it's mass and velocity. So, Newton felt the necessity of defining a quantity called linear momentum (p) as the product of mass and velocity. Mathematically, we can write

$$p = mv$$

Linear momentum, 'p' is a vector quantity in the direction of velocity. The above equation mathematically can be restated as follows:

$$F = ma$$

where 'F' is the net force acting on the body, 'm' is its mass, and 'a' is the acceleration in the direction of the net force.

According to Newton, the second law of motion is:
"The magnitude of the resultant force acting on a body is proportional to the product of the mass of the body and its acceleration. The direction of the force is the same as that of the acceleration".

The acceleration produced in a body by a force depends on the mass of the body. For example, if the same force is applied to two beds one empty and another with a patient, the empty bed is lighter and moves faster than a loaded bed. In other words, if equal forces are applied to two objects; one with a smaller mass and another larger mass, more acceleration is acquired by an object having a smaller mass. A larger force must be applied to the loaded bed for it to have the same acceleration.

So, Newton's first law of motion enables us to define inertia and the second law gives us a quantitative measure of force. In simple words, Newton's first law explains what happens to an object when no forces act on it. It either remains at rest or moves in a straight line with constant speed. Newton's second law answers the question of what happens to an object that has a non-zero resultant force acting on it.

You now know that forces cause a change in the motion of a body. But how do we exert a force on this body? Inevitably, there is an agent who makes it possible. Very often, your feet (while playing football) or hands (while playing volleyball) are the agents. That is, forces arise from interactions between systems. This information is contained in the third law of motion.

Newton's Third Law

Stated in Newton's words, the third law of motion is as follows:
"To every action, there is always an equal and opposite reaction".

An important consequence of this law is that forces always appear in pairs; a single isolated force never exists. The action and reaction forces act on different objects and must be of the same type.

If two objects interact, the force F_{12} exerted by object 1 on object 2 is equal in magnitude and opposite in direction to the force F_{21} exerted by object 2 on object 1:

$$F_{12} = F_{21}$$

Remember, the two forces in an action-reaction pair always act on two different objects.

To elaborate on the third law of motion, let us consider a book kept on a table. The book exerts a force, equal to its weight, on the table. But if this were the only force, the book would have gone through the table. Since it does not happen, the motion of the book (due to the force of its own weight) must have been resisted by an equal and opposite force exerted on it in the upward direction by the table.

Similarly, the weight of the body of a patient lying in bed pushes against the mattress. In turn, the mattress pushes him upwards. The third law helps us understand why patients in bed for a long period of time, develop bedsores. This is because the heavier parts of the body (bony parts) press more firmly against the mattress than do the lighter portions and, in turn, receive a greater reaction force. The reaction force interferes with the normal circulation of blood to the tissues and causes pressure sores.

Frictional Force

Frictional force refers to the force generated by two surfaces that contact and slide against each other. These forces are mainly affected by the surface texture and quantity of force requiring them together. The angle and position of the object affect the volume of frictional force. When an object is in motion either on a surface or in a viscous medium such as water or air, there is resistance to motion because the object interacts with its surroundings. This resistance is called the force of friction. If an object is placed against an object, then the frictional force will be the same as the weight of the object. If an object is pushed against the surface, then the frictional force will be increased and become extra than the weight of the object. The friction force is an important part of our day-to-day life activities. We cannot move, if there were no friction. However, it is undesirable in machines.

Experiments show that the friction forces come into existence from the nature of the two surfaces, because of their roughness, contact is made only at a few points of the surface where peaks of the material. The detailed analysis of friction is quite complex at the atomic level, frictional force ultimately involves an electrical interaction between atoms or molecules.

To move joints in our body, we have to overcome friction. If frictional forces become large, some diseases of joints develop. Similarly, friction can cause bedsores in a patient, particularly when he/ she is confined to bed for a long period. The synovial fluid in the joints acts as a lubricant which reduces frictional force. Similarly, saliva lubricates the mouth. Most of the large organs in the human body are in constant motion. The heart, lungs, and intestines have a rhythmic motion. In all these organs, a slippery mucous covering minimizes the friction. Further, while inserting gastric tubes, rectal tubes, and catheter, you might have used one or the other lubricant to minimize irritation of the membranes inside the body caused due to friction.

■ PRINCIPLES OF FRICTION

- Friction is the force that opposes the movement of one body over the surface of another body. The heat produced by friction is known as internal energy. Friction may be both advantageous and disadvantageous depending on the desired therapeutic effect.
- When two solid objects, slip over each other, the frictional force is called kinetic friction. When two objects do not slip over each other, the frictional force is called static friction.
- In hospitals and nursing homes, a useful safety measure is to block off areas of flooring being scrubbed and dry the floors carefully before they are walked on.
- Friction is necessary for striking a matching effect. Without friction, screws and nails would not hold wood together. Rubber tips at the bottom of crutches provide sufficient friction to keep the crutches from slipping.
- Friction may sometimes be disadvantageous. Rubber tubes such as gastric and duodenal tubes, catheters, and renal tubes may irritate the membranes over which they pass unless measures are taken to prevent friction. Therefore, the lubricant is used to minimize friction.
- Medication in tablet or capsule form is generally administered with water to prevent friction between the outer surface of the medication and the tissues of the mouth and throat.
- Frictional forces are reduced by serous fluids wherever motion occurs in the body. For example, synovial fluid in the joints and the serous fluid between the layers of the pleura, pericardium, and peritoneum. Fluid friction is a term applied to the friction of solids passing through fluids such as the blood cells through the blood.

Gravitational Force

Another very common force is the gravitational force, which the earth exerts on all bodies. The gravitational force is a force that attracts any two objects with mass. We call the gravitational force attractive because it always tries to pull masses together, it never pushes them apart. In fact, every object, including us, is pulling on every other object in the entire universe. This is called Newton's universal law of gravitation. In fact, the weight of a body is actually the force of gravitational attraction between the body and the earth. During a blood transfusion, blood gets from the hanging bag to the patient's body because of the gravitational force. The gravitational force on the skeleton contributes to healthy bones.

■ FORCES IN THE CIRCULAR MOTION

Uniform Circular Motion

The movement of a body following a circular path is called a circular motion. Now, the motion of a body moving with constant speed along a circular path is called uniform circular motion. Here, the speed is constant, but the velocity changes. You know that no force acts on a body (along the direction of motion) moving with uniform velocity along a straight line. Now consider the motion of a planet around the sun. The planet Jupiter, 300 times more massive than Earth, circles the sun at a speed of 13 km per second. Similarly, we may imagine the rotation of wheels in machinery or a merry-go-round. These are examples of circular motion. The question is: What happens to the direction of motion in such cases? The direction of motion of a body in circular motion changes continuously. Thus, a body in uniform circular motion has the variable velocity as direction is changing continuously. In other words, uniform circular motion is an example of accelerated motion. Mainly there are two forces namely centripetal and centrifugal forces, which give rise to circular motion, as detailed below:

Centripetal Force

When an object is moving in a circular path with constant speed, a constant force acts on the object. This force acts along a direction perpendicular to the direction of motion. (This is because any component in the direction of motion would also produce a change in the speed of the object and the motion will not be uniform.) The force responsible for the constant acceleration directed towards the center of the circle is called the centripetal force **(Fig. 10.1)**. You may recall playing with a top (lattu). You must have seen a cyclist turning a corner. He inclines his body

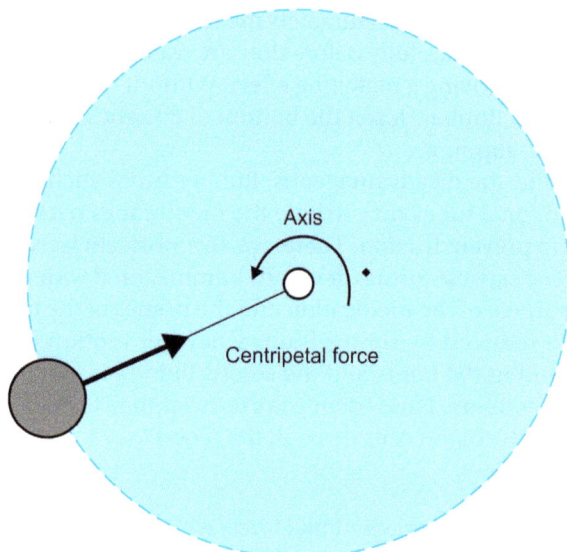

Fig. 10.1: Centripetal force.

towards the center of the curved path. By doing this, he gets the required centripetal force and ensures safety around a curve. Similarly, a racing track for motor cars is constructed in such a way that it banks inwards and provides the centripetal force.

Centrifugal Force

Tie a stone to a piece of a string and move it along a circular path around your hand. The stone moves with a constant speed along a circle. Velocity is changing because of the direction of motion is changing continuously. Hence, it is accelerated motion. Thus, a force must be acting on it. This is the force of the string pulling the stone inward. It is called the centripetal force.

Now, according to Newton's third law of motion, for every action on one body, there arises a force of reaction which is equal in magnitude but opposite in direction. In the case of uniform circular motion, a centripetal force acts on the revolving body (stone) and is directed towards the center. An equal and opposite force of reaction keeps the stone from falling inwards. This force is directed away from the center and is known as centrifugal force. If the string breaks, there will be no centripetal or centrifugal force acting on the stone or the hand respectively, and the stone would follow a straight-line path, which is tangent to the circle at the instant of time.

The centripetal force causes a body to move in a circular path of the constant radius by constantly pulling it toward the center which it describes. Since the speed is constant, this force changes only the direction of motion. The body pulls outward against this change in motion with a force called centrifugal force **(Fig. 10.2)**.

You come across a variety of situations or must have seen a variety of machines which involves circular motion and the concept of centripetal and centrifugal forces. We discuss some of them in the following:

- In the laundry, wet laundry is dried by spinning the cylinders at high speeds, which causes the drops of water to fly in front.
- In a circus, motorcyclist in death well makes use of centrifugal force to avoid fall.

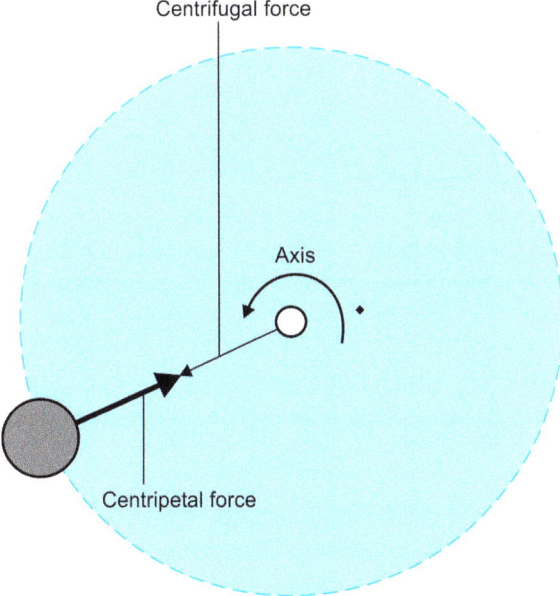

Fig. 10.2: Centrifugal force.

- When a nurse shakes down a thermometer in a circular path, she causes the heaving substance mercury to be thrown, to the bottom.
- In a chemical lab, a centrifuge is used to separate chemicals in a solution. An ultracentrifuge enables us to determine the molecular weight of large macromolecules.
- Further, you know that blood is a mixture of particles (cells, protein molecules, water molecules, etc.) of various weights and sizes. If a blood sample is placed in a centrifuge and rotated at high speeds, it separates into layers containing particles of different densities. The particles of maximum density form a layer in the bottom of the test tube (outer region of the circular path) whereas those of minimum density moves towards the top (the mouth of the tube).

WORK

When a force acts upon an object to cause a displacement of the object, it is said that work was done upon the object. There are three key ingredients to workforce, displacement, and cause. In order for a force to qualify as having done work on an object, there must be a displacement and the force must cause the displacement. In other words, work is done by a force when its point of application moves in the direction of the force. When the point of application moves against the direction of the force, work is said to be done against the force. For example, a nurse lifting a baby from the crib does some work against gravity. Similarly, work is done in shifting a patient from bed to trolley or wheelchair. Even while giving intramuscular (IM) or intravenous (IV) injection, work is done on the piston of the syringe. An important point to note here, from a physics point of view, if the point of application does not move, no work is done. Thus, in the language of physics, no work is done if you just hold a baby in your arms.

Measurement of Work

To obtain a quantitative measure of work, we define work done as follows:

The work done by a "force" is measured by the product of the force, another displacement of the point of application in the direction of the force.

Mathematically, we write

$$W = F \cdot d$$

where,
W = work done
F = force applied in the direction of motion
d = magnitude of displacement in the direction of force

In SI system, the unit of work is Joule. It is the work done by a force of one Newton when the point of application moves through one meter in the direction of the force.

$$1 J = 1 N \times 1 m$$

A smaller unit of work is 'erg' which is the work done by a force of one dyne when the body moves through a distance of one cm. The relation between Joule and erg is:

$$1 J = 10^7 \text{ erg}$$

Work is done when a person climbs a hill or walks upstairs. It is equal to the product of a person's weight (mg) and the vertical distance (h) moved. You may ask: Is work done when a person is running on a leveled smooth surface at constant speed? In the language of physics, no work is done because weight is acting along a direction normal to his motion. However, his muscles are doing (internal) work; which appears as heat and raises his body temperature. The heat generated due, to this internal work is removed from the body by the blood flow, condition of the skin, and sweating.

ENERGY

It is our common experience that we need energy in one form or the other to do work. You know that petrol burnt in a car makes the car move. A raised hammer drives a nail into the wall. A rushing stream can make a wheel rotate. In these examples, the petrol in a car, a raised hammer, and the rushing stream has the ability to work. Thus, an operational definition of energy is: *"The capacity to do work is known as energy".*

Our body gets energy from the food we eat. Food energy is used by the body to operate its various organs. Some food energy is also used in maintaining constant body temperature and some part (5%) of food energy is excreted. The remaining energy is retained as fat.

Since the energy content of a body is measured by the total amount of work it can do, the units of work and energy are the same, i.e. energy is also measured in joule (J). In nursing, we use kilocalories to measure food, energy and kilocalories per minute for the rate of heat production. The energy value of food referred to by nutritionists as a calorie is actually a kilocalorie. For example, a diet of 2000 calories per day is 2000 K cal/day.

* *Calorie:* One calorie is defined as the energy required to raise the temperature of one gram of water by 1°C.
* *Kilogram Calorie:* It is the large calorie used in nutrition and the amount of heat required to raise the temperature of 1000 cc (1 liter) of water to 1°C. It is abbreviated by K cal.
* *Kilowatt-hour (kWh):* It is a unit to measure electrical energy. 1 kWh is equal to energy consumed by 1 kW power device in one hour.
  * All these units of energy or energy consumed are related to each other. The conversion factors are given in **Table 10.1**.

Table 10.1: Energy conversion factor.

Unit	Joule (J)	Kilowatt-hour (kWh)	Calories (cal)
1 J	1	2.78×10^{-7}	0.239
1 Cal	4.186	1.16×10^{-6}	1
1 kWh	3.6×10^6	1	8.6×10^5

TYPES AND TRANSFORMATION OF ENERGY

In nature, energy exists in various different forms. Depending on its source, energy can be classified as mechanical, heat, sound, light, electrical, magnetic, chemical or nuclear. Physics in many ways is the study of energy in its various forms. But here we shall confine ourselves to different forms of energy in the body and its conversion from one form to another. For instance, chemical energy in the body is converted into mechanical work and used up in other life-preserving functions.

Kinetic Energy: It is the energy associated with motion. The kinetic energy (KE) of a moving object is calculated by:

$$KE = \tfrac{1}{2} mv^2$$

Here, m = mass of object and v = velocity.

Potential Energy: Potential energy is present in the universe in many forms, including gravitational, electromagnetic, chemical, and nuclear. It is stored energy and depends on an

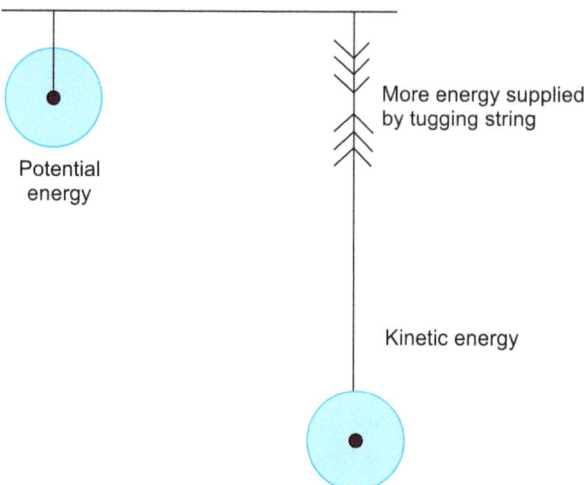

Fig. 10.3: Potential and kinetic energy

object's position or composition. The stored energy is potential energy because it is potentially available to be changed to kinetic energy **(Fig. 10.3)**. For example, in an electric motor connected to a battery, the chemical energy in the battery is converted to kinetic energy as the shaft of the motor turns. The transformation of energy from one form to another is an essential part of the study of physics, engineering, chemistry, biology, geology, and astronomy.

For gravitational systems,

$$PE = wh$$

where,
w = weight
h = height

Example: When the left ventricle forces blood into the aorta, the aorta expands and stores potential energy by virtue of the work done upon it in producing the expansion. When aorta relaxes, the potential energy is changed to kinetic energy, which aids in pushing the blood through the aorta to other arteries.

■ ENERGY IN THE BODY

Energy is a primary importance for our body. Our body requires energy for its various activities. Even while resting, about one fourth of the body energy is used by the muscles and the heart. Even in rest, body energy is used by the brain, kidneys, liver, and spleen. While working, apart from providing energy to various organs, body energy is utilized in maintaining a constant body temperature. Some parts of the body energy is excreted. If the intake of energy is more, the unused part is stored as body fat. It is for this reason that, to get rid of unnecessary body fat, doctors advise regular exercise to persons not undertaking much physical work. The basic source of body energy is the food we eat. You must realize that the food is not used directly in the form of energy. Our body converts this food into energy.

Thus, the human body derives its energy from food. This energy is released as energy for metabolism when food is oxidized in the cells of the body. The rate of oxidation is called the metabolic rate.

Table 10.2: Typical energy values of selected food types.

Food	Calorie value (kcal g−1)
Glucose	3.8
Carbohydrate	4.1
Proteins	4.1
Fats	9.3

The caloric values of some types of food converted into energy due to oxidation are given in **Table 10.2**. These are the maximum expected values. In actual practice, all this energy is not available.

This is because the oxidation may not be complete. The unutilized products are released in feces, urine, and intestinal gas.

A normal person under resting conditions requires nearly 92 kcal/hr. This so-called basal metabolic rate (BMR) signifies the minimum energy required to perform basic body functions (such as breathing and pumping blood through the arteries). The BMR primarily depends upon thyroid function, an overactive thyroid has a higher BMR. The BMR of a living being is proportional to its mass.

Suppose you are required to advise people to reduce weight or keep a constant weight. An individuals desirous of keeping a constant weight should consume just enough food to provide for BMR plus physical activities. Eating too little causes weight loss. And if continued for long, it results in starvation. However, a diet in excess of the requirements of the body causes an increase in weight. To lose weight, we should be careful about the quantity of food we eat and avoid fat-rich foods. This is because the caloric value of fats is almost twice the value of proteins or carbohydrates.

■ CONSERVATION OF ENERGY

You now know that our body gets energy from food in the form of chemical energy. The chemical energy stored in our body, in turn, changes into mechanical energy (external work, breathing, pumping blood), and electrical energy (control of muscles and organ responses). We, therefore, find that the transformation of energy from one form to another takes place in almost every physical activity. But energy is indestructible. That is, energy is never destroyed; it simply changes its form. In other words, energy is conserved. This constitutes the law governing the conservation of energy:

"Energy can neither be created nor destroyed. It can change from one form to another; the total amount of energy remains unchanged."

This is one of the most fundamental principles of science. The conservation of energy in the body can be expressed as:

Change in stored energy in the body = Heat lost from the body + Work done

Here we have assumed that no food or drink is taken in and no feces or urine is excreted during the time considered.

■ POWER

We have not yet talked about the time interval during which a task or work is done. We can define power as the rate of doing work, it is the work done in unit time. Because work is energy transfer, power is also the rate at which energy is expended. If an external force 'F' is applied to an object and work done by this force in time interval 't' is 'W', then average power during this interval is defined as:

$$P = \frac{W}{t}$$

The SI unit of power is Joules per second (J/s), also called the watt (W) (after James Watt). Another common unit of power is horsepower (hp). 1 hp is equal to 746 watt.

■ PRINCIPLES OF MACHINES

Mechanics is a branch of physics. In general, mechanics allows one to describe and predict the conditions of rest or movement of particles and bodies subjected to the action of forces. Aristotle was among the first scholars to introduce the term mechanics.

- *Simple Machines:* Machines are devices for transferring energy or transforming energy into work. Machines operate by receiving mechanical, heat, electrical, chemical, or other forms of energy, and by doing work they transfer the energy to the body upon which the work is done. For example, when a nurse injects a hypodermic medication, energy is transferred from the nurse's muscles to the syringe and needle. The muscles of the body are examples of machines that transform potential energy stored in chemicals in the muscles into kinetic energy of motion.
- Simple machines help us to get work done more easily. Usually, a simple machine helps to overcome a force applied at some point of it by means of another force applied at some other convenient point. The applied force invariably differs in magnitude or direction or both. The force that is overcome by the machine is called 'load'. It is usually the weight of a body to be lifted. The applied force to overcome the load is called the 'effort'.
- *Principles:* When work is done by the machine, the resistance (R) moves through a distance (dr). When work is done on the machine, the effort (E) also acts through a distance (de).
- Theoretically, in an ideal machine

$$\text{Input} = \text{Output}$$
$$\text{Or}$$
$$E \times de = R \times dr$$

■ EFFICIENCY AND MECHANICAL ADVANTAGE OF A MACHINE

The efficiency of a machine is the ratio of its output work to its input work expressed in percent, i.e.,

$$\text{Efficiency} = \frac{\text{Work output}}{\text{Work input}} \times 10$$

The mechanical advantage (MA) of a machine is the ratio of the resistance to the effort, i.e.,

$$MA = \frac{R}{L}$$

Mechanical advantage may also be obtained by the ratio of the distance through which the effort acts to the distance, through which the resistance moves, i.e.,

$$MA = \frac{dr}{de}$$

BODY MECHANICS

The efficiency of the human body as a machine is obtained by using the relation:

$$\text{Efficiency} = \frac{\text{Work done}}{\text{Energy consumed}}$$

Table 10.3: Mechanical efficiency of human beings.

Table	Efficiency (%)
Cycling	~20
Swimming	<2
Shoveling	~3

The efficiency of man for some activities is given in **Table 10.3**. You will note that the values are much less than 100%. One of the major reasons for the low efficiency of human beings is the presence of friction between joints. To minimize friction, the human body has an inherent mechanism of lubrication. The saliva we add when we chew food acts as a lubricant. Similarly, the heart, lungs, and intestines are lubricated by a slippery mucus covering.

Body mechanics is a term used to describe the ways we move as we go about our daily lives. It includes how we hold our bodies when we sit, stand, lift, carry, bend, and sleep.

Principles of Body Mechanics

- The wider the base of support, the greater the stability of the body.
- The lower the center of gravity, the greater the stability of the body.
- The equilibrium of an object is maintained as long as the line of gravity passes through its base of support.
- Facing the direction of movement prevents abnormal twisting of the spine.
- Dividing balanced activity between arms and legs reduces the risk of back injury.
- Maintaining good body mechanics reduces fatigue of the muscle groups.

LEVER

A lever is an example of a simple machine. It is a rigid bar that moves about a fixed axis called the fulcrum (f). The bar may be straight or bent. In addition to a fulcrum, the lever consists of two forces:
- Effort (E)
- Resistance (R)

The machine law describes the relationship between the load lifted (W) and the effort applied (P).

$$P = mW + C$$

Where,
P = Effort applied
W = Load lifted
m = Constant equal to the slope of the line
C = Exhibits mechanical friction

Holds true for all levers in the friction is neglected. Like any simple machine, a force FE is applied on one end of the bar and a load force FL is balanced. The mechanical advantage (MA) of the lever is defined as:

$$MA = \frac{FL}{EF}$$

If the MA is greater than 1, the machine helps us do work more easily. Depending upon the relative positions of the load, effort, and fulcrum, levers are classified into three classes:
1. **First class levers:** In this class of lever, the fulcrum is situated somewhere in between the effort and the resistance **(Fig. 10.4)**. Scissors, and hemostats are examples of such a machine. In the human body, a first-class lever is represented by the triceps and brachial muscles.

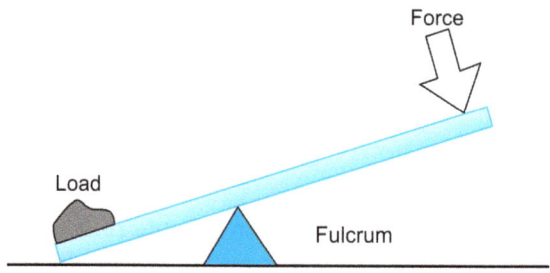

Fig. 10.4: First class lever.

2. **Second class levers:** In this class of lever, the resistance is situated between the fulcrum and the effort **(Fig. 10.5)**. Wheelbarrow and oxygen cylinder carrier are examples of second class levers.

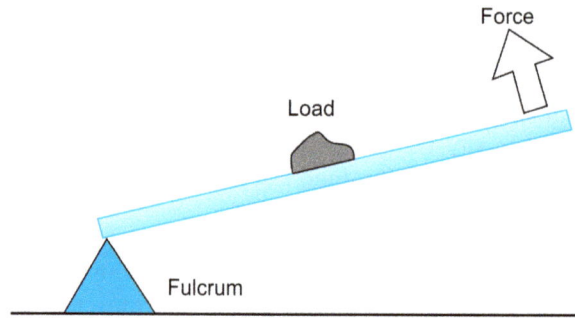

Fig. 10.5: Second class lever.

3. **Third class levers:** In a third class lever, the effort is situated between the resistance and the fulcrum **(Fig. 10.6)**. Forceps and the action of the biceps brachii are the examples of third class lever.

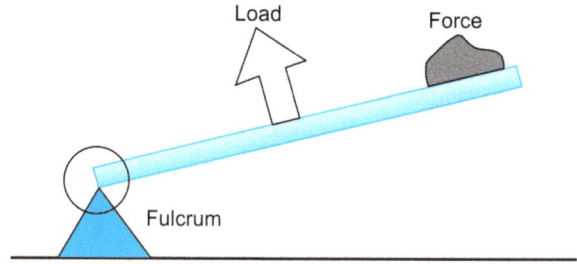

Fig. 10.6: Third class lever.

The Class III levers are most common in the human body. Class II levers are next and Class I levers are the least common. In an automobile, the force of the engine is transformed into another suitable force that rotates the wheels and makes the vehicle move.

The work done on the machine is the product of the effort and the distance through which the effort to act. The work done by the machine is the product of the load and the distance through which the output force acts. Theoretically, in an ideal machine, we expect that the work done on the machine will be equal to the work done by the machine.

■ LEVER ACTION OF JAW

The upper jaw maxilla is a fixed frame. The lower jaw mandible is movable about a fulcrum S within the skull. The effort tension E is applied by the masseter muscles situated on, both sides of the face. When we bite something using our front-cutting teeth incisors, we try to overcome the load W_1 situated between our teeth. The system acts as a Class III lever. However, when we crack a nut or chew something with deeper molars, the system is transformed into a Class II lever with muscle effort acting over the load W_2 **(Fig. 10.7)**.

Fig. 10.7: Lever action of jaw.

■ LEVER ACTION OF FOOT

When a person stands on one foot and raises his heels, a reaction force W equals the weight of the body, acts upwards at the midpoint between ball B and ankle joint of the foot. The effort required to raise the heel is applied on the heel bone as an upward pull P via tissues known as the Achilles tendon. The system may be considered equivalent, to a Class II lever with the fulcrum situated at the ball of the foot **(Fig. 10.8)**.

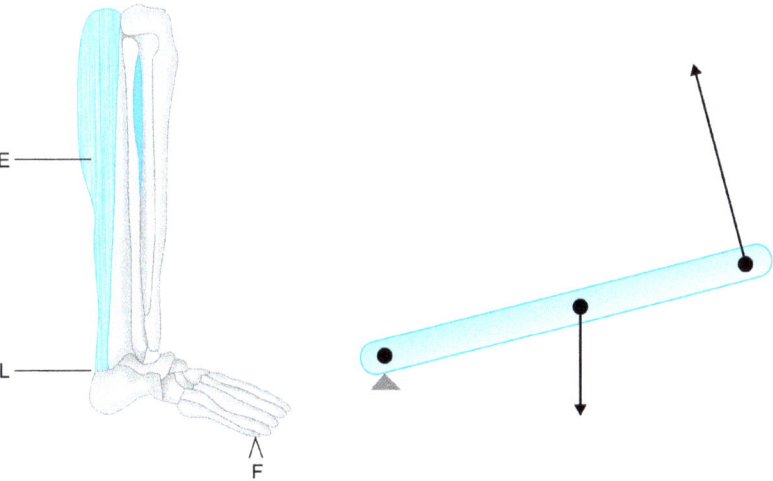

Fig. 10.8: Lever action of foot.

LEVER ACTION OF FOREARM

When we lift a load W bones known as radius and ulna constitute the lever arm BC, pivoted at the fulcrum F provided by another bone humerus. Muscles called biceps and triceps, can exert tension forces at points A and C, respectively of the bones constituting the lever BC. When we lift a load, biceps contract and the arm flexes. During this action, triceps do not act. In order to lower the raised forearm, the biceps are allowed to relax and the triceps come into action. The resulting lever action brings down the arm. When the biceps provides the effort, our forearm acts like a Class III lever and when the triceps are providing the effort force, the forearm forms a Class I lever. Note that the arm bones have two-in-one lever mechanism of action (**Fig. 10.9**).

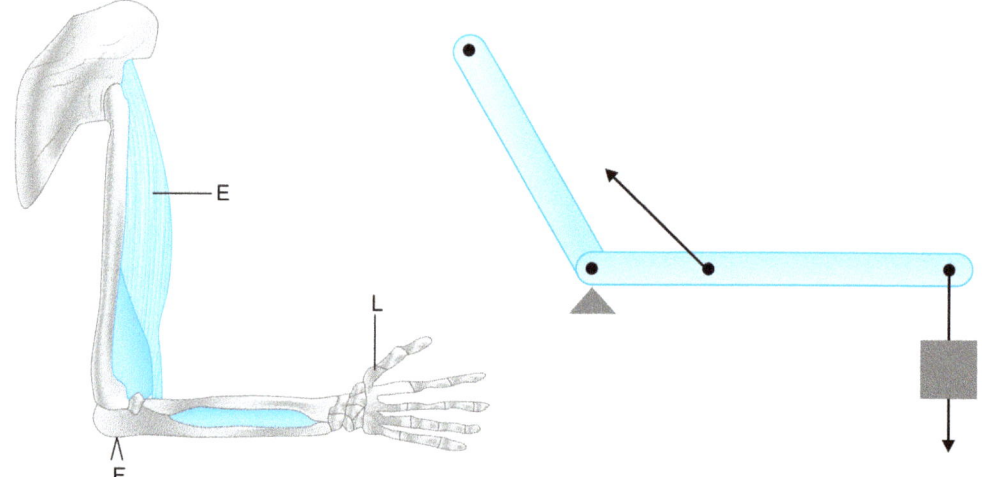

Fig. 10.9: Lever action of forearm.

They all apply forces by means of levers that have a mechanical advantage. But this arrangement provides greater speed to the limbs. A small change in the length of the muscle produces a relatively larger displacement of the limb's extremities. It seems that nature prefers speed to strength. In fact, the speeds attainable at limb extremities are remarkable. A skilled person can throw a stone at a speed in excess of 100 mph. Which was useful for survival in Stone Age.

Liver Action at Hip Joint

The hip joint for a male and its simplified lever representation, giving dimensions are stabilized in its socket by a group of muscles, represented in **Figs. 10.10A and B** as a single resultant force F_m, WL represents the combined weight of the leg, foot, and thigh. Typically, this weight is a fraction (0.185) of the total body weight (W). The weight WL is assumed to act vertically downward at the midpoint of the limb. The force on the hip joint is nearly two and one-half times the weight of the person.

Persons who have an injured hip, limp by leaning toward the injured side as they step on that foot. As a result, the center of gravity of the body shifts into a position more directly above the hip joint, decreasing the force on the injured area.

CHAPTER 10: Force, Energy and Work

Figs. 10.10A and B: (A) The hip; (B) Its lever representation.

Fig. 10.11: The bent back (Left). Lever representation (Right).

Liver Action at the Back

When the trunk is bent forward, the spine pivots mainly on the fifth lumbar vertebra. If we will analyze the forces involved when the trunk is bent at 60° from the vertical with the arms hanging freely. The lever model representing the situation is given in **Fig. 10.11**.

The pivot point A is the fifth lumbar vertebra. The lever arm AB represents the back. The weight of the trunk W_1 is uniformly distributed along the back; its effect can be represented by a weight suspended in the middle. The weight of the head and arms is represented by W_2

suspended at the end of the lever arm. The erector spinalis muscle, shown as the connection D-C attached at a point two-thirds up the spine, maintains the position of the back. This indicates that large forces are exerted on the fifth lumbar vertebra and backaches originate most frequently at this point. So the position shown in the figure is not the recommended way of lifting a weight.

■ PULLEY

A pulley consists of a wheel without a grooved rim around which a string can be passed. The pulley rotates about an axel through its center. The axle is supported by a framework called a block **(Fig. 10.12)**.

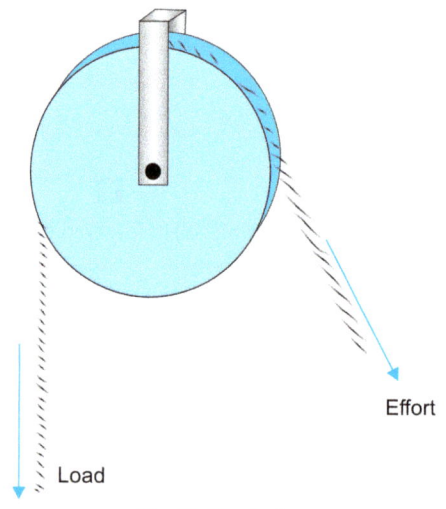

Fig. 10.12: Pulley.

Pulleys are classified as:
- *Fixed pulleys:* They are attached to some fixed support.
- *Movable pulleys:* They are attached to the resistance and move along with the resistance.

The chief function of the pulley wheel is to equalize the tension of the string on either side of it.

■ TRACTION

Traction can be used to realign a fractured bone or other dislocated body part. It uses weights, pulleys, and ropes to apply gentle pressure and pull the injured or broken part back into place. Three types of traction are there mainly: skin traction, skeletal traction, and cervical traction. The type of traction required will depend on the severity and location of the injury or broken bone.

The Purpose of Traction

Traction is used to stabilize fractures or injuries and to restore tension to surrounding tissues, muscles, tendons, and other structures. Traction can be used to:
- Stabilize and realign broken bones or dislocated parts of the body (such as the shoulder).
- Restore the bone's normal position after it has been broken.
- To reduce the pressure on the spine, stretch the neck and realign the vertebrae.
- Temporarily reduce pain before surgery.

- Reduce or eliminate muscle spasms, constricted joints, muscles, and tendonitis.
- Reduce pressure on nerves, particularly spinal nerves.
- Treat bone deformities.

Skeletal Traction

Skeletal traction can be used to treat fractures of the femur, pelvis, hip, and certain upper arm fractures. The procedure involves inserting a wire or pin directly into the bone and attaching weights using pulleys or ropes that regulate the pressure. Skeletal traction can be used to treat fractures that are more severe than others. It allows for greater weight to be added to the bone with less chance of damaging the soft tissues. Skeletal traction is performed under anesthesia to ensure that patient does not feel any pain.

Skin Traction

Skin traction is less intrusive than skeletal traction. It uses splints and bandages on the area of the fracture. The adhesive tapes are then applied to the skin. Pressure is applied by attaching weights and pulleys. The muscles and tendons pull an extremity to a shorter or bent position when a bone is broken. The traction can help to hold the fractured bone and dislocated joints in place. This can lead to painful movement and cramping at the fracture site. Buck›s traction, a form of skin traction, is used widely for hip, acetabular, and femoral fractures.

Cervical Traction

When the neck vertebrae have been fractured, cervical traction is used. This type of traction uses a device that circles the head and attaches itself to a harness that wraps around the torso. This stretch to the neck relieves pressure on the spine and aligns the vertebrae.

Risks and Contraindications

Traction poses no risk in the long-term. However, some people might experience pain or muscle spasms in the area being treated.

There are potential dangers associated with traction:
- Negative reactions to anesthesia.
- An excessive amount of bleeding at the location of a pin/screw in skeletal traction.
- Infection at the place where the screw or pin has been inserted.
- Extreme swelling can cause nerve or vascular injuries.
- In cases of skin crackle, there is damage to the surrounding tissue and skin.

Contraindications

Skin traction is not recommended for seniors as their skin may be damaged by the force of the traction. If the patient has any of the following conditions, traction may be contraindicated:
- Osteoporosis
- Rheumatoid arthritis
- Infection
- Pregnancy
- Circulatory and respiratory problems
- Claustrophobia
- Cardiovascular disease
- Joint problems

Before applying, both skin and skeletal tensions require X-rays. To ensure the correct alignment of the bones, these may be repeated throughout the treatment. The severity, location, and extent of injury or broken bone will determine how long the traction will be. The time taken to traction can range from 24 hours up to six weeks or more. Skin traction can be used temporarily to immobilize the fracture while waiting for corrective surgery.

There are many potential problems associated with prolonged immobility in traction such as bedsores also with respiratory, urinary, and circulatory problems. Various physical therapies are recommended to maintain joint and muscle movement. Regular inspections of the equipment will ensure that it is properly positioned and calibrated.

Traction can be a very challenging treatment-physically, emotionally, and psychologically, so as nursing person, we should explain and assist the person and family to cope with this challenging time.

According to balancing forces, we can also classify the tractions as follows:

- **Fixed traction:** In this, a splint such as Thomas splint is employed. In this traction the forward pull of the force (wt) is made directly on the splint **(Fig. 10.13)**.

Fig. 10.13: Thomas splint traction.

- **Balanced traction:** In this, a force is transmitted over a pulley by a cord from a weight hung at the foot, head, or side of the bed. It may be fixed to the injured part by adhesive strapping or by a pin passed directly through the bone **(Fig. 10.14)**.

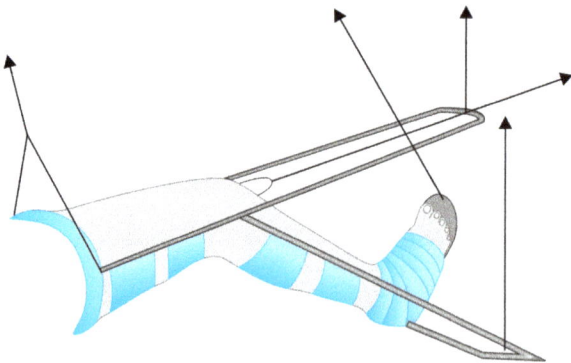

Fig. 10.14: Balanced traction.

CHAPTER 10: Force, Energy and Work

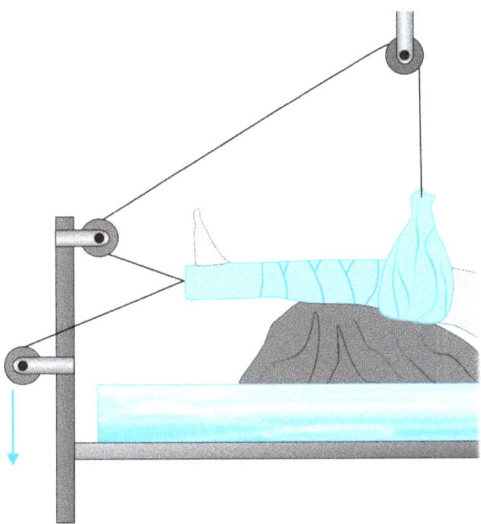

Fig. 10.15: Russell traction.

- **Russell traction:** It employs the principle of balanced traction for treating fractures of the femur. In this traction force is applied to a sling placed under the knee. This force is transmitted by a rope, which passes over a pulley to the foot of the bed. Bypassing this rope over another pulley connected to a wooden block and in the adhesive strapping below the patient's foot, the same force is applied to the lower leg (**Fig. 10.15**).
  - Russell traction is based on the concept of vector addition and equilibrium of forces. The backward pull of the muscles and the counterforce of the patient weight balance the resultant force and keep the fractured ends of the bone in alignment.

■ INCLINED PLANE

A ramp used in buildings to join floors of different levels is a practical example of a machine called an inclined plane. It is much easier to wheel a patient up a ramp (the length of the plane) than to raise him bodily from one level to the other (the height of the plane). An inclined plane can handle jobs that we might find dangerous to carry-out (**Fig. 10.16**).

Fig. 10.16: Inclined plane.

The effort (E) is the force parallel to the length of the plane necessary to move the patient and the chair. The distance the effort moves is the length of the inclined plane (l); the distance the resistance (R) is moved vertically is the height of the plane or the distance between the two floor levels (h). The law of the inclined plane is expressed as follows:

$$\text{Effort} \times \text{Length of incline} = \text{Resistance} \times \text{Height of incline}$$
$$El = Rh$$

WEDGE

It is a modified inclined plane. In this, the machine is pushed between two objects and separates them. The chief application of the wedge in nursing is its use as a mouth gag to open a patient's mouth after anesthesia or during a convulsion. The beveled edges of chisels, cutting tools, and hypodermic needles are also examples of wedges.

SCREW

The screw is also an adaptation of the inclined plane. In a sense, it is like an inclined plane that is wrapped around a cylinder. The screw is used wherever a large resistance is to be overcome by a relatively small effort. For example, jackscrew is used to lift a heavy automobile or truck. There are many pieces of equipment in the hospital that operate on the principle of screw, e.g. crank of a gatch bed, wheel of operating room tables, wheel of an autoclave door. Most common application clinically is that of the crew of a clamp used on rubber tubing. A small effort on the screw produces a large to occlude or lessen the opening of the tube.

APPLICATION OF PRINCIPLES OF GRAVITY IN NURSING

- Knowledge of the friction will help nurses to plan nursing procedures in a manner, where they can minimize the friction and irritations to patients; like the application of lubricating jelly for insertion of nasogastric tubes, endotracheal tubes, and urinary catheters.
- Nurses will understand the use of synovial fluid or other normal minimal cavity fluids to prevention of friction and smooth movements of joints or membranes.
- Newton's third law will help nurses to understand the mechanisms of development of bedsores among heavy bedridden patients and other similar entities.
- Knowledge of energy will help nurses to understand the use of energy in body functioning and the energy requirements of an individual in form of the calories.
- Nurses understanding the principles of body mechanics can utilize the energy more effectively without putting the body in much strain.
- The knowledge of the levers can help nurses to understand the mechanisms of the simple article used in clinical practices, scissors, forceps; oxygen cylinder carrying stands and so many other clinical articles.
- Knowledge of levers helps nurses understand about functioning of the different body joints and plan for physiotherapy exercises.
- Pulleys are used to lift heavy weights to open windows, and move draperies to raise heavy operating room lamps, and other apparatus in the laboratory.
- The chief use of pulleys in therapy is in balanced traction.
- Pulleys are used in the rehabilitation of patients to prevent atrophy of muscles and joints to restore motion.

QUESTIONS

Q.1: Why does a patient lying in bed for a long time develop sores? State the law that explains it.
Q.2: Explain the principles of simple machine, different types of simple machine and their applications.
Q.3: Give examples of anatomical lever and pulley in the human body.

Q.4: Traction is used in the treatment of some fractures. Explain it.
Q.5: Discuss the principles of force, energy and work in nursing.

■ BIBLIOGRAPHY

1. Alekseev GN. Energy and Entropy. Moscow: Mir Publishers, 1986.
2. Corbell HC, Stehle P. Classical Mechanics New York: Dover Publications, 1994: 28.
3. Coulomb C. "Recherches théoriques et expérimentales Sur La Force de torsion et Sur L'élasticité Des fils de metal". Histoire de l'Académie Royale des Sciences, 1784.
4. Cutnell J, Johnson KW. Physics, (6th edn). Hoboken, NJ: John Wiley & Sons Inc, 2004.
5. Drake S. Galileo At Work. Chicago: University of Chicago Press, 1978.
6. Duffin. Electricity and Magnetism, (3rd edn). McGraw-Hill, 1980.
7. Feynman RP, Leighton RB, Sands M. Lectures on Physics, Vol 1. Addison-Wesley; Kleppner, Daniel; Robert Kolenkow). An Introduction to Mechanics. McGraw-Hill, 1973.
8. Feynman, Leighton Sands. The Feynman Lectures on Physics. The Definitive Edition Volume II. Pearson Addison Wesley, 2006.
9. Halliday RD, Krane KS. Physics V. 1. New York: John Wiley & Sons, 2001.
10. Henderson T. "The Physics Classroom". The Physics Classroom and Mathsoft Engineering & Education, Inc. 2004.
11. Hetherington NS. Cosmology: Historical, Literary, Philosophical, Religious, and Scientific Perspectives. Garland Reference Library of the Humanities, 1993.
12. Land H. The Order of Nature in Aristotle's Physics: Place and the Elements, 1998.
13. Lofts G, O'Keeffe D, et al. "11-Mechanical Interactions". Jacaranda Physics 1 (2 edn.). Milton, Queensland, Australia: John Willey & Sons Australia Ltd. 2004.
14. Newton I. The Principia Mathematical Principles of Natural Philosophy. Berkeley: University of California Press, 1999.
15. Parker S. Encyclopedia of Physics, Ohio: McGraw-Hill, 1993: 443.
16. Rashed R. "The Celestial Kinematics of Ibn al-Haytham", Arabic Sciences and Philosophy. Cambridge University Press, 2007.
17. Serway RA, Jewett JW. Physics for Scientists and Engineers (6th edn). Brooks/Cole, 2004.
18. Smil V. Energy in nature and society: general energetics of complex systems. Cambridge, USA, 2008.
19. Smith C. The Science of Energy—a Cultural History of Energy Physics in Victorian Britain. The University of Chicago Press, 1998.
20. Tipler P. Physics for Scientists and Engineers: Mechanics (3rd edn). New York: W.H. Freeman, 1991.
21. Tipler P. Physics for Scientists and Engineers: Mechanics, Oscillations and Waves, Thermodynamics (5th edn). WH Freeman, 2004.
22. Verma HC. Concepts of Physics, Vol. 1, Bharti Bhavan, 2004.
23. Walding R, Rapkins G, Rossiter G. New Century Senior Physics. Melbourne, Australia: Oxford University Press, 1999.
24. Wandmacher C, Johnson A. Metric Units in Engineering. ASCE Publications, 1995.
25. Awrejcewicz, J. (2012). Fundamental Principles of Mechanics. In: Classical Mechanics. Advances in Mechanics and Mathematics, Vol 28. Springer, New York, NY. https://doi.org/10.1007/978-1-4614-3791-8_1
26. Karel Velan, A. (1992). Gravitation. In: The Multi-Universe Cosmos. Springer, Boston, MA. https://doi.org/10.1007/978-1-4684-6030-8_10
27. Alrasheed, S. (2019). Newton's Laws. In: Principles of Mechanics. Advances in Science, Technology & Innovation. Springer, Cham. https://doi.org/10.1007/978-3-030-15195-9_3

CHAPTER

Heat

Navjot Kaur, Suresh K Sharma

Chapter Outline
- Nature of Heat
- Measurement of Heat
- Transfer of Heat
- Effects of Heat on Matter
- Relative Humidity
- Specific Heat
- Temperature Scales
- Regulation of Body Temperature
- Use of Heat for Sterilization
- Application of Heat Principles in Nursing

■ INTRODUCTION

Healthcare practices are using heat and cold applications for several years for benefiting the patients suffering from several kinds of disorders. One can witness nurses providing hydrotherapies to patients having raised body temperature. Similarly, heat application has been empirically proved to be beneficial for the management of arthritis, sprains, contusions, sinusitis and back pain, etc.

■ NATURE OF HEAT

To understand the nature of heat, let us consider a cup of hot tea. From experience, we know that tea will lose energy (heat) and get cooled. Similarly, you may consider rubbing palms. The work done in rubbing produces warmth (heat). So we can say that heat is associated with the flow of energy. That is, it is energy in transit. In terms of atoms/molecules of a system (or material) we can say that:

"Heat is intimately connected with motion; it is the total kinetic energy of molecules/atoms making up a system".

How do we decide the direction of heat flow from one body to another? Before we answer this question, you should do a simple activity. "Take three cups and put hot water in one (say, cup no.1), water at room temperature in the second (say, cup no. 2), and cold water in the third (say, cup no. 3). Put your left hand in cup no.1 and your right hand in cup no. 3. Now shift both hands to the cup no. 2. How do you feel? Your left-hand feels that cup no. 2 contains cold water (heat flowing from the hand with water) while right-hand feels that the same cup (that is, cup no. 2) has hot water (heat is flowing from the water to the hand). This activity shows that we cannot rely on our senses for deciding the direction of flow of heat energy. We must look for a more precise parameter.

A *quantitative measure of heat/thermal energy of the system is given by temperature.* It determines the direction in which heat energy is transferred from a system when it is placed in contact with another. (It arose from the physiological sensation of hotness.) For example, when we touch a hot cup, our fingers register a feeling of warmth physically; it means that the energy is flowing from the cup to our fingers. The cup is said to be at a higher temperature than the finger (which is at 98.6°F). We may, therefore, conclude that:

"Temperature characterizes the thermal state of a body and determines whether energy will flow from or towards it from another body in thermal contact".

Heat and temperature are not the same in nature:
- Heat is the total energy content of a system, whereas temperature is a measure of this energy and decides the direction of the flow of energy.
- You can imagine that heat is analogous to the quantity of water. Can you think of a similar astrology of temperature? It is analogous to the level of water.
- Two bodies having the same temperature can have different quantities of heat. For example, a spoonful of a sweet liquid taken from a jug is as sweet as the liquid in the jug, though it does not contain as much sugar. Similarly, the temperature of boiling water in a tea cup may be the same as that in a big bucket, but the heat content of the water in the bucket will be much greater.

■ MEASUREMENT OF HEAT

- As a form of energy, heat has the unit joule (J) in the International System of Units (SI). However, in many applied fields in engineering, the British thermal unit (BTU) and the calorie are often used. The standard unit for the rate of heat transferred is the watt (W), defined as one joule per second
- Quantity of heat is defined as the sum of the kinetic energy of all the molecules of which an object is composed of.
- The temperature of an object is a measurement of the speed of its molecules (i.e. hotness).
- Any form of energy that increases the speed of the molecules of an object will raise the temperature of the object. For example, if the pitcher of water is heated by a gas flame or by an electric hot plate, energy is transmitted from the gas flame or the hot plate to the molecules of the water in the pitcher. The resulting increase in the temperature of the water is actually due to the increase in the motion of the molecules of water.
- You can get an idea about the body temperature of a person by your sense of touch. In this case, your hand acts as a temperature sensor and compares the person's body temperature with yours. But this method is not reliable; it provides only a qualitative measure. To get a better measure of temperature, we must know to express it quantitatively. The device that gives a quantitative measure of temperature is called a thermometer. The earliest thermometer was developed by Galileo.
- In a thermometer (**Fig. 11.1**), we make use of some temperature-dependent and measurable properties like length, volume, or electrical resistance of matter. We know that most substances expand when heated and contract when cooled. In principle, any such substance could be used as an indicator in a thermometer. But the most commonly used substance in an ordinary thermometer is mercury. However, nowadays uses of mercury thermometer is banned in a healthcare setting due to their deleterious effects on health and therefore digital thermometer is recommended for clinical uses.

Fig. 11.1: Thermometer.

Advantages of Mercury as the Thermometric Substance
- Mercury is easily visible through glass because it is opaque to light.
- It can conduct heat rapidly.
- It does not wet glass.
- It has a low freezing point and high boiling point so that the range of temperature for which it is used is large.
- It expands uniformly with rise in temperature.

Construction of Mercury Thermometer
A typical thermometer consists of a thin-walled glass bulb, attached to a capillary tube of the uniform bore. The bulb and capillary tube are filled with mercury and heated to a temperature a few degrees above the maximum temperature thermometer is designed to measure. The mercury rises in the tube and overflows. The open end is then sealed. The tube is now marked with reference points called fixed points. These points are usually the position of the mercury in the tube when it is placed in melting ice (lower fixed point) and steam (upper fixed point). The intervening distance between these two fixed points is then graduated into a number of equal intervals, and a scale is thus devised.

■ TRANSFER OF HEAT
Heat can be transferred from one surface to another in several ways. We now know that when an object is at a temperature higher than its surroundings; energy is transferred to the surroundings. This is analogous to the flow of fluid from a region of higher pressure to a region of lower pressure. The human body uses a variety of mechanisms to transfer heat produced due to various internal functions of the body and maintain an average temperature of 98.6°F. In the same way, the skin of the whole body also loses heat by conduction, convection, and evaporation. Following are the main ways to transfer heat.

Conduction
Heat conduction is the transfer of thermal energy between neighboring molecules in a substance due to a temperature gradient. It always takes place from a region of higher temperature to a

region of lower temperature and acts to equalize temperature differences. Conduction needs matter and does not require any bulk motion of matter. For conduction two surfaces must come in contact with other.

Substance conducts heat at different rates. Metals are considered as good conductors and nonmetals as poor conductors. For example, if one has to touch metal door knobs and a wooden door simultaneously on a cold day, the metal knob would feel much cooler than the wooden door. This sensation is due to the ability of metals to conduct heat from the body much more rapidly than wood.

Applications of Conductors

- Mercury is a good conductor of heat. So it expands rapidly with a slight increase in temperature.
- Conductors play an important part in nursing and therapeutics. When it is necessary to release heat slowly to an external portion of the body, a poor conductor is used. Rubber is one such poor conductor. It conducts heat more slowly than does a metal. Therefore, it is used in the manufacturing of hot water bottles, icecaps, and ice collars.
- Air, which is a mixture of gases, is a poorer conductor than rubber. A layer of air between a piece of equipment and the body acts as an insulator to prevent heat from passing too rapidly. So a hot water bottle is usually placed in a cloth cover such as flannel, which encloses a layer of air that separates the hot water bottle from the patient. The air slows the passage of heat energy, prevents burning the patient, and prolongs the therapeutic effect.

Convection

This mode of transfer of heat is possible in fluids (liquids and gases) and that too is because of gravity. When a fluid is heated, the hotter part expands, and the density of this portion of the liquid decrease. Due to the buoyancy force; the hotter part, being lighter, tends to rise and its place is taken by the colder and heavier fluid from the top and sides. This, in turn, gets heated and rises up, and so on. *The movement of the hotter part of the liquid upwards and the colder part towards the bottom constitutes the convection current and the transfer of heat due to this process is called convection.*

This can easily be seen by coloring water by keeping a crystal of potassium permanganate at the bottom of the flask. During pathological testing of urine using a spirit lamp and test tube we can observe the, effect of convection. So we can say that: *In convention, heat is transferred by the actual movements of matter.*

The process of convection is entirely different from conductions where heat energy is transmitted by atoms/molecules via collisions without being drifted. Some familiar examples of convection are given below:

- You must have seen the rising smoke up a chimney of oil lamps: Hot air above the flame rises up the chimney, its place being taken by cold air from below drawn from the room.
- Wind blows due to convection currents set up in the atmosphere due to, unequal heating of land and sea breezes, and trade winds are caused by convection currents in the atmosphere.
- The effectiveness of ventilation in our homes, hospitals, and public buildings depends upon convection currents.
- For clinical purposes, a thermos bottle is used and a sedative bath is prescribed to help emotionally disturbed patients.

- Steam inhalations and colonic irrigations transfer heat by convection.
- Natural convection and anomalous expansion of water play a very important role in saving the lives of aquatic animals when the atmospheric temperature goes below 0°C on winter days. When water at the surface is cooled, it becomes denser and goes down. Less cold water from the bottom, comes up to the surface and gets cooled and so on. This way the entire water is cooled to 4°C. Further, water at the surface gets cooled; it expands and its density decreases. So, it remains on the surface only and gets cooled further, and then it starts freezing. As ice is a poor conductor, so freezing to downwards is very slow and the temperature at the bottom remains 4°C for long times.

Radiation

Heat is transferred from the sun to the earth without requiring any material medium. Heat energy can be transmitted through a vacuum from some source of heat. The process of emitting energy is called the radiation of an object. Highly polished objects, such as a mirror and light-colored objects reflect radiant energy. For example, the use of lasers.

Evaporation

Heat from the human body is also lost through breathing, by perspiration, by urination, by defecation and through exposed body parts. Loss of heat in these processes is due to evaporation or vaporization. Vaporization takes places in all liquids due to the movement of molecules from the liquid surface. The slow and spontaneous change from the liquid to the vapor or gaseous state of matter is called evaporation. As evaporation takes place, it results in cooling. The use of ecu-de-cologne on your body gives a cooling sensation due to evaporation.

A newborn baby loses (transfers) heat by all four mechanisms **(Fig. 11.2)**.

Fig. 11.2: Illustration on different Modes of Heat Transmission.

■ EFFECTS OF HEAT ON MATTER

There is known effect of heat of different matters like with lower temperature liquids change in solid and with increased temperature solid changes to liquid or gases. Following are some of the physical technicalities need to learn to understand the effect of heat on different matter.

Freezing and Melting Points

The temperature at which a liquid changes to a solid is called its freezing point. The temperature at which the same solid is changed back to a liquid is its melting point **(Fig. 11.3)**.

CHAPTER 11: Heat

Fig. 11.3: Freezing and melting points.

Vapor Pressure

When a liquid is heated, its molecules leave the surface of the liquid. The pressure developed by the molecules of the liquid as it is changed into a gas is known as the vapor pressure of that liquid **(Fig. 11.4)**.

Fig. 11.4: Vapor pressure.

Boiling Point

The boiling point of a liquid is the temperature at which its vapor pressure is equal to atmospheric pressure. A certain quantity of heat is absorbed by the molecules of a liquid when it changes from a liquid to a vapor at the boiling point, this same amount of heat is lubricated when the vapor (gas) condenses to a liquid. The boiling point of water is 100°C.

Heat of Fusion

The heat of fusion is the number of calories needed to produce molecular separation so that material will pass from the solid to the liquid state at the melting point. When ice changes into water at 0°C, approximately 80 calories of heat are absorbed before the ice melts to form 1 gm of liquid water. Ice-filled caps and collars are effective is reducing fever because of the heat of fusion of ice.

Heat of Solidification

When a liquid is changed into a solid, the liquid liberates the same number of calories, that is absorbed in changing from a solid to a liquid. Water releases 80 calories when 1 gm of water is at 0°C changes to ice at the same temperature.

Heat of Vaporization

The number of calories needed to change 1 gm of liquid at a particular temperature to a vapor (gas) at the same temperature is called the heat of vaporization of that substance. The heat of vaporization of water is about 538 cal/gm at 100°C.

Heat of Condensation

When steam at 100°C condenses to form water at 100°C it liberates the heat absorbed when it is changed from a liquid at 100°C to a gas at 100°C. The heat of condensation is the number of calories liberated when a gas condenses to form 1 gm of a liquid at a particular temperature.

Heat of Combustion

It is the quantity of heat in calories given off during the combustion of 1 gm of a substance. It is also measured in kcal/gm.

Sublimation

It is a direct change from the solid to the vapor phase. Dry ice (solid CO_2), camphor, iodine and naphthalene passes directly from the solid to the gaseous phase.

■ HUMIDITY

The concentration of water vapor present in the air is known as humidity. The widely employed primary measurements of humidity are: absolute humidity, relative humidity and specific humidity

Absolute Humidity

Absolute humidity describes the water content present in the air and is expressed in either grams per cubic meter or grams per kilogram. The absolute humidity in the atmosphere ranges from near zero to roughly 30 grams per cubic metre.

Mathematically absolute humidity is defined as mass of the water vapor divided by the volume of the air and water mixture, which is expressed as

The absolute humidity varies with respect to air temperature and pressure changes, if the volume is not fixed. The mass of water vapor per unit volume in the equation is also defined as volumetric humidity.

Relative Humidity

The relative humidity of an air water mixture is defined as the ratio of the partial pressure of water vapor in the mixture to the equilibrium vapor pressure of water over a flat surface of pure water at a given temperature. It is normally expressed as a percentage. Higher percentage indicates that the air-water mixture is more humid.

Relative humidity is a crucial metric that is used in weather forecasts as it is an indicator of the likelihood of precipitation, dew or fog. In hot summer weather, a rise in relative humidity increases the temperature of humans by hindering the evaporation of perspiration from the skin. Relative humidity is expressed as a percentage. For example, if relative humidity on a given day (that is, at a given temperature) is 60%; it means that 60 units of water vapors are present per cubic meter of air which saturates with 100 units of water vapor.

Importance of Relative Humidity

- A high humidity is maintained in operation theaters as it prevents the drying of the exposed tissues. It also reduces the hazard of explosion due to ether fumes.
- Premature infants also require a high humidity environment so that evaporation from the nasal passage can be minimized. If the air at 68° F has a vapor pressure of 8.7 mm Hg and the normal vapor pressure at 68° F is 17.4 mm Hg and the relative humidity is 50%.

$$\frac{8.7 \text{ mm Hg}}{17.4 \text{ mm Hg}} \times 100 = 50\%$$

If the same air containing 8.7 mm Hg of vapor pressure were reduced in temperature to 49° F, the relative humidity would be nearly 100%. The temperature at which the existing water vapor that produces saturation is called the dew point. A slight decrease in temperature below this point may produce a condensation of water vapor in the form of dew or frost.

Specific Humidity

The ratio of mass of the mass of water vapor to the total mass of the air parcel is known as specific humidity

SPECIFIC HEAT

The specific heat of a substance denotes the amount of heat required to raise the temperature of a unit mass of a substance by 1°C.
- Specific heat of a substance is the ratio of its thermal capacity to that of water at 15° C.
- If the thermal capacity(s) of a substance is known, the heat (H) necessary to change temperature of mass (m) from an initial temperature (t_1) to a final temperature (t_2) can be calculated by the following formula:

H = ms (t_2-t_1) or   H = msDt

Since by definition the thermal capacity of water is 1, specific heat is quantitatively equal to the thermal capacity. The thermal capacity of common substances is given in **Table 11.1**.

Table 11.1: Thermal capacity of common substances.

Substance at 20° C	In cal/gm/ °C/ BTU/ lb/ °F
Blood (37°C)	0.80
Water	1.00
Alcohol	0.58
Mercury	0.03
Ice	0.51

TEMPERATURE SCALES

Two commonly used scales for measuring temperature are **(Fig. 11.5)**:
* The Fahrenheit scale, which was devised by German scientists Gabriel Heit (1714).
* The Celsius scale (also called the Centigrade scale). The Celsius scale was proposed by a Swedish scientist, Anders Celsius (1742).

Fig. 11.5: Celsius and Fahrenheit scale.

* On Celsius scale, the freezing point of water is 0° and the boiling point of water is 100°. The interval between the two fixed points is divided into one hundred equal parts.
* In the Fahrenheit scale, the freezing point of water is 32° and the boiling point of water is 212°. The interval between the two fixed points is divided into 180 equal parts.
* Thus, 32°F = 0°C and 212°F = 100°C. Clearly, the Celsius scale is more convenient.

$$\frac{F-32}{C-0°} = \frac{212-32°}{100-0°} = \frac{180°}{100°} = \frac{9}{5}$$

* In order to convert a reading of temperature from one scale to the other, following equation is used:

$$\frac{F-32}{9} = \frac{C}{5}$$

By this equation, the human body temperature of 98.6°F corresponds to 37°C.
* Besides the Fahrenheit and Celsius scales, the absolute or Kelvin scale is also used in physics. The lowest fixed point on this scale is known as absolute zero, which is equivalent to –273°C (–459.6°F) conversions from the absolute scale, i.e. in K, to the Celsius scale is:

$$C° = K - 273$$

Whereas, the conversion from the Celsius scales to the Kelvin scale is:

$$K = C° + 273$$

Relation between Celsius Fahrenheit and Kelvin scales

In order to convert a reading of temperature from one scale to the other, following equation can be used OSC Equation:

Clinical Thermometer

This thermometer is used to record the temperature of the body. In a clinical thermometer, the temperature is recorded in degrees Fahrenheit (or degrees Celsius). In very precise thermometers, each degree is further subdivided into two or more equal parts. Parts of the clinical thermometer are as follows **(Fig. 11.6)**:

- The stem of the thermometer usually has a curved surface that magnifies the numbers on the scale and a flat surface that prevents it from rolling. A white backing is placed behind the mercury column to make reading easier.

Fig. 11.6: Oral thermometer.

- Oral thermometers are usually made with a long, slender *bulb*, so the mercury in the bulb is exposed to a large surface, the mercury absorbs heat rapidly and registers quickly is a maximum reading thermometer. This means that the column of mercury continues to show the maximum.
- Rectal thermometers have a shorter, thicker-walled bulb and register more slowly than oral thermometers.
- The clinical thermometer temperature level even remains the same after use. So, before using it again, it is reset by shaking the mercury down into the bulb. This is made possible by constriction in the bore of the tube immediately above the bulb.

■ REGULATION OF BODY TEMPERATURE

- Basal metabolism of the body causes heat production. Over and above the basal metabolism, there are other factors that contribute to heat production in the body. A healthy body functions best at an internal temperature of about 37°C (98.6°F). But everyone has their own individual "normal" body temperature, which may be slightly higher or lower. Our bodies also constantly adapt their temperature to environmental conditions. It goes up when we exercise, for instance. And it is lower at night, and higher in the afternoon than in the morning.

- Our internal body temperature is regulated by hypothalamus. The hypothalamus checks our current temperature and compares it with the normal temperature of about 37°C, when body temperature increases, due to heavy exertion: the hypothalamus initiates sweating and vasodilatation. On the other hand, when the body temperature drops, the hypothalamus initiates shivering, which tends to restore body temperature.
- The main heat loss mechanisms are conduction, convection, radiation and evaporation (perspiration). The rate of heat production in the body for a 2400 kcal per day diet is about 120 W. For the body temperature to remain constant, the heat should be lost at the same rate. Generally, the human body employs more than one of these mechanisms to transfer heat to the surroundings.
- For example, the therapeutic effect of cold sponging for a high fever patient is achieved due to the transfer of heat by conduction, convection, and evaporation. The cold sponge placed over the groins, axilla, neck, and forehead of the patient takes the heat off the circulating blood and brings down the fever (heat) to a safer range. In the same way, the skin of the whole body also loses heat by conduction, convection, and evaporation.
- The temperature of the human body is the result of a balance between heat energy produced and heat energy is lost. Heat energy is produced in the body mainly due to the oxidation of foodstuffs in the tissues, and the heat energy is lost from the body by conduction, convection, radiation, and evaporation. If a person weighing 70 kg is sitting quietly at rest, she expends nearly 100 kcal per hour. However, the same person will expend 1100 kcal per hour to walk up a flight of stairs. The expenditure of energy for various activities is given in **Table 11.2**.
- Most of the heat of the body is lost through the skin. The rate at which heat is lost depends on the temperature difference between the skin and the environment. Nearly half of the heat produced in the body is lost by a person sitting comfortably in a room at a temperature of 22°C. This means that even at room temperature, heat loss (mostly due to radiation) is significant.
- The death of a person with heat or sunstroke happens because external heat is applied to the body exceeds the amount normally lost. This upsets the total heat balance of the body and the person collapses.

Table 11.2: Relative expenditure of thermal energy per hour.

Activity	Expended energy
Sitting quietly	1.00
Sleeping	0.65
Lying quietly	0.77
Dressing/undressing	1.18
Typing	1.40
Light exercise	1.70
Walking slowly	2.00
Active exercise	2.90
Severe exercise	4.50
Swimming	5.00
Running	5.70
Walking fast	6.50
Walking upstairs	11.00

CHAPTER 11: Heat

■ USE OF HEAT FOR STERILIZATION

- Sterilizers are based on the Charles's law that states: the temperature of a gas increases as the pressure increases when the volume is kept constant. The increased temperature of the gas resulting from increased pressure destroys the microorganism. Steam at 100°C in contact with boiling water is called moist heat.
- Nonspore-forming bacteria are killed at from 52 to 70°C; the boiling water is sufficient to kill them, whereas spore-forming bacteria require temperatures from 110 to 72°C to kill them. Hence, 120°C for 30 minutes is the ideal temperature for actual sterilization.
- Sterilizers that are used for sterilizing glassware and powders are based on dry heat. Dry heat with a temperature of 160°C is effective to kill bacteria, but its penetration is less than with steam.
- An autoclave is the equipment used for sterilization of surgical tools and other items.. An autoclave is a device that contains steam in a closed chamber of constant volume and the temperature of the steam is increased. Steam is heated to 121–134°C (250–273°F). To achieve sterility, a holding time of at least 15 min at 121°C (250°F) at 100 kPa (15 psi) or 3 min at 134°C (273°F) at 100 kPa (15 psi) is required. Due to such high temperature of the steam, microorganisms present in the tools kept in autoclaves are destroyed.
- Additional sterilizing time is usually required for liquids and instruments packed in layers of cloth, as they may take longer to reach the required temperature. Following sterilization, liquids in a pressurized autoclave must be cooled slowly to avoid boiling over when the pressure is released.

■ APPLICATION OF HEAT PRINCIPLES IN NURSING

Study of heat and principles of heat helps the nurses to understand:
- Understanding the temperature regulation of the body will help the nurses to understand the basis of pathophysiology of some of the human disease process such as neonatal hypothermia, heatstroke, frost bite, etc.
- Use of heat and cold applications in healthcare practices to manage several types of disorders such as fever, arthritis, pain, inflammation, injury, etc.
- Accurate measurements of the body temperature and working of clinical thermometer.
- Temperature scales and conversion of one type of temperature scale in another like Centigrade to Fahrenheit Scale or vice versa.
- Transfer of heat from body to surrounding or vice versa, as well as understand about the regulation of body temperature by losing the heat by different means like conduction, convection, radiation and evaporation.
- Use of heat in sterilization for effective destruction of microorganisms including spores.
    - **Use in environment preparation:** To prepare the soothing environment in wards and home environmental temperature and humidity is a big concern. Now a days this is maintained by air conditioning units and a nurse should know adequate setting for them. If air conditioning is not available proper ventilation should be maintained, during summer cooler or clay pitcher or any water filled open utensil can be kept to maintain humidity.
    - **Use in care of neonate and old person**
        - Both neonate and old age person are prone to suffer from hypothermia that may lead to pneumonia, so extra care should be taken care while carrying them. For neonate at birth there should be provision of radiant warmer, clothes should be pre-warmed and placed in skin to skin contact of mother as soon as possible.

- Older people often have diminished temperature sensation and impaired mobility and communication, so they have a tendency to remain in a cool environment. These impairments combined with diminished subcutaneous fat may contribute to hypothermia. For old age person there should be a provision of heater in the room and he or she should wear multilayer cloths instead of single thick cloth as air between layers act as insulator and keep them warm.
- **Use in care during disease condition**
    - *Hypothermia:* Hypothermia is a core body temperature less than 35°C. This is diagnosed by core temperature by rectal and esophageal probes not by oral temperature, electronic thermometers are preferred. Symptoms progress from shivering and lethargy to confusion, coma and death. Mild hypothermia requires a warm environment and insulating blankets (passive rewarming). Severe hypothermia requires active rewarming of the body surface with forced-air warming systems, radiant sources and rewarming of core by inhalation of steam, heated infusion and lavage, extracorporeal blood rewarming.

        During major surgery, if broad area is exposed and also internal organs are exposed then the nurse should aware about the risk of hypothermia and keep the heater and warm infusion ready.
    - *Hyperthermia:* Hyperthermia is defined as a temperature greater than 37.5–38.3°C, (99.5–100.9°F) such elevations range from mild to extreme; body temperatures above 40°C (104°F) can be life-threatening. This can be diagnosed by a clinical thermometer. Symptoms progress from heavy sweating, rapid breathing, fast, weak pulse then hot, dry skin to confusion and aggressive behavior having tachycardia and tachypnea. Eventually, organ failure, unconsciousness and death will result.

        When body temperature is significantly elevated, mechanical cooling methods are used to remove heat and to restore the body's ability to regulate its own temperatures. Passive cooling techniques, such as resting in a cool, shady area and removing clothing can be applied immediately by convention and radiation. Active cooling methods, such as sponging the head, neck, and trunk with cool water, remove heat from the body using latent heat of vaporization and thereby speed the body's return to normal temperatures. Drinking water and turning a fan or dehumidifying air conditioning unit on the affected person may improve the effectiveness of the body's evaporative cooling mechanisms.

        When the body temperature reaches about 40°C (104°F), or if the affected person is unconscious or showing signs of confusion, hyperthermia is considered a medical emergency more aggressive cooling measures are used, including intravenous hydration through cool normal saline gastric lavage with iced normal saline, and even hemodialysis to cool the blood.
    - *Pain:* Heat increases the blood circulation and dilates blood vessels in a particular area so prevents ischemic pain. It also softens the proteins in ligaments to provide relief for stiffed joints and muscles. Increased temperature causes increased movement of molecules of applied oil or medication which cause deeper penetration for local effect during massage. It is used in specific disease conditions such as Arthritis, Stiffness of joints and muscles.

        Opposite to heat cold application causes shrinkage of blood vessels with decrease in blood circulation to a particular area, so it is used to prevent edema and associated pain as at the intra muscular injection site.

- Heat is used during various procedures such as steam inhalation, normal bath, sitz bath, sponging, sterilization, hot water bottle, infrared lamp, massaging, poultice, rubbing of palms.

QUESTIONS

Q.1: Use of bath blanket in bed bath.
Q.2: Effects of steam inhalation in patient with common cold.
Q.3: Why autoclaving is a better sterilization method than simple boiling?
Q.4: Explain difference between heat and temperature. What is the difference between clinical thermometer and laboratory thermometer?
Q.5: Explain the mechanism of temperature regulation by human body and discuss its limitations.
Q.6: Methods of local heating.
Q.7: Running hot water over the medicine bottle metal cap.
Q.8: Heat therapy is given to patients in shock.
Q.9: Use of heat for sterilization.
Q.10: Use of heat in abdominal distension.
Q.11: Sources of heat energy in the hospital setting.

BIBLIOGRAPHY

1. Baierlein R. Thermal Physics. Cambridge University Press, 2003.
2. Cengel YA. Boles M. Thermodynamics—An Engineering Approach (4th edn). McGraw-Hill, 2002.
3. Clark, JOE. The Essential Dictionary of Science. Barnes and Noble Books, 2004.
4. Clausius R. The Mechanical Theory of Heat—with its Applications to the Steam Engine and to Physical Properties of Bodies. London: John Van Voorst, 1 Paternoster Row, 1865.
5. Perrot P. A to Z of Thermodynamics. Oxford University Press, 1998.
6. Reif. Fundamentals of Statistical and Thermal Physics. Singapore: McGraw-Hill, Inc, 2000.
7. Schroeder DV. An introduction to thermal physics. San Francisco, California: Addison-Wesley, 2000: 18.
8. Smith JM, Van Ness HC, Abbot MM. Introduction to Chemical Engineering Thermodynamics. McGraw-Hill, 2005.
9. InformedHealth.org [Internet]. Cologne, Germany: Institute for Quality and Efficiency in Health Care (IQWiG); 2006-. How is body temperature regulated and what is fever? 2009 Jul 30 [Updated 2016 Nov 17]. Available from: https://www.ncbi.nlm.nih.gov/books/NBK279457/
10. Osilla EV, Marsidi JL, Sharma S. Physiology, Temperature Regulation. [Updated 2021 May 7]. In: StatPearls [Internet]. Treasure Island (FL): StatPearls Publishing; 2022 Jan-. Available from: https://www.ncbi.nlm.nih.gov/books/NBK507838/

CHAPTER 12

Light

Suresh K Sharma, Navjot Kaur

Chapter Outline

- Nature of Light
- Law of Reflection and Refraction of Light
- Lenses
- The Physics of Vision
- Defects of Vision and its Corrections
- Biological Effects of the Light
- Uses of Light in Therapy
- X-rays
- Photosensitivity
- Application of Principles of Light in Nursing

■ INTRODUCTION

Almost all life on earth depends on light. Plants convert light energy into chemical energy via photosynthesis: the most basic foundation of almost all food and life cycles. Along with this, light is responsible for the sense of sight. Light and sound are responsible for our communication with the external world. Just as the ear enables us to apprehend sound waves, the eye is the sense organ that enables us to see the objects around us. Light energy from the external environment is transformed into nerve impulse, which is in turn interpreted in the occipital region of the cerebral cortex. Just as the human body is able to detect and interpret sound waves only within a definite range of frequencies, so it is able to detect and interpret as a vision within a certain range of light waves.

■ NATURE OF LIGHT

The nature of light has been a subject of great interest and research since ancient times. We begin with the historic models for light and then will discuss the modern theory.

Corpuscular Theory of Light

Philosophers of the middle ages imagined that luminous bodies emit a stream of particles or corpuscles that produce the sensation of light when they enter the eye. In line with this point of view, Sir Isaac Newton developed the corpuscular theory of light (**Fig. 12.1**).

Fig. 12.1: Light as a particle.

Failures of Corpuscle's Theory of Light

These particles travel without being affected by the earth's pull and produce the sensation of light when they enter the eye. But it failed to explain:
- Light bends around corners (diffraction)
- Light travels faster in a vacuum than in a material medium.
- Light redistributes on superposition.

Wave Theory of Light

Huygens conceived the idea that light is transmitted by waves through a material medium. To explain how light waves could pass from the sun to the earth through apparent space: Huygens postulated that hypothetical luminiferous ether filled all of space. He showed that a wave theory of light could also explain reflection and refraction. In 1801, Thomas Young provided a clear demonstration of the wave nature of light, showing that light rays interfere with each other.
- In 1864, Jams Clark Maxwell proposed the electromagnetic theory of light.
- In 1888, Henrich Hertz measured the electromagnetic waves described by Maxwell.
- In 1895, Hendrick Antoon Horentz advanced the idea that the source of electromagnetic light waves are the motion of the electrons in the atoms of elements, and that as the electrons oscillate or revolve, they emit electromagnetic energy of definite wavelength and frequency (**Fig. 12.2**).

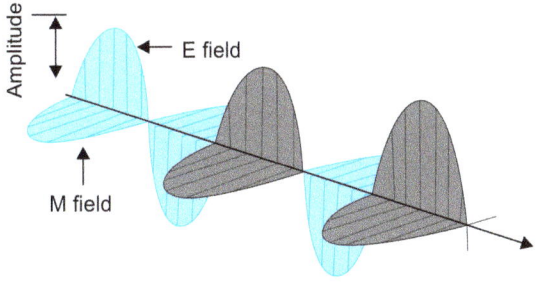

Waves of electromagnetic radiation

Fig. 12.2: Light as a wave.

Failures of Wave Theory of Light

It cannot explain the photoelectric effect. The photoelectric effect is a phenomenon in which ultraviolet light incident on a piece of material causes the ejection of electrons from the surface of the material **(Fig. 12.3)**.

The most remarkable fact about this process is that the energy of electrons emitted by the metal depends on the intensity of the incident light.

Quantum Theory of Light

To explain this, in 1990, Max Planck advanced the quantum theory of light. The quantum theory applied to light waves, states that electron emits energy discontinuously in units of energy called quanta **(Fig. 12.4)**.

Fig. 12.3: Photoelectric effect.

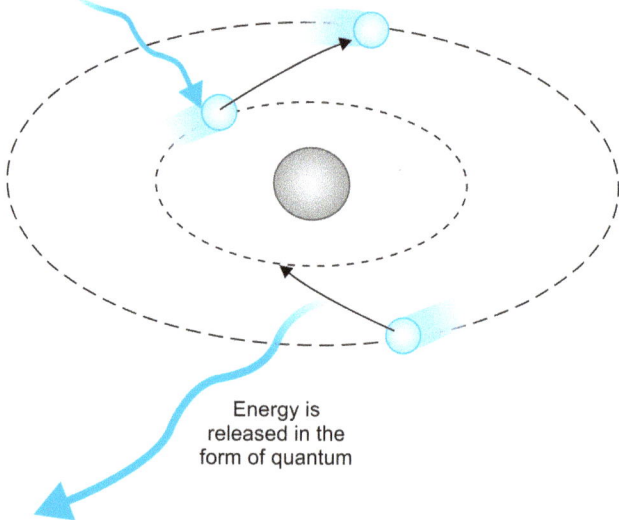

Fig. 12.4: Light in form of quantum.

In 1905, Albert Einstein introduced the use of the term photon, a unit of measurement of quanta of energy. The amount of energy (E) per quantum or photon increases directly as the frequency of light. The frequency (n) may be obtained when the values for velocity of light and the wavelengths are known as

$$n = v/\lambda$$

The energy of a single quantum (photon) is obtained from the following question:

$$E = hn$$

In this relationship, 'h' is known as Planck's constant. It has a value of 6.6256×10^{34} joule-second. For practical purposes, 6.65×10^{34} joule-sec may be used.

If one of these photons is absorbed by an atom of substance, electrons of the atom receive sufficient energy to get ejected from the surface of the substance. The success of Einstein's postulates in explaining experimental observations of the photoelectric effects revealed that light behaves as particles. Thus, you may be tempted to ask how can light behaves as a wave as well as a particle? The answer to this question is yes, light does exhibit dual character. As a wave, it produces interference and diffraction. (These phenomena are not of much interest in medicines) and as particles, it can be absorbed by materials and cause chemical and electrical changes. In fact, the particle character of light is responsible for seeing things when a light photon is absorbed in one of the sensitive cells of the retina. Chemical changes in it induce an electrical signal to the brain.

Light at an Interface

Light is invisible, but makes us to see things. Even the act of reading this text involves images made within our eyes. Before we understand the mechanism for seeing things let us learn what is responsible for the formation of images? To explain optical phenomena, like the formation of images; it is sufficient to assume that light travels in straight lines. That is, we can specify the direction of (Light) wave propagation by a straight line. Such a straight line with arrowheads is referred to as a ray of light **(Fig. 12.5)**.

You are familiar with the reflection and refraction of light. These can and should be explained on the basis of the wave nature of light. But for the present, we shall assume that light travels in straight lines and discuss this phenomenon using the concept of rays of light.

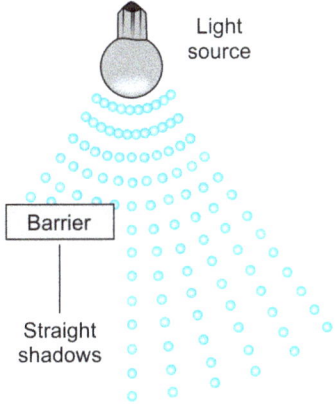

Fig. 12.5: Casting of shadow.

By suitable placement of a source of light energy, the object can be made to cast a sharp shadow. This is the most common illustration of the rectilinear propagation of light. A shadow is formed when an opaque object is placed in the path of light. It intercepts the rays of light and the region in space where light does not reach is termed as a shadow.

■ LAW OF REFLECTION AND REFRACTION OF LIGHT

When light falls on the interface separating two media, one or all of the three following processes can occur **(Fig. 12.6)**:
- The incident light or a part of it is turned back; that is reflected into the first medium.
- The incident light is partly or completely absorbed by the second medium.
- A fraction of the incident light is transmitted, i.e. refracted into the second medium as in the case of air-water interface.

Reflection of Light

A light ray is reflected from a smooth surface according to these two laws of the reflection:
- The angle of incidence is equal to the angle of reflection.
- The incident ray, the reflected ray, and normal to the reflecting plane or surface are coplanar.

If you know the angle of incidence, you can predict the direction of the reflected ray using these laws **(Fig. 12.7)**.

The reflection of light from a smooth surface is called specular reflection **(Fig. 12.8B)**. If the surface is rough, the reflecting rays will not be parallel, but in various random directions, such reflection is called diffuse reflection **(Fig. 12.8A)**.

The difference between the two kinds of reflections explains why it is difficult to drive on a rainy night. When the road is wet, the smooth surface of water specularly reflects most of the headlight beams away from our car and when the road is dry, its surface diffusely reflects part of the headlight beams back towards us, enabling us to see the highway clearly.

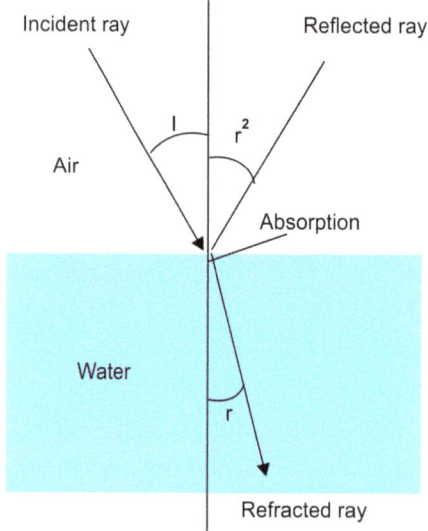

Fig. 12.6: Reflection and refraction of light.

Fig. 12.7: Reflection of light.

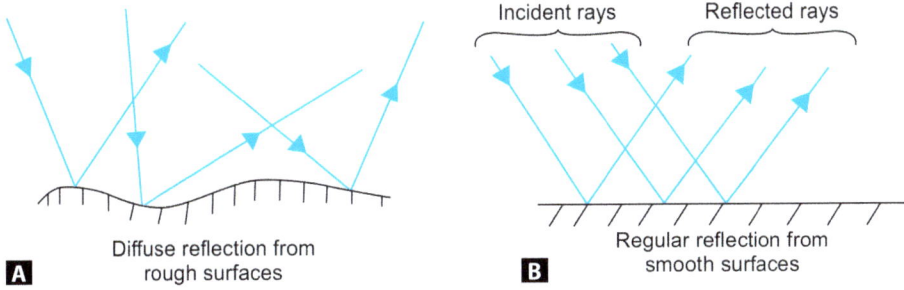

Figs. 12.8A and B: Diffuse and Smooth Reflection of Light.

The process through which light rays fall on the surface and get bounced back is known as a **reflection of light.**

Types of Reflection

Regular Reflection

The plane mirrors with a smooth surface produce this type of reflection. In this case, the image is clear and is very much visible. The images produced by plane mirrors are always virtual, that is they cannot be collected on a screen.

In the case of curved mirrors with a smooth surface, we can see the images of reflection either virtually or really. That is, the images produced by curved mirrors can be either real (collected on a screen and seen), or virtual (cannot be collected on a screen, but only seen).

Irregular Reflection

Unlike mirrors, most natural surfaces are rough on the scale of the wavelength of light, and as a consequence, parallel incident light rays are reflected in many different directions irregularly, or diffusely. Hence, diffuse reflection helps in seeing the objects and is responsible for the ability to see most illuminated surfaces from any position.

Uses of Reflection

- Reflection is used in periscopes to view advancing enemies on the battlefield from a safe position.
- Reflection is the reason why we see objects.
- Reflection by a concave mirror and a convex mirror has many uses.
- Reflection helps in medical diagnosis and optical communications.
- Light and sound both follow the law of reflection, both being waves.
- Using the law of reflection for sound and light, we can measure the distances accurately to objects.
- Reflection is the reason why we hear the echo of sound.

Refraction of Light

When a ray of light is incident on a plane or surface separating two transparent media, ray bends at the time of changing the medium.

"Refraction is the change in the direction of a wave passing from one medium to another." For a given pair of media (for example air or water) the ratio of the sine the angle of incidence to the sine of the angle of refraction is constant for all angles of incidence. This constant is known as the refractive index of one medium with respect to another. We denote it by the symbol μ.

$$\mu = \sin i / \sin r$$

The above relation is called Snell's law. Since refractive indices of different optical media are different, the speed of light changes when it goes from one medium into another. Thus, an alternative definition of the refractive index of a medium is the ratio of speed of light in a vacuum to its speed in a given medium.

Since velocity of light $c = \nu\lambda$ refractive indices for lights of different colors will have different values. The value increases from the red end of the visible spectrum to the violet. This suggests that refraction index is essentially a property of the medium since velocity of the same light is different in different media.

Refractive index of ordinary glass is 1.3, whereas that of water is 1.5, i.e. glass is denser than the water.

Further, a ray of light bends towards the normal when it goes from a rarer to denser medium **(Fig. 12.9)**. Further extent of bending is a function of wavelength of light. That is why sunlight which consists of seven colors (wavelengths), is split into a spectrum of seven colors when it passes through a prism.

Refraction of Light in Real Life

- Mirage and looming are optical illusions resulting from the refraction of light.
- A swimming pool always looks shallower than it really is because the light coming from the bottom of the pool bends at the surface due to refraction of light.
- Formation of a rainbow is an example of refraction as the sun rays bend through the raindrops resulting in the rainbow.
- When white light passes through a prism it is split into its component colors—red, orange, yellow, green, blue and violet due to refraction of light.

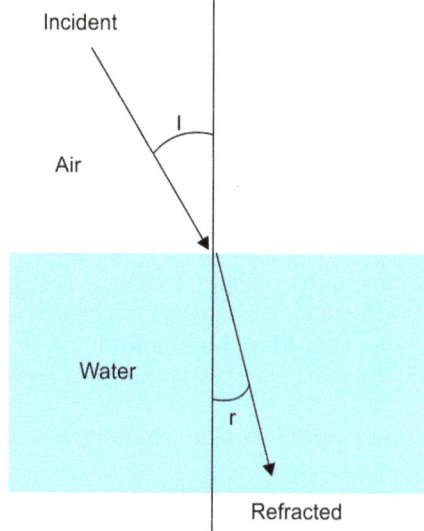

Fig. 12.9: Refraction of light.

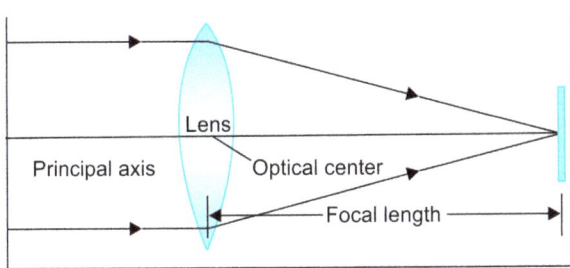

Fig. 12.10: Basic features of a lens

LENSES

All of us are familiar with the lenses. We all have lenses in our eyes, some of us have lenses in our spectacles. A lens is made of transparent material and is bounded by two spherical surfaces. Lenses are commonly used to form images via refraction in cameras, microscopes, etc. Light passing through a lens experiences refraction at two surfaces.

Features of Lens

Following are the basic features of the lens (**Fig. 12.10**):
- **Principal axis/optic axis:** It is a line that passes through the center of curvature of the lens and is perpendicular to the surface.
- **Optical center:** This is a point on the principal axis of equidistance from both surfaces of the lens. Rays of light passing through the optical center do not change their direction and pass through the lens undeviated.
- **Principal focus:** Rays parallel to the principal axis of the lens, after refraction converges to (or appears to diverge from) a point. This point is called the principal focus.
- **Focal length:** The distance from the optical center of the lens to the principal focus.

Lenses and Images

To locate an image made by some object in front of a thin convex lens graphically. Only a few rays need to be drawn through many others exist. The essential rays that are drawn are one along the principal axis, one parallel to it, and one along the secondary axis (**Fig. 12.11**).

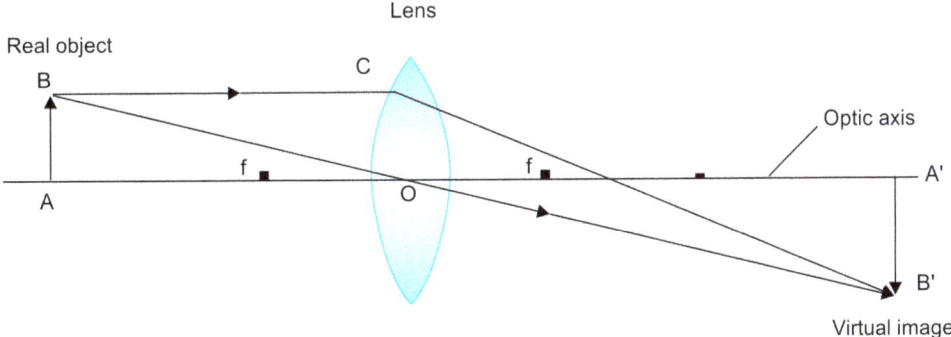

Fig. 12.11: Formation of an image in case of a convex lens.

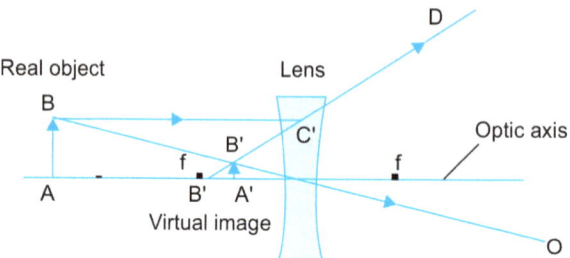

Fig. 12.12: Formation of an image in case of a concave lens.

When an object is placed on the principal axis at a distance from the lens greater than its focal length, (in the diagram object is represented by AB), Ray BC from the tip of the arrow is drawn parallel to the principal axis.

The ray is refracted and passes through the principal focus (FL) to form ray CB'. Another ray (BO) passes through the optical center. It is not refracted and continuous on as ray CB' and OB' meet an image of arrow tip will be formed. If point B' is now connected to the principal axis by a perpendicular line at point A' an image of the arrow will be formed. A screen placed at this point will reproduce on its surface a real and inverted image of the arrow.

In the case of a concave diverging lens, if the source of light is far away and all the rays enter the lens parallel to the principal axis, the rays will be refracted outward and diverge. No real image can be obtained behind the lens was the case with a converging lens, like ray AO is drawn again along the principal axis. Ray BO is parallel to the principal axis. It is bent outwardly and diverges, however from C'D. Ray BO passes through the optical center. In this case, if ray C'D is extended, it meets BO at point B' where the image of the tip appears. As before, if a line is drawn perpendicular from B to the principal axis, the vertical image of the arrow A'B' appears erect and reduced in size **(Fig. 12.12)**.

■ THE PHYSICS OF VISION

The eye is one of the most important human organs. It is responsible for visual contact with nature and all its creations. The helplessness we feel in the dark, particularly in the unfamiliar surroundings, only brings out our dependence on vision. The processes involved in producing the functioning of three major components; the eyes, optic nerves, and visual cortex. In case of dysfunction of any of these parts, blindness results.

Structure of Eye

The basic components of the structure of the eye are following **(also Fig. 12.13)**:
- The eye is like a thick convex lens, which forms images on the retina.
- A white membrane called the sclera covers the eye externally. Its front portion is transparent and more convex than the rest of the eye. It is called the cornea.
- Internal to the cornea is a dark brown membrane called choroids.
- In the front portion of the choroids is a sheath of muscles called the ciliary muscle.
- A circular diaphragm perforated at the center hangs from the ciliary muscles. This diaphragm is called the iris.
- The focusing lens of the eye, which is a biconvex lens is suspended behind the iris. The color of the iris gives color to the eye.

Fig. 12.13: Structure of the eye.

- A purple-red membrane stretches at the internal back portion of the choroids. It is light sensitive and is known as the retina. The retina contains light receptor nerve cells, which receive the light waves.
- The optic nerve fibers carry light sensations from the nerve cells to the visual center of the brain.

The Action of the Eye

Light enters the eye through the hard and transparent cornea into a fluid called aqueous humor. It then passes through the eye lens and vitreous humor via the iris. The combination of the cornea, aqueous humor, lens, and vitreous humor focuses the incoming light on the retina, in the normal eye, the principal focal point coincides with the retina so that all objects are focused on it. The real inverted image formed on the retina is transmitted to the brain. Most of the refraction, which causes image formation in the retina, actually takes place at the cornea and vitreous humor. But the focal length of the lens is adjustable and enables fine adjustment in our vision.

Power of Accommodation

When an image is formed by a lens, the image distance (distance of the image from the optical center of the lens) varies with the object distance (distance of the object from the center of the lens).

We know that image is formed on the retina by the eye lens and the distance of the retina from the eye lens is fixed. So the image distance from the human eye is fixed. Thus to see the objects, at varying distances from the eye, the focal length of the eye lens must change. The change in the focal length of the eye lens is involuntary, the image, however, is always formed on the retina. This capacity of the eye lens to change its focal is called the power of accommodation.

The normal eye can focus on near as well as infinitely remote objects on the retina. The power of accommodation lies in the ciliary muscles, which are connected to the suspensory ligaments in such a way that when the muscles contract, the ligaments relax, releasing the tension on the lens. The lens rounds are in position for near vision and vice versa.

Least Distance of Distant Vision

For every eye, there is a limit to its power of accommodation. This power ceases for objects beyond a certain minimum distance from the eye. The nearest distance up to, which a small object can be seen distinctly, is called the near point of the eye. The distance of the near point from the eye is called the least distance of distant vision. For a normal eye, it is about 25 cm.

We may, therefore, conclude that the human optical system has the following features, which are not available in the most expensive cameras.

- The eye can observe events over a very large angle even while looking intently at an object directly ahead of it.
- Blinking provides the cornea with a built-in lens a cleaner and lubricator vision.
- A rapid automatic focusing system permits viewing objects at far away distances as well as near objects at a short interval.
- The eye can operate over a wide range of light intensities; daylight and dark light.
- The eye has a self-regulating pressure system that maintains internal pressure (20 mm Hg) and keeps the eye in shape.
- The images are blended perfectly giving a good depth perception.

DEFECTS OF VISION AND ITS CORRECTIONS

Defects of the vision are as follows:
- Hypermetropia or long-sightedness
- Myopia or short-sightedness
- Presbyopia or far-sightedness
- Astigmatism

Hypermetropia or Long-sightedness or Hyperopia

Hyperopia is a very common refractive condition in childhood and adults. A long-sighted person cannot see near objects distinctly. For long-sighted persons, the distance of near point is greater than 25 cm. This is because the image of an object is placed at the near point from the eye is formed behind the retina.

Conventionally the hyperopia is etiologically classified into:

Axial hyperopia (most common-simple hyperopia): It is due to anterior-posterior axial shortening of the eyeball. Genetic predisposition plays an important role. Retinal edema can cause a hyperopic shift. A 1 mm decrease in axial length leads to 3 diopters of hyperopia.

Curvature hyperopia: It is due to flattening of the cornea or the lens or both. A radius of curvature increases by 1 mm leads to 6 diopters of hyperopia.

Index hyperopia: It is due to the change in the refractive index of the crystalline lens, which occurs in old age or diabetics. The refractory index gradually increases from the center to the periphery.

Positional hyperopia or **absence of the lens (aphakia)** or **ocular pathologic conditions**: This condition occurs due to malposition or absence of the crystalline lens (congenital or acquired) or intraocular lens owing to the creation of an aphakic zone in refractive media. Post-traumatic or post-surgical aphakia is not an uncommon cause of hyperopia.

This defect arises because:
- The eyeball is too short.
- The focal length of the lens is elongated.
- This is normally seen in elderly persons.
- To correct this defect, we interpose a convex lens (converging lens). As a result, the focal length of the combination (eye and lens) decreases and the image is formed on the retina **(Fig. 12.14)**.

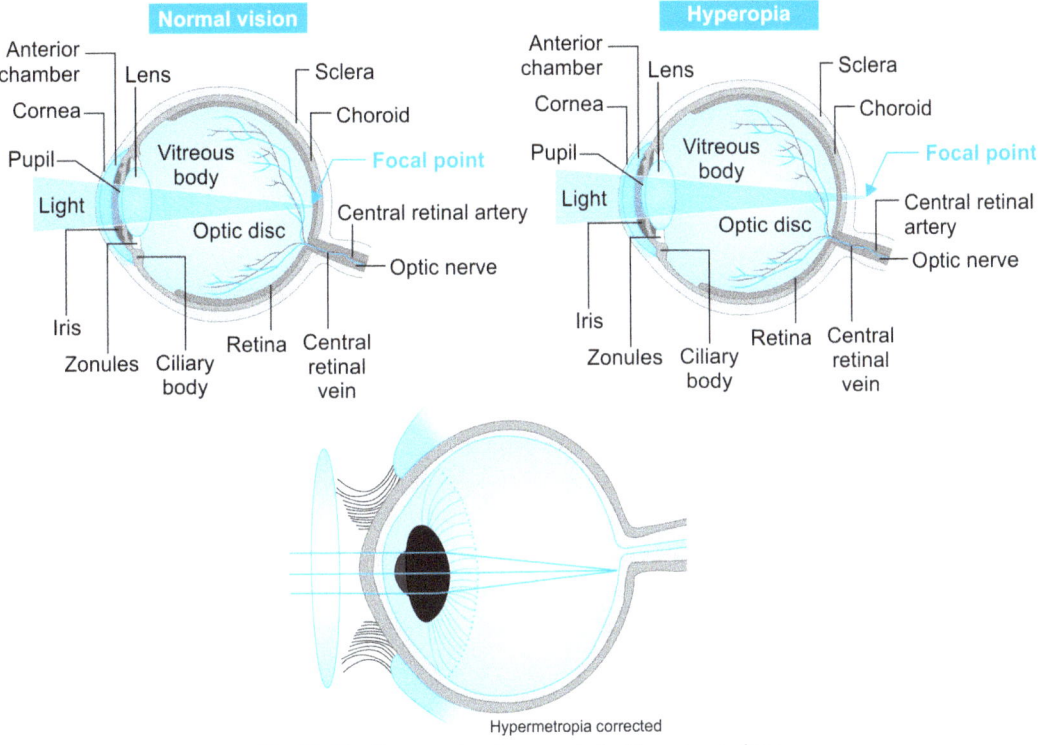

Fig .12.14: Hypermetropia corrected with a convex lens.

Myopia or Short Sightedness

A shortsighted person cannot see distant objects distinctly. The image is formed in front of the retina.

This defect can arise due to:
- Elongation of the eyeball.
- The focal length of the eye lens is too short.
- It is seen in school or college- going children.
- To correct this defect, a concave (diverging) lens is used **(Fig. 12.15)**.

Presbyopia or far Sightedness

This defect is long-sightedness caused due to old age. A progressive decrease in the accommodative capacity of the lens is the major cause of presbyopia. The lenses of the eye, which are crystalline, lose elasticity gradually with age, and the accommodation power of ciliary muscles decreases. Thus, the short-sighted eye in childhood tends to become normal in later years, but the defect of long-sightedness is sure to increase gradually. This defect is corrected by the use of the bifocal lens.

Astigmatism

It is an optical defect, whereby vision is blurred due to the inability of the optics of the eye to focus a point object into a sharp focused image on the retina. This image may be due to an irregular or toric curvature of the lens or cornea.

Fig. 12.15: Myopia corrected with a concave lens.

It is of two types:
1. **Irregular:** It is caused by corneal scar or scattering in the crystalline lens. It cannot be corrected by a spectacles lens but by a contact lens.
2. **Regular:** It is due to a toric surface like a doughnut, where there are two regular radii, one smaller than the other. It can be corrected by a spectacles lens.

■ BIOLOGICAL EFFECTS OF THE LIGHT

Light may regulate a number of biological processes and also the structural as well as behavioural characteristics of animals. The important effects of light on animals are as given below: :

Effect on Metabolism

The absorbed radiant energy heats the tissues and causes protoplasm ionization. This improves enzyme activity and overall metabolic rate. Cave animals, which have little light, have a slower metabolism. The amount of absorption of calcium is influenced by the amount of light to which a person is subjected. It was seen that 15% absorption of calcium was increased when a person was exposed 8 hours daily for 4 weeks to 500-foot candles of broad-spectrum fluorescent light.

Effect on Locomotion

Many lower organisms are controlled by light to control their speed of locomotion (Photokinesis). Studies on blind mussel crab larvae (Pinnotheres maculatus), have shown an increase in swimming speed with increasing illumination. The role of light is often important in orientating locomotion. Phototaxis is the movement of animals in response to light. Positive phototactic is when an animal moves toward the source of light, e.g. Euglena. If it moves away, it is called negative phototactic. (e.g., earthworms, slugs). This can also be noticed that children are active in daytime or in bright light and less active in darkness.

Effect on Development

Some animals have accelerated or retarded development due to light as Salmon larvae develop normally when there is enough light. The absence of light causes abnormal egg development and results in a high mortality rate for larvae. The larvae of Mytilus grow larger in darkness than in the light. The intensity of the light in the environment affects the development of the eyes in many cave-dwelling animals, such as Proteus eyes are either missing or very basic. The eyes of deep-sea fishes and nocturnal animals are larger in size.

Pigmentation Effects

Different light conditions can affect the pigmentation of plants and animals. Due to lack of light, cave animals are often devoid of pigments. Many animals have pigmentation that gives them protection against enemies. This is known as "protective coloration". The body color of a leaf insect is, for example, similar to a leaf. Melanocytes in human skin produce melanin stimulated by Ultraviolet radiations. This is a protective mechanism against further injury to DNA of cells.

Photoperiodicity and Photosensitivity

Photoperiodism is the organism's response to day length. Many organisms have a 24-hour cycle of activity. This is known as diurnal periodicity or circadian rhythm. Photosynthesis, which is subject to fluctuations due to light changes daily, is the most important diurnal rhythm. Copepods, and other planktonic creatures, move toward the surface of the water at night while moving downwards during the day. Some animals are more active in daylight than in darkness, and vice versa. Many organisms' activities in relation to their reproductive cycle are closely related to the moon. This phenomenon is called lunar periodicity. This is when the biological rhythm occurs once or twice per lunar month. Semilunar rhythms occur in 15 days. Lunar rhythms occur in 30 days.

* Sometimes interaction of light with some chemicals results in toxic substances in the body that may produce a rash. This photosensitizing property is beneficial in the treatment of some skin disorders such as skin cancer, herpes, psoriasis, etc.
  * In the case of malignancy, photosensitizing agents seem to inactivate DNA in unwanted cells.
  * In herpes and psoriasis, these agents inactivate DNA in the protoplasm of causative organisms.
* Light is effective in treating jaundice in infants.

Influence on Reproduction and Gonads

Light is the key too many animals, including birds, launching their annual breeding activities. In summer, birds' gonads are more active due to increased light. Animals can be classified into short, long, or indifferent day animals. Short-day animals such as deer, sheep, and goats are sexually active during decreased exposure to daylight. Birds that breed in spring experience a lengthening day and are also known as long-day animals. Guinea pigs and squirrels are not affected by daylight. They are therefore indifferent day animals. Light may have a significant influence on the sexual maturity of humans as it has been proven that girls who are blind have an earlier menarche than girls who are normally sighted.

Endocrines: Effect

Evidence suggests that there is a circadian rhythm in the secretion of thyrotrophin-releasing factor and rhythmic variation in ACTH secretion and corticotrophin-releasing factor from the hypothalamus. When rats are continuously exposed to light for a prolonged period of time, the cyclic pattern in gonadotrophins release is eliminated and the normal cycle of the oestrus is replaced with a state of constant oestrus. The constant light stimulus may inhibit the activity of pineal glands, according to some theories. Ultraviolet radiations act on the skin and are effective in the synthesis of vitamin D. In animal experimentation, it is found to inhibit ovulation and modify the secretions of other hormones such as serotonin.

Diapause

A type of dormancy in animals is called diapause. It can occur at any stage of the animal's life cycle, such as egg, larvae, pupa, or adult. Diapause has the same causative mechanisms as plants, i.e. Hormones that are regulated by environmental stimuli.

Below a certain threshold, diapause can occur. Insect to insect, the critical amount of daylight is different. It takes approximately 12 hours for cabbage white butterflies. The pupae go into diapause when the light drops below this level. They do not resume their development until the next spring. Experimentally, it has been proven that light does not stimulate the eyes. Covering them does not stop the diapause response. The light stimulates the brain directly, and possibly produces other substances that inhibit growth-stimulating hormones. In some species, the end of diapause and the transition to longer days could be the most effective stimulant. However, in insects, a certain period of cold is required before growth can be resumed. This is similar to stratification in seeds or buds.

Circadian Rhythm and Health Aspects

Circadian rhythm coordinates a wide variety of body processes, including sleep. The circadian pacemaker is a tiny part of the brain that is strongly influenced by light exposure. Human biology evolved to sleep according to the daily cycles of daylight and darkness. A person's circadian rhythm is closely controlled by sunrise. This allows them to stay awake during daylight hours and sleep when it gets dark. Modern society has many light sources, which can affect the brain's circadian rhythm maker.

The amount of light that we are exposed to each day, as well as the time and duration, can have a significant impact on our sleep quality. Understanding the intricate links between light exposure and sleep will help us to set up our bedroom for consistent, high-quality sleep for patients.

A person's circadian rhythm can be disrupted by excessive or inappropriate artificial light exposure. This can disrupt their sleep and cause other health effects such as eye strain, weight gain, metabolic problems, cardiovascular problems, and even a higher cancer risk. The mood and mental health of people are affected by their circadian rhythms. Seasonal effective disorders, for example, is a form of depression that affects those who live in areas with very short winter months. The winter season can bring about mood changes by reducing daylight.

Melatonin, a hormone naturally produced by the body and closely linked to light. The pineal gland in the brain produces melatonin when it is dark. Light exposure can slow down or stop this production. The hormone is known to increase sleepiness when melatonin levels rise. Daily cycles of melatonin release help to maintain a steady sleep-wake rhythm by normalizing the circadian rhythm. Some people may need synthetic melatonin to regulate their sleep time.

Each sleep cycle has its own characteristics. A person will go through between 70 and 120 minutes of sleep each night. These cycles include multiple stages of sleep, they also include rapid eye movement (REM), and non-REM sleep. Night-time light exposure can slow down transitions between sleep cycles and reduce the quality. Repeated awakenings can disrupt the sleep cycle, resulting in a decrease in time spent in deep, more restorative stages.

Jet lag occurs after long-distance flight travel. Because the body's internal clock remains attuned to the departure time zone, it is most common after crossing five to more time zones. A person might have difficulty falling asleep, wake up early, or feel tired during the day. Jet lag is usually addressed by adjusting to the new time zone. This can be done by getting sunlight at certain times or avoiding light at other times. This will help to align your circadian rhythm. This can take up to two weeks and may take several days.

Shift workers are often devoid of sleep during the night, which puts them at risk for a misaligned circadian rhythm or the development of shift work disorder. This disorder of the circadian rhythm can lead to insufficient sleep, excessive sleepiness at inappropriate times, mood problems, and increased risk for workplace accidents.

Blue light has a shorter wavelength and is emitted from many LEDs. It has been shown to have a greater effect on melatonin and the circadian rhythm than light that emits a longer wavelength. Many electronic devices such as cell phones, tablets, and laptops emit blue light. This can lead to sleep problems.

Although blue light can be reduced by many phones and tablets, it may still cause sleep disturbances due to stimulation from the screen. Some people are not able or willing to sleep in the darkness. They can use a dim red light source as red light can increase levels of melanin and helps our bodies prepare for bed.

To promote sleep, the first thing that should be done in the bedroom is to make it dark. To create a dark environment, blackout curtains block most of the light from outside. Keep lights dimmed when getting ready to go to bed. A small, low-power lamp may help in the transition to sleep and pitch darkness. Warm color temperature and low illuminance can help to relax and get into the right frame of mind for sleep. Healthy sleep can be supported by routines and habits.

Light therapy is one treatment for many circadian disorders. This involves sitting near a powerful lamp at set times to reset the body's internal clock. To normalize circadian timing, the strong lamp mimics daylight. It is commonly used in the morning. Although all lighting can impact sleep, not all lights have the same effect. Direct sunlight can produce up to 10,000 lux. This is more than bright office lighting, which only rarely exceeds 500 lux. Daylight has a significant influence on sleep and circadian timing. Current studies are being conducted in which human beings are exposed to constant artificial light (absence of normal cyclic exposure) for months. In these cases, the body rhythms become circadian or approximately 24 hours in length.

■ USES OF LIGHT IN THERAPY

The light has significance in medical science.. Some of the common diagnostic and therapeutic uses of light are discussed below **(Fig. 12.16)**.

Visible Light in Medicine

❖ Visible light is responsible for visual information about the patient, e.g., colors of the skin, to detect the presence of abnormal structures.

Fig. 12.16: Application of visible light in diagnostic tools.

- ENT specialist examines internal parts of the ear, nose, or throat by using a curved mirror with a hole in the middle and another lighted instrument called an examination otoscope.
- An ophthalmoscope is used by ophthalmologists for examining the eye.
- Endoscopes-like cystoscopes, proctoscopes, bronchoscopes that are rigid are used to view internal body cavities. Flexible endoscopes by the use of fiber optic techniques are also being discovered. These are mainly used to view the small and large intestines.
- Transillumination (in which light is passed into the body through the skin) is used to study hydrocephalus and pneumothorax in infants. The sinuses, breasts and testes are also examined by this method.
- Visible light is a form of energy and is selectively absorbed by certain molecules. This enables us to use visible light for therapy, particularly in infants, it is successfully used to treat jaundice and maintain their body temperature.

Infrared Radiation

- The transfer of heat energy by radiation from the surface of hot objects is in the form of infrared rays.
- Infrared rays are invisible; penetrate mist, fog, and the tissues of the body better than visible light does.
- Special film sensitive to infrared rays can be used on foggy days to produce photographs. By using visible light, infrared light or black light, as it is sometimes called, photographs can be taken in complete darkness. Infrared photography is especially useful in certain cardiovascular conditions. The light penetrates the skin, permitting the veins under the skin to be photographed.
- Baking lamps used to produce invisible infrared rays in the home or hospital may give visible light and orange light in addition.
- Infrared light is emitted by incandescent lamps, steam pipes, hot stoves, heating pads, and hot water bottles.

- Infrared radiation is classified into two categories mainly near-infrared and far-infrared. Near-infrared radiation has a wavelength range from 700 A to 5,000 A and far-infrared radiation has a wavelength range from 25,000 A to 200,000 A.
- The warmth due to the radiation from the sun is most beneficial for the human body. They can penetrate through the tissues of the body from 1 to 10 mm.
- Infrared radiation heat lamps and heating pads to heat tissues for relieving pain due to muscle ligaments, backache, spondylosis, etc.
- Another clinical application of infrared radiation in medicine is thermography.

Thermography

- It is a method of recording photographically, the heat emitted through the skin at various points on the body **(Fig. 12.17)**.
- Thermograph is an infrared camera that in addition to being extremely sensitive to heat emitted by an area of the body is able to transfer heat into an electric current. The current then operates a visible light of variable intensity that is recorded on a photographic film. The resulting pictorial representations are called thermographs.
- Because most tumors have temperatures 1 or 2°C higher than those of surrounding areas, they can be detected by thermography. On the thermogram, the relatively warmer tumor appears lighter in color than the cooler surrounding area.
- Several principles of physics explain medical thermography. The law that describes the relationship between temperature and radiation is the 'Stefan-Boltzman law'.
  - Total radiations emitted from a surface is proportional to the fourth power of its absolute temperature.
  - Although, variations within the range of 23 to 36°C occur normally.

Uses

- Diagnosis of tumor and arthritis.
- Effects of drugs or other agents on the body.
- In the diagnosis and treatment of rheumatic diseases.
- Detection of breast cancer and ocular diseases.

Fig. 12.17: Thermography.

SECTION 2: Biophysics

ULTRAVIOLET RADIATION

They are basically of two types:
- Near UV radiation: 2,900 to 3,900 A wavelength.
- Far UV radiation: 1,800 to 2,900 A wavelength.
  - Both types of radiation are superficial. Both produce chemical changes in the tissues. UV radiations are produced artificially by solids heated to a very high temperature of approximately 3,000°C by either establishing an electric arc between metal and carbon electrodes or by producing glowing mercury vapors.

Uses

- Production of erythema
- Exfoliation
- Activation of ergosterol in the skin to form vitamin D.
- Bactericidal effects due to changes in the protein molecules of organisms at 2,650 A wavelength.
- Radiations are also used for sterilization of air using 2,500 A wavelength radiations.
- It improves general body resistance.
- In the treatment of rickets and tuberculosis.
- As a counterirritant in neuritis, lumbago, and fibrositis.
- In the treatment of skin conditions such as psoriasis, acne vulgaris, etc.

Dangers and Precautions

- Many lamps known as sun lamps produce UV radiation. Their use is prohibited by the Council on Physical Medicine of the American Medical Association because it can cause conjunctivitis and other abnormal conditions of the eye.
- It results from the snow that in bright sunshine reflects a large amount of UVsradiation, electric welding arcs, and other sources of UV rays.
- When UV rays are administered, the eyes of the operator should be protected by clear or dark glasses and the eyes of the patient by pledgets of cotton or gauze moistened with water, which absorbs the radiations.
- Water has an absorption spectrum of 1,800 to 3,000 A in the UV region. This limits the amount of radiation that reaches the organism immersed in water. Similarly, the amount of water vapor in the air limits these radiations from reaching the earth's surface.

X-RAYS

- X-rays are electromagnetic waves of an extremely short wavelength of approximately 0.01 nm up to 10 nm and of high frequency.
- They were discovered by roentgen in 1895. He discovered it while he was considering the question of luminescence from the cathode tube with which he was experimenting. He discovered in his studies that an invisible penetrating radiations came from the tube and affected a photographic plate. Because the tube was covered by an opaque shield and because the electron in the tube could not penetrate the glass, he concluded that the unknown radiations were coming from the walls of the tube where the electrons were striking the glass. In addition, because the waves could pass through the glass, roentgen considered these unknown X-rays to be very penetrating. Roentgen further studies on the nature of X-rays led to their use medically within three months after discovery.

- The type of tube used to produce X-rays was refined by Coolidge in 1913. X-rays may be produced in a vacuum tube by the bombardment of a metal target with a stream of electrons moving at high speed. The metal target is usually made up of tungsten or molybdenum. When the electrons strike the target, they are stopped and about 99% of the energy of the electrons is converted to heat. The remaining 1% of energy is converted to X-rays.
- X-rays have great power of penetration and when passed through the body, affect a photographic plate and produce a "negative picture" or a "shadowgraph". Structures and tissues that allow the rays to pass through them easily appear dark on the developed film and those that do not allow the rays to pass appear as lighter areas on the film.
- X-rays, as it is frequently referred to result from photons of electromagnetic energy. As we know,

$$E = hn$$
$$E = c/\lambda$$
$$\lambda = hc/E$$

So wavelength can be known.

Types

- Hard or high energy X-rays
- Soft or low energy X-rays

The relationship between the energy and wavelength is
$$\lambda = 1/E$$

- So those with high energy are of shorter wavelength and vice versa. Hard X-rays that are used for deep therapy have an average wavelength of 0.14 A. They are generated at about 200 kV. Softer X-rays used for diagnosis or superficial therapy have wavelengths of about 0.7 to 0.5 A and are generated by the voltage of 75 to 100 kV, respectively. The voltage applied in generating the radiations controls the hardness and softness of the X-rays.

Units

The unit of dosage used in X-ray therapy is the roentgen. It is defined as the amount of radiation that the associated corpuscular emission in 1 ml of air at a temperature of 0°C and a pressure of 760 mm of Hg produces in air ions carrying electrostatic units of electricity of either sign. The roentgen refers to ionization produced in the air.

Uses

- When the X-rays pass through the body tissues, ionization of the matter occurs and the position of the electrons within the body tissues changes, producing chemical changes that are destructive to the cells. Cells of malignant tumors are more susceptible to the effect than are the normal cells X-rays are useful in the treatment of superficial lesions of skin cancer and also in irradiatinggdeep-lying tumors of visceral organs.
- When it is necessary tos X-ray the ventricle of the brain, the ventricles are tapped and cerebrospinal fluid is removed. The ventricles are then filled with air. When X-rays are passed through the skull and brain, the air in the ventricles retards their passage and the ventricles are outlined on the photographic plate.
- Certain chemicals such as barium sulfate and diodrast are opaque to X-rays. They are used when it is necessary to outline an organ such as the stomach, kidney or urinary bladder. Since the X-rays do not pass through the organs caused by these chemicals, the organs appear as light shadows on the developed plate.

Fig. 12.18: Photosensitivity.

- By the same principle, air O_2, CO_2, etc. may be injected into the fascial spaces around the kidneys to mark the adrenal glands.
- A miniature radiographic tube for intracavitary insertion has been reported to be used in dentistry to obtain an 'inside-out' wide-angle picture of teeth and jaw.

■ PHOTOSENSITIVITY

It has been seen that administration of dye substances such as methylene blue and other drugs such as quinine to the patients has sometimes resulted in sensitivity reactions to light and possess a potential danger to human life. It is due to the production of the toxic material as a result of the interaction of drugs or dye with light. This phenomenon is known as photosensitivity reactions. An explanation for this reaction is related to the activation of molecules by light energy when a photon of light is absorbed by a molecule, such as dye, energy is transferred to the molecule and raises it to the level of energy above that which it had originally. This increase in energy may appear as heat because of the many collisions of the "activated" molecules with others or the energy may be emitted again from the molecules as another form of light. In still other situations, the molecule may retain the excess energy and remain in the activated state for some time. Most of these reactions are limited to the light of shorter wavelengths. Now in the case of dye, activated dye molecules react with the molecules of the substrate in which they are located (this may be the protoplasm of the cell) to form a substance that is capable of being oxidized. According to one theory, this oxidation product is abnormal and harmful to the organisms and is responsible for the production of symptoms of hypersensitivity (**Fig. 12.18**).

■ APPLICATION OF PRINCIPLES OF LIGHT IN NURSING

Study of principles of lights nurses will be able to understand:
- Nature of light, will enable nurses to understand the use of light in different healthcare practices.
- Refractive errors of the eye and will understand the corrective measures by using a different type of lenses.

- Use of light in different diagnostic tools like an otoscope, ophthalmoscope, proctoscope, cystoscope and colonoscope, etc.
- Use of light in the management of different medical disorders like treatment of malignancies, skin problems, etc.
- Nurses will be able to understand the biological effect of the light on the human body.
- Understand the mechanism of the photosensitivity.

QUESTIONS

Q.1: Write two applications of infrared rays in nursing practice.
Q.2: Define power of accommodation. Name the defect of vision related to it and how it is corrected.
Q.3: Use of laser in the repair and treatment of detached retina.
Q.4: Diverging lens to treat Myopia.
Q.5: Explain how X-rays can be used in medicine. What are the limitations of conventional X-rays and how they can be overcome?
Q.6: What is ionizing radiation and how does it damage living organisms? What measures are taken to re- duce exposure to X-rays in hospital?
Q.7: When we enter the dark room, why we have to wait for sometime to see the things in the room.
Q.8: Describe the main features of eye and show how it forms images.
Q.9: Barium sulfate is used to outline organs. Explain.
Q.10: Irradiation by UV rays in case of neonatal jaundice.
Q.11: Lens of the eye and accommodation.
Q.12: Causes of blackout of vision at high angular acceleration.

BIBLIOGRAPHY

1. Cassidy D, Holton G, Rutherford J. Understanding Physics. Birkhäuser, 2002.
2. Hallo GH. Camera lenses: from box camera to digital. SPIE Press, 2006.
3. Hamarneh S. Review of Hakim Mohammed Said, Ibn al-Haitham, Isis, 1972; 63 (1): 119.
4. InformedHealth.org [Internet]. Cologne, Germany: Institute for Quality and Efficiency in Health Care (IQWiG); 2006-. Presbyopia: Overview. [Updated 2020 Jun 4]. Available from: https://www.ncbi.nlm.nih.gov/books/NBK423833/
5. Kalumuck KE. Human body explorations: hands-on investigations of what makes us tick. Kendall Hunt, 2000.
6. Kumar N. Comprehensive Physics XII. Laxmi Publications, 2008.
7. Longair, Malcolm. Theoretical Concepts in Physics, 2003: 87.
8. MacKay RJ, Oldford RW. "Scientific Method, Statistical Method and the Speed of Light", Statistical Science, August 2000, 15 (3): 254–78.
9. Majumdar S, Tripathy K. Hyperopia. [Updated 2022 Feb 21]. In: StatPearls [Internet]. Treasure Island (FL): StatPearls Publishing; 2022 Jan-. Available from: https://www.ncbi.nlm.nih.gov/books/NBK560716/
10. Nichols EF, Hull GF. The Pressure due to Radiation, The Astrophysical Journal, 1903;17 (5):315–51.
11. Ptolemy, Smith AM. Ptolemy's Theory of Visual Perception: An English Translation of the Optics with Introduction and Commentary. Diane Publishing, 1996.
12. Rashed, Roshdi. "The Celestial Kinematics of Ibn al-Haytham", Arabic Sciences and Philosophy. Cambridge University Press, 2007.
13. Singh P, Tripathy K. Presbyopia. [Updated 2022 Feb 21]. In: StatPearls [Internet]. Treasure Island (FL): StatPearls Publishing; 2022 Jan-. Available from: https://www.ncbi.nlm.nih.gov/books/NBK560568/
14. Verma RL. Al-Hazen: father of modern optics, 1969.
15. Vyasa, Krishna-Dwai. The Mahabharata of Krishna-Dwaipayana Vyasa 1st Book Adi Parva, The Echo Library, 2000.

CHAPTER 13

Pressure and Fluid Mechanics

Navjot Kaur, Shiv Kumar Mudgal

Chapter Outline
- Importance of Pressure in the Human Body
- Atmospheric Pressure
- Applications of Atmospheric Pressure
- Hydrostatic Pressure
- Applications of Pascal's Law
- Pressure in Flowing Fluids
- Osmotic Pressure
- Applications of the Osmotic Pressure
- Measurement of Pressures
- Applications of these Principles in Nursing

■ INTRODUCTION

In day-to-day life, we use the word pressure in a number of different contexts. Students feel the pressure of work during examination days. Many a time we talk of political pressure. When the water coming out of our taps has low-speed, we say that water pressure is low. The steam pressure is used to cook food. Air pressure in car tyres permits safe driving. The weather man tells us the atmospheric pressure and the doctor measures our blood pressure. In physics, like work, pressure has a definite meaning. It is defined as follows:

"Pressure is the force on a unit surface area".

If the force F is acting on a surface of area A, the pressure P is given by:

$$P \frac{F}{A}$$

- ❖ The pressure exerted by fluids is called fluid pressure.
- ❖ The SI unit of pressure is called Pascal and is denoted by the symbol 'Pa'.
- ❖ Pressure has no fixed direction and is therefore a scalar quantity.
    - You probably know that atmospheric pressure is about 10^5 Pa. In medical practice, the most common method of indicating pressure is by the height of a column of mercury. The pressure of a column of liquid can be calculated using the relation:

$$P = hdg$$

- Where 'd' is the density of the liquid, 'g' is the acceleration due to gravity and 'h' is the height of the liquid column.

IMPORTANCE OF PRESSURE IN THE HUMAN BODY

Knowledge of pressure is needed to understand the functioning of the human body. Body cavities and organs are affected by pressure both in health and in disease. For example:
- Normal breathing depends partially on differences in intrapleural and intrapulmonic pressures and changes in pressure may produce respiratory distress.
- The effectiveness of treatments such as enemas and other irrigations depends on pressure.
- Many body functions depend on fluid pressure. For example, the heart pumps blood through the arteries at quite high-pressure (100-140 mm Hg). The returning venous blood is at quite low-pressure and has to be helped to go from the legs to the heart. Some typical values of the fluid pressures in the body are given in **Table 13.1**.

ATMOSPHERIC PRESSURE

The air around us has weight, and it presses against everything it touches, that pressure is called atmospheric pressure, or air pressure. It is the force exerted on a surface by the air above, it as gravity pulls it to Earth. Atmospheric pressure drops as altitude increases.

As the pressure decreases, the amount of oxygen available to breathe also decreases. At very high altitudes, atmospheric pressure and available oxygen get so low that people can become sick and even die.

The atmospheric pressure was first measured by Torricelli nearly three centuries ago following some observations of the Duke of Tuscany (Italy). The Duke got a deep well dug and found that the suction pumps available at that time failed to lift water to a height of more than

Table 13.1: Typical pressure in a normal and healthy human body.

Body/organ pressure	The typical value of pressure (in mm Hg)
Arterial blood pressure	
Maximum	100–140
Minimum	60–90
Venous blood pressure	3–7
Intrathoracic pressure (between lung and chest wall)	10
Capillary blood pressure	
Arterial end	30
Venous end	10
Middle ear pressure	<1
Urinary bladder	<2
Eye pressure—aqueous humor	20
Cerebrospinal fluid pressure in brain	5-12
Gastrointestinal pressure	10-20

Fig. 13.1: Torricelli experiment.

about 34 feet (10 m). To discover the answer to this curious phenomenon, Torricelli took a long glass tube open at one end and filled it with mercury. He closed the open end of the tube with his finger and inverted it into a vessel containing mercury. When he removed his finger, he observed that the level of mercury dropped to a certain height, leaving an empty space at the top. This empty space is known as the Torricellian vacuum (**Fig. 13.1**).

The length of the column of mercury was found to be nearly 30 feet, i.e., 76 cm. It was also found that the level of mercury in the tube is independent of its cross-section as well as its inclination.

By performing this experiment, Torricelli showed that the height of a liquid column cannot rise beyond a certain height because, it is experimentally determined by the atmospheric pressure. Thus, the water from the well got dug by the Duke of Tuscany did not rise beyond on and mercury in Torricelli's experiment did not rise beyond 76 cm. In this way, Torricelli was able to clear the confusion of the Duke of Tuscany.

Above the earth's surface, there is a vast quantity of air which is a mixture of many gases, is termed as atmosphere. The weight of the atmosphere exerts a force on the surface of every object on or near the surface of the earth. At sea level, this force produces a pressure of 14.7 lb/in^2. Torricelli found that at sea level the atmospheric pressure is sufficient to maintain the mercury column at 76 cm above the surface of the mercury in the container. Atmospheric pressure is sometimes expressed in terms of cm of mercury as 76 cm Hg or 760 mm Hg. This is equivalent to a pressure of 14.7 lb/in^2.

Mountain climbers use bottled oxygen when they ascend very high peaks. They also take time to get used to the altitude because quickly moving from higher pressure to lower pressure can cause decompression sickness. Decompression sickness also called "the bends", is also a problem for scuba divers who come to the surface too quickly. Aircraft create artificial pressure in the cabin so passengers remain comfortable while flying.

Atmospheric pressure is an indicator of weather. When a low-pressure system moves into an area, it usually leads to cloudiness, wind, and precipitation. High-pressure systems usually lead to fair, calm weather.

The Instrument for Measuring Atmospheric Pressure

An instrument used for measuring the atmospheric pressure is called a barometer. It is made up of a glass tube closed at one end, and it is filled up with mercury and inverted into a bowl of mercury. When atmospheric pressure increases, the level of the mercury column in the tube rises, when pressure decreases the level of the column falls.

Let us further elaborate on the inferences, of Torricelli's experiment with respect to fluid pressure. You can visualize this as follows: When a glass tube is inverted in a vessel containing mercury, Pascal's law implies that the pressure exerted by the atmosphere on the free surface of mercury is transmitted equally over its entire volume. This gives us an upthrust base of the inverted glass tube and pushes mercury upwards. As a result, mercury rises in the tube till the weight of the mercury column balances the up-thrust. Therefore, the height of this column is equivalent to the pressure of the atmosphere on the free surface of the mercury in the vessel. If the height of the mercury column in the tube above the free surface of the mercury in the container is 'h' and the density of mercury is 'd', then the atmospheric pressure is given by:

$$P = hdg$$

Thus, the normal atmospheric pressure is written as 760 mm Hg (or 76 cm Hg). If the pressure is below 760 mm Hg, it is said to be sub-atmospheric (that is, less than atmospheric pressure).

You may ask: Can we create sub-atmospheric pressure? Yes; if all gases are confined in a container could be recovered from it so that a perfect vacuum is created, then pressure becomes zero. However, practically it is not possible to create a perfect vacuum, and only a partial vacuum can be created. These partial vacuums give rise to a sub-atmospheric pressure. Since fluids (liquids and gases) flow from points of higher pressure to those of lower pressure, fluids above atmospheric pressure will flow into a vessel that is at sub-atmospheric pressure.

Applications of Atmospheric Pressure

- Suction is a process by which a region having sub-atmospheric pressure can be created. It is employed during surgical operation for the removal of blood and serosanguineous fluids from the region of the human body being operated.
- Many kinds of aspirators in the hospital wards work on the application of controlled suction.
- Water-seal drainage used after thoracic operations works on controlled suction and gravity.
- Suction apparatus for drainage in the postoperation treatment of patients with alimentary tract disorders are commonly observed in surgical wards.
- Tidal drainage by means of gravity flow and siphonage initiates the natural physiological process of the urinary bladder.
- Pressure greater than atmospheric pressure is applied by numerous mechanical devices to alleviate disturbing pulmonary functions (Birds Respirator Oxygen Tent).
- Pumps are dependent on their functioning on atmospheric pressure. A pump operates on the principle of pressure gradients, i.e., that fluids move from places of greater to those of lesser pressure.
- In hospitals, pumps can be used to fill air rings and air mattresses or to remove fluids from body cavities.
- The human heart operates in many ways like a pump. The right and left ventricles of the heart function like two synchronized pumps. They keep the flow of blood streaming continuously in one direction. The right ventricle pumps venous blood to the lungs. At the same time, the left ventricle pumps oxygenated blood to the tissues of the body. The ventricles are equipped

Fig. 13.2: Siphon.

with two sets of valves, the atrioventricular valve, and the semilunar valves. As the ventricles fill, the pressure within them increases. When the ventricles contract, the increased pressure closed the atrioventricular valves and opens the semilunar valves.

- **Siphon:** It is a device made of glass or rubber tubing with one short and long arm. It is used to move a liquid, the surface of which is exposed to the atmosphere, from a higher to a lower level. The siphon is so arranged that the shorter arm is placed in the liquid to be emptied and the longer arm is placed in a container at a lower level **(Fig. 13.2)**. The decompression apparatus for emptying the urinary bladder and the munro tidal drainage apparatus operate partially by siphon. A siphon is also the basis of action in gastric lavage. A rubber tube is passed into the stomach. After the stomach is filled with fluid, the funnel and tube are turned downward to form the long arm of the siphon. When there is no air in the system fluid will flow out of the stomach.

HYDROSTATIC PRESSURE

Hydrostatic pressure refers to the pressure that is exerted, due to the force of gravity, by a fluid at equilibrium at any particular point of time. Furthermore, hydrostatic pressure is proportional to the depth whose measurement takes place from the surface as the increase in weight of the fluid happens. Moreover, this increase in weight happens when a downward force is applied.

This very important property of all fluids (gases and liquids) was discovered by Pascal. He observed that when pressure is applied to a confined fluid, it is transmitted uniformly throughout its volume. He stated this observation in the form of a law, which is known as Pascal's law. We may state it as:

"Any change of pressure applied at any point in an enclosed fluid at rest is transmitted undiminished and uniformly to all its parts transpose".

Liquids that are enclosed in a vessel produce pressure by virtue of their weight. The pressure at any point below the surface is proportional to the weight of the column of liquid above that point. If a substance is twice as heavy as water, the pressure will be doubled. The pressure at any point below the surface can be determined by knowing the height of the liquid column and the density of the liquid, i.e.

$$P = hdg$$

Where,
- P = pressure
- h = height
- d = density
- g = acceleration due to gravity (is constant for a particular place)

For example:
Fluid in an enema container or in irrigating equipment exerts pressure by virtue of the weight of the column of fluid above the point of exit of the fluid. The greater the column of fluid is an enema container the greater the pressure at the level where it enters the body. The same principle applies to intravenous infusions and other parenteral fluids.

Applications of Pascal's Law

Pascal's law has been put to a variety of uses in day-to-day life as well as healthcare practices.
- In medicine, the use of water-mattress and air-rings work on the same principle. These mattresses are used to prevent bedsores in bedridden patients.
- The amniotic sac enclosing the fetus in the uterus is filled with amniotic fluid, which is a confined fluid and serves as a protection to the fetus. Any pressure exerted against the abdominal wall will be transmitted to the amniotic fluid to all surfaces of the fetus. To avoid unequal pressure, which may cause fetal deformity, the patient is usually cautioned against wearing tight clothing during pregnancy.
- Lumbar puncture and spinal fluid flow test to locate the blockage in the flow of CSF is also based on this principle only.
- In sphygmomanometer, the mercury manometer operates on the principle of Pascal's law. The flow of blood in the artery is occluded by the pressure of the enclosed air in the airtight cuff. The pressure supports a column of mercury in the manometer. When the air in the cuff is released slowly, the blood just begins to flow again; the pressure is measured by the height of this mercury column **(Fig. 13.3A)**.
- Medicine droppers and rubber bulb syringes enclose a fluid also work on the principle of Pascal's law. Pressure applied against the rubber bulb is transmitted to the enclosed liquid and caused it to flow from the open end of the dropper or syringe **(Fig. 13.3B)**.

Figs. 13.3A and B: Working applications of Pascal's law.

- Hydraulic brakes, are used in aircraft, automobiles, and trucks.
- The hydraulic press, is used to compress metal sheets, wool, or bales of cotton.
- Hydraulic carjacks, these are collectively referred to as hydraulic machines. A hydraulic jack is used to lift heavy vehicles in an automobile workshop. A force is applied on the piston of a smaller area of cross-section. The piston is gradually pushed inwards and the automobile moves upwardly.
- The dentist's chair also works on the same principle. The seat of the chair is placed over the larger piston and the smaller piston is operated by a foot pedal.
- Heavy lids of some sterilizers are lifted by using the same principle.
- The latest technology hospital beds also work on the sample principle, where the position of the patient can be changed very easily by a small piston operated by hand or foot.

PRESSURE IN FLOWING FLUIDS

You now know that some of the observed properties of fluids at rest can be understood in terms of simple concepts like pressure, density, and Pascal's law. You can now ask: What happens when fluids are in motion? The knowledge of the dynamics of the flowing fluid is important to understand the flow of blood in the circulatory system, in the preparation and administration of blood transfusions, intravenous infusions, etc.

An important requirement for the flow of fluids in a system is pressure gradient, i.e., difference in pressures at the ends of the system:

"Fluid flows from a region of higher pressure to that of lower pressure".

Breathing (that is, the flow of air in and out of the human body) is possible due to pressure differences. Further, the flow rate, i.e., volume of liquid flowing out per second, through a straight tube of the uniform cross-section is directly proportional to the pressure gradient across it. During internal hemorrhage, blood flows out of the blood vessel, and the pressure drops within the circulatory system.

Other factors being equal, the flow of fluid through an orifice depends on:
- ***Area of the orifice:*** The larger the orifice, the greater is the fluid flow.
- ***The pressure gradient:*** The greater the pressure gradient; the greater is the rate of flow.

However, when a fluid flows through a pipe of varying cross-section, irregular motion or turbulent flow occurs and the speed of flow in a pipe increases at a constriction. This suggests a connection between high blood pressure and the thickening of arteries. For flowing the same amount of blood in a narrowed artery, more pressure is required. Normally, the flow of blood in blood vessels of our body is laminar (uniform). But when blood vessels develop roughened walls or linings, or there is some bulging, turbulent flow of blood may rupture the delicate platelets in the blood and initiate the formation of blood clots in the vessel or bloodstream. Such internal hemorrhages possess a serious threat to life.

Some of the important relations among various physical parameters of fluids are known as different laws given below:
- ***Boyle's law*** states that the volume of a gas varies inversely with the pressure if the temperature is constant. This law is the basis of the working of a sphygmomanometer (BP apparatus).
- ***Charles's law*** states that the pressure of a gas is directly proportional to its temperature if the volume is kept constant. Many of the pressure cookers and autoclave machines work on these principles.

- ***Dalton's law*** states that in a gas mixture, the pressure exerted by each individual gas in space is independent of the pressures of other gases in the mixture. This principle is used while giving general anesthesia.

OSMOTIC PRESSURE

- Osmosis is the process by which solvent moves from a region of lesser concentration of solutes to a higher concentration of solutes through a semipermeable membrane.
- It may be defined as the equivalent of the external pressure that must be applied to a solution in order to prevent the passage of the solvent into it through a perfect semi-permeable membrane.
- The osmotic pressure of a solution is proportional to the concentration of the solute particles that cannot cross the membrane. The higher the solute concentration, the higher the solution's osmotic pressure.
- In the case of substances that ionize, the osmotic pressure that would be expected from the concentration alone will actually be greater because of a larger number of particles per molecule than one.
- Osmotic pressure is the pressure caused by water at different concentrations due to the dilution of water by dissolved molecules (solute), notably salts and nutrients.

For example:
- Sodium chloride solution will contain two particles, one sodium ion, and one chloride ion, for each molecule of sodium chloride. Osmotic pressure from substances such as sodium chloride that are strong electrolytes (i.e., ionize to a great extent) will be higher than that produced by substances that ionize weakly or not at all, other things being equal. In addition, the size of the molecules in the solution has an effect on osmotic pressure.
- Osmotic pressure is closely related to some other properties of solutions, the colligative properties. These include the freezing point depression, the boiling point elevation, and the vapor pressure depression, all caused by dissolving solutes in a solution.

Measuring Osmotic Pressure

Osmotic pressure can be measured in various ways which are described below: 1. Mechanical Methods, 2. Biological Methods, 3. Physical Methods.

Mechanical Methods

By Putting Weights

The simplest way is to apply adequate pressure (i.e., weight) upon the stronger solution to prevent any rise of volume. That pressure, which is just needed to stop the increase of volume of a particular solution is the measure of its OP. If a piston is used to apply more pressure to the fluid in the right arm, with enough pressure, the volume of pressure in each arm could be restored to the starting volume and the concentration of the solute in the right arm would be the same as it was in the beginning. The amount of pressure needed to restore the starting condition equals the osmotic pressure **(Fig. 13.4)**.

By a Manometer

The same thing can be done by connecting the apparatus with a suitable manometer, in which the pressure will gradually rise till it equalizes with the osmotic pressure of the solution, at which point further rise will stop (Pfeffer's method)

Fig. 13.4: Measurement of osmotic pressure.

Biological Methods

Hamburger's Red Corpuscle Method:

Red cells are kept in the unknown solution for some time, after which the cell volume is noted. If the cell volume is reduced, the solution is hypertonic than plasma (hence, water has been drawn out), if the cells swell up, the solution is hypotonic (so that water has entered), and if no change—the solution is isotonic, if sufficiently hypotonic the red cells will gradually swell up and ultimately burst (Hemolysis) **(Fig. 13.5).**

Physical Methods

By noting depression of freezing point. Higher the concentration, lower will be the freezing point, and therefore higher will be the osmotic pressure.

By Noting the Vapor Tension
Higher the concentration, lower will be the rate of evaporation from the solution and higher the osmotic pressure.

Fig. 13.5: Fate of RBC in different solution.

Hill's Method
Using thermopile; the higher the rate of evaporation more will be the fall of temperature and less will be the osmotic pressure. Comparison is made with a solution of known osmotic pressure.

Burger's Capillary Glass Tube Method
Alternate drops of known and unknown solutions separated by air bubbles are drawn in a standard capillary glass tube and after some time the edges of the solutions are noted. The edges will shift according to the rate of evaporation. From these data, Osmotic Pressure can be calculated.

Applications of the Osmotic Pressure

- Blood albumin helps to maintain the colloidal pressure of the blood. At the capillaries, this pressure is effective in maintaining the normal fluid content of the blood. If a patient loses blood albumin which may happen in nephrosis the colloidal osmotic pressure will drop and fluid remains in the tissues. This results in edema.
- Sometimes infusion of a hypertonic solution is useful to treat patients who have cerebral edema, and excess interstitial fluid in the brain like mannitol. It relieves such fluid overload by causing osmosis of water from the interstitial fluid into the blood. Then the kidneys excrete excess water from the blood into the urine.
- Administration of hypotonic solutions either IV or oral, can be used to treat people who are dehydrated. The water in the hypotonic solution moves from the blood into the interstitial fluid and then into the body cells to rehydrate them.
- In dialysis along with diffusion, osmosis also works.

MEASUREMENT OF PRESSURES

Arterial Pressure

The cardiovascular system has three types of pressures: hemodynamic, kinetic energy, and hydrostatic. Hemodynamic pressure is the energy imparted to the blood by the contraction of the left ventricle. This type of pressure is preserved by the elastic properties of the arterial system. Kinetic energy is the energy associated with motion and affects the pressure measured during direct arterial BP monitoring. Fluid density and gravity contribute to hydrostatic pressure, which is the pressure a column of fluid exerts on the container's wall. For example, in a column of fluid, the pressure at a given level in the container is proportional to the height of the fluid column above that level. The pressure is highest at the bottom of the column. In the vascular system, hydrostatic pressure is proportional to the height of the column of blood between the heart and the peripheral vasculature. In a standing person, the pressure in the leg is higher than the pressure in the arm by the difference in hydrostatic pressure. In summary, arterial blood pressure represents the force exerted by the blood per unit area on the arterial wall and is the sum of hemodynamic, kinetic, and hydrostatic pressure.

Measuring Arterial Pressure
The arterial pressure is measured using a sphygmomanometer (i.e., blood pressure cuff) on the upper arm, the systolic and diastolic pressures that are measured represent the pressure within the brachial artery, which is slightly different from the pressure found in the aorta or the pressure found in other distributing arteries. As the aortic pressure pulse travels down the aorta and into distributing arteries, there are characteristic changes in the systolic and diastolic pressures, as well as in the mean pressure. The systolic pressure rises and the diastolic pressure

falls, therefore, the pulse pressure increases, as the pressure pulse travels away from the aorta. This occurs because of reflective waves from vessel branching, and from decreased arterial compliance (increased vessel stiffness) as the pressure pulse travels from the aorta into systemic arteries. There is only a small decline in mean arterial pressure as the pressure pulse travels down distributing arteries due to the relatively low resistance of large distributing arteries. Arterial blood pressure also can be measured by placing an intra-arterial catheter and directly attaching it to a monitor through a transducer.

Central Venous Pressure

Central venous pressure, which is a measure of pressure in the vena cava, can be used as an estimation of preload and right atrial pressure. Central venous pressure is often used as an assessment of hemodynamic status, particularly in the intensive care unit. The central venous pressure can be measured using a central venous catheter advanced via the internal jugular vein and placed in the superior vena cava near the right atrium.

Measuring Central Venous Pressure (CVP)

The CVP can be measured either manually using a manometer or electronically using a transducer. In either case, the CVP must be 'zeroed' at the level of the right atrium. This is usually taken to be the level of the 4th intercostal space in the midaxillary line while the patient is lying supine. Each measurement of CVP should be taken at this same zero position. Trends in the serial measurement of CVP are much more informative than single readings. However, if the CVP is measured at a different level each time, then this renders the trend in measurement inaccurate. CVP can be measured in two ways as described below:

- **Using the manometer:** A 3-way tap is used to connect the manometer to an intravenous drip set on one side, and via extension tubing filled with intravenous fluid, to the patient on the other. It is important to ensure that there are no air bubbles in the tubing, to avoid administering an air embolus to the patient. You should also check that the CVP catheter tubing is not kinked or blocked, that intravenous fluid can easily be flushed in and that blood can easily be aspirated from the line. The 3-way tap is then turned so that it is open to the fluid bag and the manometer but closed to the patient, allowing the manometer column to fill with fluid. It is important not to overfill the manometer, so preventing the cotton wool bung at the manometer tip from getting wet. Once the manometer has filled adequately the 3-way tap is turned again—this time, so it is open to the patient and the manometer, but closed to the fluid bag. The fluid level within the manometer column will fall to the level of the CVP, the value of which can be read on the manometer scale which is marked in centimeters, therefore giving a value for the CVP in centimeters of water (cm H_2O). The fluid level will continue to rise and fall slightly with respiration and the average reading should be recorded.
- **Using the transducer:** The transducer is fixed at the level of the right atrium and connected to the patient's CVP catheter via fluid-filled extension tubing. Similar care should be taken to avoid bubbles and kinks, etc. as mentioned above. The transducer is then 'zeroed' to atmospheric pressure by turning its 3-way tap so that it is open to the transducer and to the room air, but closed to the patient. The 3-way tap is then turned so that it is now closed to room air and open between the patient and the transducer. A continuous CVP reading, measured in mm Hg rather than cm H_2O, can be obtained.

Intraocular Pressure

Intraocular pressure (IOP) is the fluid pressure inside the eye. As pressure is a measure of force per area, IOP is a measurement involving the magnitude of the force exerted by the aqueous humor on the internal surface area of the anterior eye. Intraocular pressure is measured with a tonometer.

Tonometry is the measurement of tension or pressure within the eye. A tonometer is an instrument for measuring tension or pressure., Tonometry is the procedure, that eye care professionals perform to determine the intraocular pressure (IOP), the fluid pressure inside the eye. It is an important test in the evaluation of patients with glaucoma. Most tonometer's are calibrated to measure pressure in mm Hg.

Measuring Intraocular Pressure

There are three basic methods to measure intraocular pressure. A brief description of these methods are as follows:

- **Applanation method:** It measures the intraocular pressure either by a force required to flatten a constant area of the cornea (Goldmann tonometry) or by the area flattened by a constant force.
    - In applanation tonometry, a special calibrated disinfected probe attached to a slit lamp biomicroscope is used to flatten the central cornea by a fixed amount. Because the probe makes contact with the cornea, a topical anesthetic, such as oxybuprocaine, tetracaine, etc. is introduced onto the surface of the eye in the form of one or two eye drops. A yellow fluorescein dye is used in conjunction with a cobalt blue filter to aid the examiner in determining the IOP.
- **Dynamic contour tonometry:** Dynamic contour tonometry (DCT) is a novel method that uses the principle of contour matching instead of applanation.
- The pascal tonometer is currently the only commercial DCT tonometer available. It uses a miniature pressure sensor embedded within a tonometer tip contour matched to the shape of the cornea. The tonometer tip rests on the cornea with a constant appositional force of one gram. When the sensor is subjected to a change in pressure, the electrical resistance is altered and the pascal's computer calculates a change in pressure in concordance with the change in resistance.
- **Pneumatonometry:** A pneumatonometer utilizes a pneumatic sensor (consisting of a piston floating on an air bearing). It is touched to the anesthetized cornea. A precisely regulated flow of filtered air (from an internal air pump) enters the piston. A small (5 mm dia.) fenestrated membrane at the end of the piston reacts to both the force of the air blowing through it and to the force represented by the pressure behind the cornea, against which it is being pressed. The precise balance between these two forces represents the precise intraocular pressure.

Intracranial Pressure

Intracranial pressure (ICP) is the pressure in the cranium and thus in the brain tissue and cerebrospinal fluid (CSF); this pressure is exerted on the brain's intracranial blood circulation vessels. ICP is maintained in a tight normal range dynamically, through the production and absorption of CSF and pulsates approximately 1 mm Hg in normal healthy adults. CSF pressure has been shown to be influenced by abrupt changes in intrathoracic pressure during coughing (intra-abdominal pressure), Valsalva maneuver, and communication with the vasculature (venous and arterial systems). ICP is measured in millimeters of mercury (mm Hg) and, at rest, is normally 7-15 mm Hg for a supine adult, and becomes negative (averaging −10 mm Hg) in the vertical position. Changes in ICP are attributed to volume changes in one or more of the constituents contained in the cranium.

Measuring Intracranial Pressure

There are two basic techniques or methods of measuring intracranial pressure.

❖ **Noninvasive methods**
- Clinical deterioration in neurological status is widely considered a sign of increased ICP. Bradycardia, increased pulse pressure, and pupillary dilation are normally accepted as signs of increased ICP. The clinical monitoring is age-old and time tested.
- Transcranial Doppler, tympanic membrane displacement, and ultrasound 'time of flight' techniques have been advocated. Several devices have been described for measuring ICP through open fontanel. Ladd fiber optic system has been used extracutaneously.
- Manual feeling of the craniotomy flap or skull defect, if any, gives a clue.

❖ **Invasive methods**
- Intraventricular monitoring remains one of the popular techniques, especially in patients with ventriculomegaly. The additional advantage is the potential for draining CSF therapeutically. Insertion of the ventricular catheter is not always simple and can cause hemorrhage and infection (5%).
- Other most commonly used devices are the hollow screw and bolt devices, and the subdural catheter. Richmond screw and Becker bolt are used extradurally. A fluid-filled catheter in the subdural space, connected to an arterial pressure monitoring system is cost-effective and serves the purpose adequately.
- The Ladd device is currently in wide use. It employs a fiberoptic system to detect the distortion of a tiny mirror within with balloon system. It can be used in the subdural, extradural, and even extracutaneously.
- A mechanically coupled surface monitoring device is the 'cardio search pneumatic sensor' used subdurally or extradurally. These systems are not widely used.
- Electronic devices (Camino & Galtesh design) are getting popular the world over. Intraparenchymal probes, the measured pressure may be compartmentalized and not necessarily representative of real ICP. In addition to ICP monitoring, modern intraparenchymal sensors help study the chemical environment of the site of pathology.
- Fully implantable devices are valuable in a small group that requires long-term ICP monitoring for brain tumors, hydrocephalus, or other chronic brain diseases. Common intracranial pressure tele sensor can be implanted as a part of the shunt system. Ommaya reservoir is an alternative that can be punctured and CSF pressure readings are obtained.
- Lumbar puncture and measurement of CSF pressure for obvious reasons are not recommended.

■ APPLICATIONS OF THESE PRESSURES IN NURSING

Applications of different types of pressures in healthcare practices and nursing procedures are discussed with the description of each type of pressure. Therefore, you can refer to the application of different pressures as discussed individually in the chapter.

■ QUESTIONS

Q.1: State Pascal's law. Give two examples of its application in the human body.
Q.2: How can we create sub-atmospheric pressure? Give two applications from the nursing procedure.
Q.3: Force acting on the unit surface is called as…………..
Q.4: Mouth to mouth respiration in respiratory distress. Explain.
Q.5: What is pressure, osmotic diuresis, and diffusion?

Q.6: What are the physiological functions of the human body that depend upon the osmotic pressure and dialysis for their normal function?
Q.7: Occurrence of edema in nephrosis. Discuss.
Q.8: Why a chronic bedridden patient is advised to use an air-mattress instead of an ordinary mattress?
Q.9: Heart as a double compression pump. Discuss.
Q.10: Positive pressure is applied to patients with pulmonary edema. Discuss.
Q.11: When the normal breathing stops in a drowsed person, artificial respiration helps to restore it?
Q.12: Factors affecting pressure and the two pressures in the human body. Explain.

■ BIBLIOGRAPHY

1. Atkins P, J de Paula. Elements of Physical Chemistry, Fourth edition, WH. Freeman, 2006.
2. Cotterill RMJ. Biophysics: An Introduction. Wiley, 2002.
3. Dogonadze RR, Urushadze ZD. "Semi-Classical Method of Calculation of Rates of Chemical Reactions Proceeding in Polar Liquids". J Electroanal Chem, 1971; 32: 235-45.
4. Giancoli, Douglas G. Physics: Principles with applications. Upper Saddle River, NJ: Pearson Education, 2004.
5. Hobbie RK, Roth BJ. International Physics for Medicine and Biology (Fourth edition). Springer, 2006.
6. Perutz MF. Proteins and Nucleic Acids: Structure and Function. Amsterdam: Elsevier, 1962.
7. Roland G. Biophysics: An Introduction (Corrected edition). Springer, 2004: 11-23.
8. Sneppen K, Zocchi G. Physics in Molecular Biology, First edition. Cambridge University Press, 2005:10-17.
9. Volkenshtein MV, Dogonadze RR, Madumarov AK. Theory of Enzyme Catalysis. Molekuliarnaya Biologia (Moscow)1972; 6: 431-39 (In Russian, English summary).
10. Darwish A, Lui F. Physiology, Colloid Osmotic Pressure. [Updated 2021 Oct 1]. In: StatPearls [Internet]. Treasure Island (FL): StatPearls Publishing; 2022 Jan. Available from: https://www.ncbi.nlm.nih.gov/books/NBK541067/
11. Joseph Feher. Osmosis and Osmotic Pressure. Quantitative Human Physiology (Second Edition) Academic Press, 2017 Pages 182-198. Available from https://doi.org/10.1016/B978-0-12-800883-6.00017-3.
12. Shah P, Louis MA. Physiology, Central Venous Pressure. [Updated 2021 Sep 14]. In: StatPearls [Internet]. Treasure Island (FL): StatPearls Publishing; 2022 Jan. Available from: https://www.ncbi.nlm.nih.gov/books/NBK519493/
13. Machiele R, Motlagh M, Patel BC. Intraocular Pressure. [Updated 2021 Jul 31]. In: StatPearls [Internet]. Treasure Island (FL): StatPearls Publishing; 2022 Jan. Available from: https://www.ncbi.nlm.nih.gov/books/NBK532237/

CHAPTER 14

Sound Waves

Rakhi Gaur, Navjot Kaur

Chapter Outline
- Mechanism of Propagation of Waves
- Types of Waves
- Types of Wave Motion
- Sound Waves
- Some Important Terms Connected with Wave Motion
- Wave Phenomenon
- Characteristics of Sound
- Vocalization and Hearing
- Doppler Effect
- Applications
- Noise Pollution and its Prevention

■ INTRODUCTION

You must have seen that when we throw a piece of stone into the water in a pond, we observe ripples traveling on the surface of the water in concentric circles of ever-increasing radius, till they strike the boundary of the pond. When we put a piece of cork on the surface of this water, we observe that the cork piece moves up and down as the wave passes, but the piece does not travel along with the waves. Thus, the particles of the medium certainly oscillate about their mean position, but their displacement away from their mean position is not there. The water waves carry energy but there is no transfer of water. So, wave motion is the propagation of disturbances—that is, deviations from a state of rest or equilibrium—from place to place in a regular and organized way. Most familiar are surface waves on water, but both sound and light travel as wavelike disturbances and the motion of all subatomic particles exhibits wavelike properties.

So we can define, "wave motion as a kind of disturbance which travels through a material medium (having property of elasticity and inertia) or account of repeated periodic vibrations of the particles of medium about their mean position, the disturbance being handed on from one particle to the adjoining particle and so on, without any met transport of the medium".

The central feature of wave motion is "Energy is transferred over a distance but the matter is not".

■ MECHANISM OF PROPAGATION OF WAVES

Let us look at some of the important terms before understanding the mechanism of propagation of waves.

❖ **Kinetic energy:** It is the energy associated with motion.
$$KE = \tfrac{1}{2} mv^2$$
❖ **Potential energy:** It is stored energy and depends on an object's position
$$PE = mgh$$
- *Inertia:* It is the property by which particles can store energy and overshoot their position.
- *Elasticity:* It is the property by which particles can return to their mean position, after having been disturbed.

'XY' represents the horizontal surface of the water when a stone hits a particle of water at 'O', the particle moves down to 'A' **(Fig. 14.1)**. During the motion of particles from 'O' to 'A', a restoring force develops on account of the elasticity of the water. Work done against the restoring force while the particle moved from 'O' to 'A' is stored in the particle at 'A' in form of potential energy. From 'A', the particle moves towards 'O', under the action of restoring force. The potential energy of the particle is converted into kinetic energy at 'O'. On account of inertia, therefore the particle cannot stop at 'O'. It overshoots its mean position 'O' and goes over to B, the particle then moves back to 'O', under the action of restoring force again and so on. Thus, the particle of water at 'O' executes periodic vibrations due to elasticity and inertia.

This disturbance is communicated to the adjoining particles which also start vibrating simply harmonically about their mean positions. Hence, wave motion travels on and on at the water surface.

■ TYPES OF WAVES

❖ **Elastic waves or mechanical waves:** Waves that can be produced or propagated only in a material medium are called elastic waves or mechanical waves. For example, waves on the water surface, sound waves, etc.

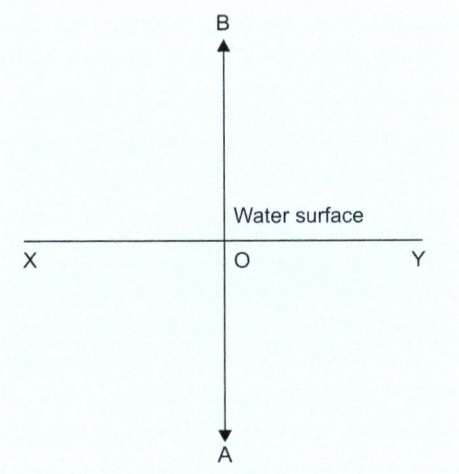

Fig. 14.1: Mechanism of propagation of waves.

❖ **Electromagnetic waves or non-mechanical waves:** The waves which can pass even through vacuum; for example, light waves from the sun, radiowaves, microwaves, X-rays, etc.

■ TYPES OF WAVE MOTION

The wave motion is primarily classified into two broad categories, i.e., transverse wave motion and longitudinal wave motion. The details are given below:

Transverse Wave Motion

Let us consider a rope with one end fixed to a wall and another end held by a child. When a child flicks the rope, a bump (technically called 'pulse') is formed in the rope and this pulse travels along the rope with some definite speed. A rope is the medium through which pulse travels. If the child moves the end of the rope up and down continuously, this would create a pulsating wave.

For this pulsating wave, the wave's propagation direction is from the child's hand towards the wall, i.e., along the rope, and each disturbing element of the rope moves upwards or downwards, i.e., perpendicular to the direction of the propagation. This kind of wave motion is called transverse wave motion **(Fig. 14.2)**.

A transverse wave motion is a motion in which individual particles of the medium execute simple harmonic motion about their mean position in a direction perpendicular to the direction of propagation of wave motion. For example, movement of rope or string as described above.
❖ A transverse wave travels through a medium in the form of crests and troughs.
❖ The crest is a portion of the medium, which is raised temporarily above the normal position of the rest of the particles of the medium when a transverse wave passes through it.
❖ A trough is a portion of the medium, which is depressed temporarily below the normal position of the rest of the particles of the medium when a transverse wave passes through it.

Another example of transverse wave is a light wave. In light waves, electric and magnetic fields move perpendicular to the direction of propagation of light.

Longitudinal Wave Motion or Pressure Wave

A longitudinal wave motion is that wave motion in which individual particles of the medium execute simple harmonic motion about their mean position along the same direction along

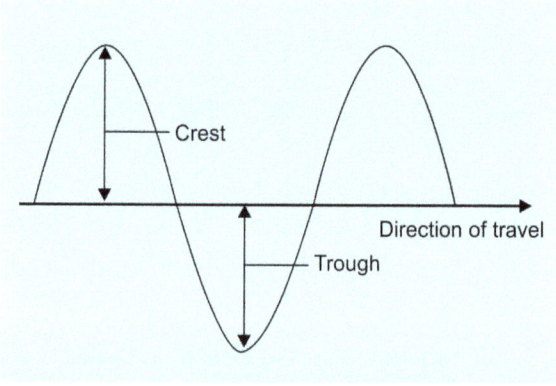

Fig. 14.2: Transverse wave motion.

Fig. 14.3: Longitudinal wave motion.

which the wave is propagated, for example, sound waves travel through the air in the form of longitudinal waves **(Fig. 14.3)**.

A longitudinal wave travels through a medium in the form of compressions or condensations (C) and rarefactions (R).
- **A compression:** It is a region of the medium in which particles are comprised, i.e., particles come closer (distance between the articles becomes less than the normal distance between them). Thus, there is a temporary decrease in volume and a consequent increase in the density of the medium in the region of compression.
- **A rarefaction:** It is a region of the medium in which particles are rarefied, i.e., particles get farther apart than they normally are. Thus, there is a temporary increase in volume and a consequent decrease in the density of the medium in the region of rarefaction.

A mechanical wave shall be transverse or longitudinal depending on:
- Nature of the medium.
- Mode of excitation of vibration

Example: In solid, mechanical waves can be either transverse or longitudinal. In strings, mechanical waves are always transverse. In liquids and gases, mechanical waves are generally longitudinal.

Though, all the waves cannot be characterized as longitudinal or transverse waves. For example, when a steady surface of the water is disturbed, waves are produced on the surface. Water particles move in a circular or elliptical fashion when a wave passes through them. An elliptical motion has both components, i.e., along and perpendicular to the wave motion.

SOUND WAVES

When we listen to a guitar or sitar sound, no material particle is ejected from the guitar or sitar and falls on our ears. It is just a disturbance in the part of the air close to the sitar. Energy is transferred to these air particles by pushing or strumming sitar wires. The disturbed air particles exert force on the next layer. In this way, the disturbance proceeds in medium (here air), and finally the air near our ear gets disturbed.

Hearing is one of the primary sensations. The physical cause that produces the sensation of hearing is the vibration of the source, e.g., when we listen to a sitar recital, the sitar wire vibrates. Sound is derived from objects that vibrate producing pressure variations in a sound-transmitting medium, such as air. A pressure wave is propagated outward from the vibrating source. When the pressure wave encounters another object, the vibration can be imparted

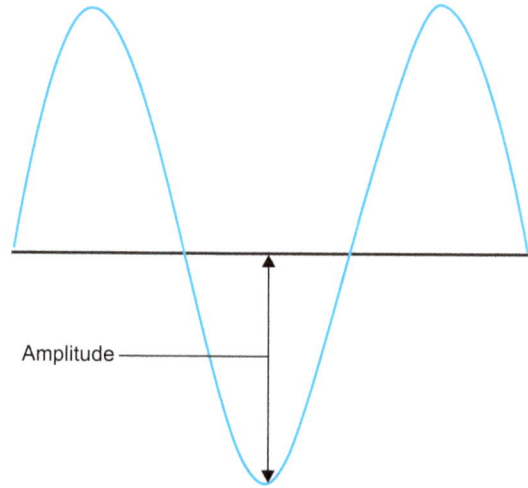

Fig. 14.4: Amplitude.

to that object and the pressure wave will propagate in the medium of the object. The sound wave may also be reflected from the object or it may diffract around the object. Thus, a sound wave propagating outward from a vibrating object can reach the eardrum of a listener causing the eardrum to vibrate and initiate the process of hearing. Our ear is sensitive only to those vibrations whose frequency lies between 20 and 20,000 Hz. This frequency range is called the audible range.

"A vibration whose frequency is greater than 20,000 Hz is called ultrasonic vibration. The sound waves which have a frequency less than the audible range are called infrasonic waves. These cannot be heard by the human ear".

The velocity of sound in air at room temperature and normal pressure is roughly 332 ms^{-1} which is approximately 1200 kmh^{-1}. This is much greater than the speed of the fastest car. That is why the horn of a motor car approaching us is heard much before the car reaches us.

Now we know that a longitudinal wave motion travels in the form of compressions and rarefactions which involve changes in the volume and density of the medium. As air possesses volume elasticity therefore sound comes to us from the source in the form of longitudinal waves only. As crests and troughs cannot be sustained in air, therefore sound cannot travel through the air in the form of transverse waves.

Sound waves are longitudinal mechanical waves that cannot travel in a vacuum. For example, two persons on the the surface of moon cannot talk to each other, as the moon has no atmosphere through which sound would travel **(Fig. 14.4)**.

■ SOME IMPORTANT TERMS CONNECTED WITH WAVE MOTION

- **Amplitude:** It is the maximum displacement that the particle of the medium in which the wave moves are displaced from their resting position as the wave train passes, it is equal to the half of the distance through with the particles vibrate.
- **Frequency:** The frequency of a particle is defined as the number of vibrations completed by a particle in one second or it is the number of waves (a pair of compression and rarefaction)

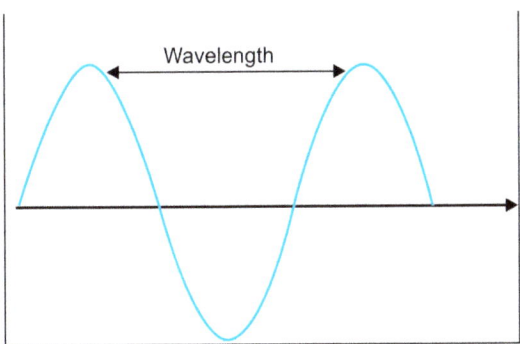

Fig. 14.5: Wavelength.

crossing a point in one second. It is measured in cycles/second or Hertz and it is donated by (ν).

- **Time period:** In wave motion, particles of medium execute simple harmonic motion or oscillatory motion, i.e., repeats its motion after a regular interval of time. This interval of time is called the time period. The time period of a wave is reciprocal to its frequency. In other words, it is the time taken by the wave to travel a distance equal to one wavelength. It is donated by 'T'. During one time period (T), the wave moves through a distance equal to one wavelength. Therefore the velocity (v) of wave.

$$\frac{V - \lambda}{T} = \lambda \upsilon$$

- **Wavelength:** Wavelength of a wave is equal to the length of one wave. It is defined as the distance between any two particles of the medium vibrating in the same phase. In the other wards, distance between two successive compressions or rarefaction is called the wavelength of the wave **(Fig. 14.5)**.
- **Velocity (V):** The velocity of waves varies with the medium through which the waves are passing and with the temperature of the medium. For Example, at 0°C, the velocity of sound waves in dry air is 1089 Ft/sec and at 200°C, it is 1126 Ft/sec.
  - In a rigid solid such as ivory, the sound travels at 3000 m/sec. In water at 190°C, the velocity of sound is 4794 Ft/sec.
  - The velocity of sound depends on the pressure and density of the medium through which it travels, i.e.,

$$V = \frac{P}{d}$$

here   P = Pressure, d = density
And   V = λ ν

If 'V' remains fixed, the wavelength will increase at increased temperature. Conversely, if the wavelength remains fixed, the frequency will increase with an increase in temperature. Out of three phases, solids metal conducts sound wave best and gases conducts sound waves poorly.

- **Intensity:** The intensity of sound depends on the amount of energy with which the sound waves strike the tympanic membrane of the intensitysity of sound is defined as the energy flow across a unit of area in a unit of time. In the MKS system, the unit of intensity of sound is watts per square meter.

The intensity of sound is inversely proportional to the square of the distance from the source, i.e.,

$$I \alpha 1/D^2$$

Where D is the distance from the source

Variations in the sound level are expressed in decibel (dB), i.e., intensity of sound with respect to various levels is expressed in dB.

The basic unit of sound intensity is 10^{-12} W/m² which is audible to the normal ear. Normal conversation is in the range below 60 dB and 70 dB, and heavy traffic produces a sound intensity of about 80 dB. At 120 dB a person feels discomfort whereas at 140 dB pain is experienced. A normal person can detect the sound of intensity between 10^{-12} W/m² and 1-12 W/m² (i.e., in the range of 0 to 120 dB).

WAVE PHENOMENON

Regardless of type, transverse or longitudinal, waves exhibit similar behavior. When any wave strikes a surface, the wave may be reflected, refracted, absorbed, transmitted, or diffracted or it may exhibit interference.

- **Reflection:** When waves or rays hit a flat surface they may be reflected back. For example; the echo exemplifies this phenomenon in sound waves **(Fig. 14.6)**.
  In the case of perfect reflections, $\theta_1 = \theta_2$
- **Refraction:** When a wave or ray passes from one medium to another, its velocity may change, causing a change in the direction of the wave. The change in the direction is known as refraction **(Fig. 14.7)**.
- **Absorption:** When a wave strikes a medium or a surface, some of the energy is absorbed and changed to heat. A piece of black cloth placed on snow on a bright sunny day may absorb sufficient radiant energy from the sun to melt the snow. For example, special materials used in the construction of soundproof rooms absorb rather than reflect the sound energy, transforming it into heat energy.
- **Transmission:** Waves or rays passing from a source of energy in a given medium move outward and are transmitted by the molecules of the medium. When the waves strike another medium, they are transmitted unchanged, if both media have the same refraction index.
- **Diffraction:** It is a term used to mean a departure from a straight line when waves meet

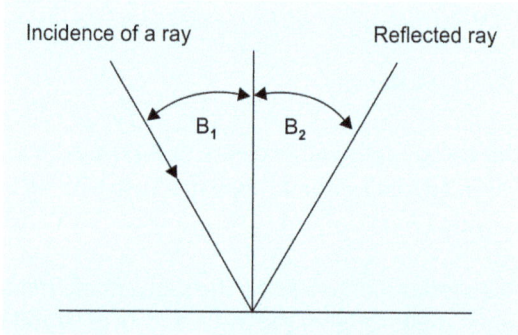

Fig. 14.6: Reflection of a ray.

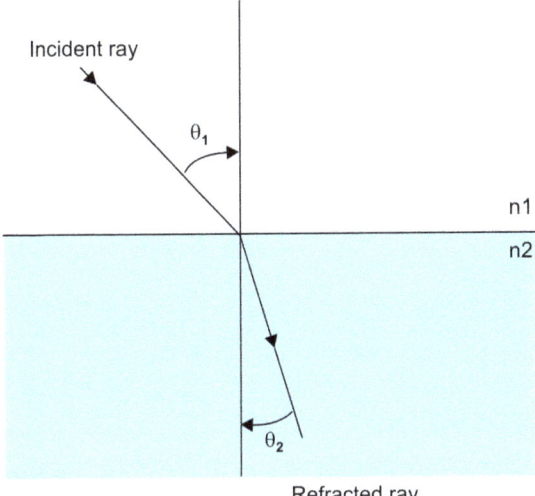

Fig. 14.7: Refraction of a ray.

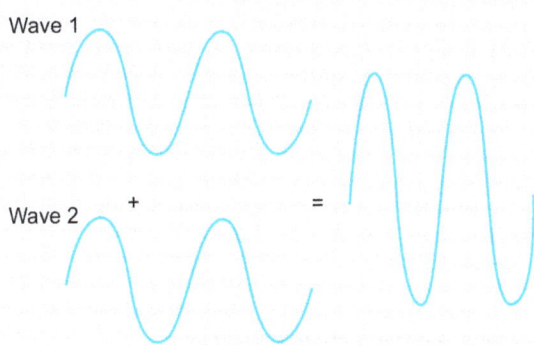

Fig. 14.8: Constructive interference.

and pass an obstacle or go through an aperture. In everyday speech, diffraction refers to the property of waves being able to "bend around corners".

❖ **Interference:** Interference may occur when more than one wave train is moving through the same medium. The effect can be demonstrated experimentally by propagating two wave trains in water that moves from opposite directions through an intervention. In the intersection area, the wave patterns are disrupted, but after passing the intersection the wavefront reappears in this original form.
- **Constructive:** When two small waves coming from opposite directions combine to form a large pulse and then reappear in their original form, it is called a constructive interference pattern **(Fig. 14.8)**.
- **Destructive:** When two transverse waves that are equal and opposite in direction meet, the upward and downward wave pulses cancel each other temporarily and a destructive interference pattern is formed **(Fig. 14.9)**.

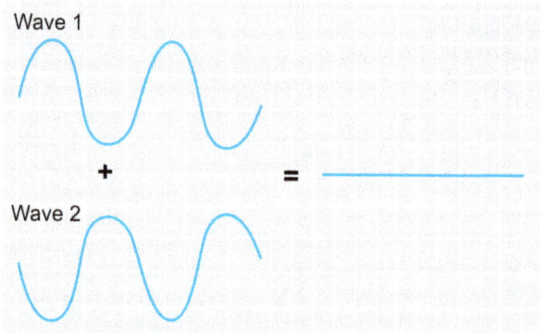

Fig. 14.9: Destructive interference.

CHARACTERISTICS OF SOUND

In our everyday life, we hear different types of sounds. Broadly, sound may be divided into two classes:

- **Musical sound:** Musical sound is a continuous and pleasing sound. It is produced by regular periodic vibrations. The sound produced by violin, guitar, piano, *ektara, tabla*, etc. is musical in nature.
- **Noise:** Every sound other than musical sound is noise. While the musical sound is pleasing, noise such as automobile horn is irritable and can adversely affect us. You may beware that the noise level in all metropolitan cities of or country has increased to alarming levels.

How do we differentiate among a variety of musical sounds such as from guitar, *sitar, veena*, tabla, etc? It can be done on the basis of three parameters, i.e., intensity, pitch, and quality (timber) as discussed below:

- **Intensity:** Intensity is defined as the energy carried by a wave in a unit of time across a unit area normal to the direction. It is measured in W/m^{-2}. Qualitatively, it is a measure of loudness. As we know,

$$I \propto 1/r_2$$

For example, if 'r' increase, intensity decreases.

It is for this reason, that chirping of birds, the sound of the vehicle, or a cracker fad out **(Table 14.1)**.

Table 14.1: Intensities of sound waves generated from different sources.	
Source	Intensity (wm^{-2})
Threshold of hearing	10^{-12}
Rusty waves	10^{-11}
Whisper, the intensity at eardrum	10^{-10}
Home	10^{-8}
Office	10^{-7}
Ordinary conversation	3.2×10^{-6}
Street traffic	10^{-15}
Busting cracker, at 1 m	8×10^{-5}
Jet take-off, at 7.8 m	105 W/m²

- **Pitch:** The pitch of the sound is related to frequency. The greater the frequency of the sound waves the higher the pitch. If one inhales a quantity of helium and talks while exhaling it the voice sounds thin and piping. The velocity of sound in helium is greater than that in air and since the wavelength of the sounds produced by the vocal cords does not change, the frequency of the sound increases, and the pitch is raised.
- **Quality/Timber:** The quality of timber is the most important characteristic of a musical sound because it enables us to distinguish a sound produced by one musical instrument from that of another instrument. The quality of a tone is dependent upon the frequencies that are integral multiples of the fundamental frequency. These frequencies are called harmonics. A "pure" tone depends upon the fundamental frequency only. The presence of different harmonics and their relative intensities introduce uniqueness in the sound produced by a particular source.

VOCALIZATION AND HEARING

Human beings have the ability to produce a variety of sounds. Physically this is possible because the vocal cords produce vibrations of various frequencies. Also air currents passing over the cords can produce a variety of intensities.

Vocalization

During normal breathing, the vocal cords are relaxed and air can pass easily through the larynx. A voiced sound is produced when the cords close off the larynx. As air is exhaled, pressure builds up behind the cords and escapes through them. This reduces the pressure on the back of the cords. When the pressure is reduced, the cords again close, the pressure again increases and the action is repeated. By the action of a series sound waves are produced, each with a specific frequency depending on the tension on the mass of the cord.

The character of the voice is influenced by the tension, thickness, and size of the cords as well as the size and shape of the throat, thorax, and paranasal sinuses. Thus in general, the frequency of sound is higher in women. This is because their vocal cords are lighter. Similarly, change of voice in adolescence is connected to the increase in mass that accompanies growth and development.

Hearing

Ear is responsible for hearing. The ear can be divided into three parts the external ear, the middle ear, and the inner ear The external ear is shaped like a cone, fixed at the periphery. At the end of the external ear lies the tympanic membrane, commonly called the eardrum. The middle ear contains the three ossicles the malleus, the incus, and the stapes. They stretch across the middle layer from the eardrum to the membrane of the head of the first ossicle. The hearing starts with the outer ear. When a sound is made outside the outer ear, the sound waves, or vibrations, travel down the external auditory canal and strike the eardrum (tympanic membrane). The eardrum vibrates. The vibrations are then passed to three tiny bones in the middle ear called the ossicles. The ossicles amplify the sound. Hearing results from stimulation of the nerve cells of the inner ear and the interpretation of these impulses in the brain.. The three ossicles are so mounted that the vibrations of the eardrum are transmitted to the last ossicles and at the oval window. This rocking motion, in turn, sets up pressure waves in the cochlear fluid in the inner ear. The cochlear of the inner ear is like a tapering coil.

This tube is divided into three canals which are filled with fluid. The partition between the two canals is madeup of the organ of Corti, which contains the sensory cells. Impulses from the nerve fibers, which are connected to sensory cells, project into the auditory center of the cerebrum.

Thus, the structure of the ear allows sound waves from the outside air to travel right up to the inner ear, where these vibrations are converted into nerve impulses. The external ear acts like a trumpet because of its conical shape and thus produces greater pressure on the eardrums. The middle ear exerts amplifying action, i.e., increases the intensity of the sound wave. The inner ear changes the vibrations in the fluid to specific increased impulses that are translated by the brain into the sound of varying pitch and loudness.

DOPPLER EFFECT

It was first described (1842) by Austrian physicist Christian Doppler. The apparent difference between the frequency at which sound or light waves leave a source and that at which they reach an observer, is caused by the relative motion of the observer and the wave source. You all must have heard the whistle of a moving train. What do you feel if the train approaches you? The pitch of the whistle seems to rise and when it goes away, the pitch appears to decrease. These apparent changes in the sound heard are caused due to Doppler effects.

In general, when the source approaches the listener or the listener approaches the source, or both approach each other, the apparent frequency is different than the actual frequency of the sound produced by the source. This change in frequency is known as the Doppler shift. Doppler shift can be used to measure the rate of blood flow. It is also used by obstetricians to detect fetal heartbeat or pulsation in the umbilical cord.

To detect the blood flow, a continuous ultrasound beam is sent to blood cells in an artery that is moving away from the source. The frequency of ultrasound received by the blood cells appears lower. The apparent lowering of frequency is detected by the echoes sent by the blood cells, this helps estimate the rate of blood flow in an artery or any other organ of the human body and the heart rate of the fetus.

APPLICATIONS

Hearing Aids

Hearing aids are electronic devices consisting of a minute microphone that picks up sound waves and converts them into electric current. The current is amplified and passes to a miniature loudspeaker that fits into the ear.

Stethoscope

- The stethoscope is a familiar instrument for listening to sounds in the human body. This simple "hearing aid" permits a physician or nurse to listen to sounds made inside the body, primarily in the heart and lungs. This is called auscultation.
- The main parts of a modern stethoscope are the bell, which is either open or closed by a thin diaphragm, the tubing, and earpieces **(Fig. 14.10)**.
- A closed bell is an impedance matcher between the skin and the air and accumulates sound from the contact area. The skin under the open bell acts as a diaphragm. The skin diaphragm has a natural resonant frequency at which it most effectively transmits sounds. It is used to hear the low-frequency heart murmurs.

Fig. 14.10: Stethoscope.

- A crude open system used in midwifery is called a fetoscope and is used to hear the heart beats sounds of the baby in the pregnant uterus.
- In a stethoscope, we are dealing with a system that is closed at the far end by a pressure-sensitive diaphragm. It is desirable to have a bell with as small a volume as possible. The smaller the volume of gas, the greater the pressure changes for a given movement of the diaphragm at the end of the bell.
- The volume of tubes should also be small and there should be minimum frictional loss of sound due to the walls of tubes. Typically the length of the tube is 25 cm and its diameter is 0.3 cm.

Symbalophone

This instrument is made of two stethoscopes, one going to one ear, the other to the ear. Sounds coming from two regions may be heard at the same time and compared. An example of its use is the simultaneous comparison of the heart sounds of the fetus and mother.

Audiometry

- Audiometry is an apparatus for measuring the ability of the human ear to hear. Basically, measurements are made by determining the minimum intensity of sounds of various frequencies that are just distinguishable by the ear. The minimum intensity obtained is compared with that of the normal ear and is expressed in decibels.
- The audiometer is made to produce sounds of known frequency and intensity that are controlled by the operator. The patient is allowed to hear a sound at higher intensity, and then the intensity is gradually reduced to below the threshold for the patient. The intensity is then increased slowly until the patients just hear it. At that point, the patient signals the operator.
- Separate measurements are made for each ear and by the use of some special audiometers measurements of both air and bone conduction are made for each ear. The patient is tested throughout at intensities between 15 dB below the level which is the threshold for a normal

ear and 95 dB above this level. The results of the measurements are recorded on a chart called an audiogram. Deviations from the zero point on these charts give a measure of hearing loss.
- ❖ Audiometers are of two types
    - Type 1 or Step Type: It has a limited number of specific discrete frequencies.
    - Type 2 or Sweep Type: It has a continuous range of frequencies.
    - Frequencies frequently used in testing hearing are 125, 250, 500, 750, 1000, 2000, 3000, 4000, 6000, 8000 cps.

Speech Audiometry

- ❖ In order for a person to understand the spoken word he must be able to hear at least in the middle of the audiometer range, that is 500, 1000, and 2000 cps. The hearing level for these three frequencies is close to a person's hearing level for speech.
- ❖ The hearing level for speech can be measured by a test that uses tape-recordings of certain selected words of syllables, such as railroad, in which six such words are presented to the person being tested each time at a successively lower intensity level of 4 dB until the words are no longer heard by him.
- ❖ The intensity at which the person can repeat one-half of the words is accepted or is considered to be his speech reception threshold (SRT). The difference between this intensity level and the normal average SRT gives an indication of the person's hearing level of speech.
- ❖ By using a risk of phonetically balanced (PB) monosyllabic words, more information about a person's hearing may be obtained. The PB lists contain 50 words each and represent a frequency of sounds of speech that approximate those found in normal English conversation. A list of words is presented to the person at a uniform intensity. The percentage of words that the person can repeat correctly is called the discrimination score (DS). The average DS for loud sounds (85 dB), for normal sounds (70 dB), and for faint sounds (55 dB) is a practical measure of a person's ability to hear in everyday situations. The score is known as Davis Social Adequacy Index (SAI). The hearing ranges between 94 and 1000. The SAI score that represents the lower limit for social adequacy of the hearing is considered to be 33. A person within this range can understand that only amplified shouted speech may not be understood **(Table 14.2)**.

Applications

- ❖ Ear covers are recommended for employers who work in nosy locations.
- ❖ Airplane field attendants wear covers during landing and take-off of airplanes. Hearing protection is exposed for prolonged period to noises louder than 85 dB for frequencies above 150 cps.

Sonar Navigation and Ranging

During World War I, a technique called sound ranging was developed to locate the position of enemy guns by using a technique to detect the sound of cannon in action. This has led to the development of sonar (sound) navigation and ranging. In sonar, high-frequency sound waves

Table 14.2: Interpreting the hearing loss based on audiometry results.

Results	Interpretation
> 25 dB but not > 40 dB	Slight hearing loss
>40 dB but not > 55 dB	Mild hearing loss
>55 dB but not > 90 dB	Marked hearing loss
70 dB but not > 90 dB	Severe hearing loss

Fig. 14.11: Sonar navigation.

are sent towards the target, and reflected sound is detected. The time taken by sound wave in this round trip gives an idea about the distance of the target (**Fig. 14.11**).

$$V = \frac{x + x}{t}$$
$$v \times t = 2x$$
$$x = \frac{vt}{2}$$

Since velocity is known, distance can be calculated by measuring time.

Ultrasonic Sound Waves

Ultrasonic wave is defined as inaudible sound with high frequency for human, the frequency of which generally exceeds 20 kHz. Ultrasonic waves penetrate tissue and are scattered and absorbed within it. The scattered and reflected ultrasound contains information about the form and structure of the tissue. This ultrasound signal is converted into a visible image using specialized computer techniques, which is called ultrasound imaging.

Production of ultrasonic sound waves: These waves are produced by:
- Magnetostrictive devices depend upon changes in the length of metals such as nickel when magnetized.
- Devices that utilize a crystal depend upon the crystal's exhibiting a piezoelectric reaction. This reaction is the movement of the crystal when a current is passed into it. The device, whether a moving crystal or metal, has a vibrating head known as the transducer, which produces the beam of ultrasonic sound waves.
  - **Adverse effects of the ultrasonic sound waves:** In brief, the effects of high-frequency ultrasonic sound are heating, paralytic and lethal effects.
  - **Heating:** Lipids and proteins have been shown to exhibit an increase in temperature when subjected to ultrasonic sound waves.
  - **Paralytic:** Paralysis of hind legs has been reported. Human beings exposed to ultrasonic fields for long periods of time may develop a loss of equilibrium and an inability to concentrate.
  - **Lethal:** Lethal effects have been reported in studies on large protozoa, red blood cells, and some bacteria.

Uses of Ultrasound

- **Ultrasound diathermy** is helpful in the treatment of joint disease and joint stiffness (**Fig. 14.12**). Ultrasound waves interact with tissue primarily by microscopic motion of tissue particles. As these waves move through the tissue, the regions of compressions and rarefaction cause pressure differences in adjacent regions of the tissue. This results in stretching of stiff

Fig. 14.12: Diathermy.

regions and gives relief to the patient. However, one has to be careful because if the stretching exceeds the elastic limit of the tissue, it may rupture. That is why the eardrum can be ruptured by a very intense sound.

❖ **Ultrasound:**
- It mainly works upon the transmission and reflection properties of sound waves.
- The other thing is change in velocity of sound waves in different mediums thus changing frequency, pitch, and direction.
- Physics of ultrasound used in sonography: In general, pulses of ultrasound are transmitted into the body by placing the vibrating crystal in close contact with the skin, using water or a jelly paste to eliminate the air between the crystal and skin. This gives the good coupling at the skin and greatly increases the transmission of the ultrasound the pulse serves as a detector. The signals received are amplified and displayed on an oscilloscope. This procedure is called the A scanning method of ultrasound diagnosis. For many clinical purposes, A scans have been largely replaced by B scans. The B scan method is used to obtain two-dimensional views of the internal organs or the body. The principles of the B scan are the same as for the A scan except that the transducer is moved. A storage oscilloscope is used so that is lasting image can be formed and photography can be made.
- **The main uses of ultrasound in healthcare practices are:**
  - Sonography is used to assess the fetal well-being during pregnancy as well as used to diagnose several medical illnesses like cirrhosis of the liver, tumors of organs in the abdominal or pelvic cavity, obstruction of intestine, etc.
  - **Echocardiography:** A technique that transmits ultrasonic signals into the tissues and utilized a receiver that record changes in blood velocity have been employed to diagnose heart conditions.
  - Use in diagnosing eye diseases like cataract, measuring the thickness of cornea, the thickness of vitreous humor, etc.
  - **Fetal heart monitoring:** Fetal heart monitor has the ability to reflect ultrasonic sound signals so that the fetal heart beat in as early a period as the 12th week of pregnancy can be detected.
  - **Echoencephalography:** This technique is based on partial reflection of sound at the interface of two media. It is used to detect brain tumors. In this process, the ultrasound

pulses are sent in the skull slightly above the ear, and echoes from the left side of the head are compared with those from the right side.

■ NOISE POLLUTION AND ITS PREVENTION

Noise is often defined as 'unwanted sound' but this definition is subjective to the fact that one man's sound may be another man's noise. Perhaps a better definition of noise is "wrong sound in the wrong place, at the wrong time." Man is living in an increasingly noisy environment. Noise pollution is displeasing human, animal or machine-created sound that disrupts the activity or balance of human or animal life. The word noise comes from the Latin word nausea meaning seasickness.

Sources of Noise

The source of most outdoor noise worldwide is transportation systems, including motor vehicle noise, aircraft noise, and rail noise. Poor urban planning may give rise to noise pollution since side-by-side industrial and residential buildings can result in noise pollution in the residential area.

Other sources of indoor and outdoor noise pollution are car alarms, emergency service sirens, office equipment, factory machinery, construction work, groundskeeping equipment, barking dogs, appliances, power tools, lighting hum, audio entertainment systems, loudspeakers, and noisy people.

Human Health Effects of Noise

Noise health effects are both health and behavioral in nature. The unwanted sound is called noise. This unwanted sound can damage physiological and psychological health. Noise pollution can cause annoyance and aggression, hypertension, high-stress levels, tinnitus, hearing loss, sleep disturbances, and other harmful effects. Furthermore, stress and hypertension are the leading causes of health problems, whereas tinnitus can lead to forgetfulness, severe depression, and at times panic attacks.

Chronic exposure to noise may cause noise-induced hearing loss. Older males exposed to significant occupational noise demonstrate significantly reduced hearing sensitivity than their non-exposed peers, though differences in hearing sensitivity decrease with time and the two groups are indistinguishable by age 79. A comparison of Maaban Tribesmen, who were insignificantly exposed to transportation or industrial noise, to a typical US population showed that chronic exposure to moderately high levels of environmental noise contributes to hearing loss.

High noise levels can contribute to cardiovascular effects and exposure to moderately high levels during a single eight hour period causes a statistical rise in blood pressure of five to ten points and an increase in stress and vasoconstriction leading to the increased blood pressure noted above as well as to the increased incidence of coronary artery disease. Noise pollution is also a cause of annoyance. A 2005 study by Spanish researchers found that in urban areas households are willing to pay approximately four Euros per decibel per year for noise reduction.

Hearing Loss

Hearing loss is inability to partially or completely hear sound in one or both of ears. Hearing loss typically occurs gradually over time. It can be Mild (26-40 decibel), Moderate (41-55 decibel), and Severe (more than 71 decibels) hearing loss.

A person's auditory system consists of the outer ear, middle ear, inner ear and acoustic nerve. The sound wave comes to outer ear then hit on eardrum causing vibration to the drum. This vibration moves to inner ear through bones of middle ear. Where it is converted in nerve impulse by organ of Corti. From there these impulses carried to brain via acoustic nerve. When one of these parts is not working in an optimal way, a hearing loss can occur. While hearing loss can range from mild to profound, there are four classifications that all hearing losses fall under.

There are four types of hearing loss sensorineural, conductive, mixed (sensorineural and conductive) and auditory neuropathy spectrum disorder.

Sensorineural Hearing Loss

Sensorineural hearing loss happens when there's damage to inner ear (cochlea) structures or in the acoustic nerve pathways to the brain. Damage to these structures can occur due to exposure to loud noises, illness (meningitis), ototoxic medications, or it can happen simply due to genetics or the aging process(Presbycusis).

Sensorineural hearing loss is permanent, and treatments include the use of hearing aids and cochlear implants.

Conductive Hearing Loss

A conductive hearing loss occurs when something prevents sound from passing through the outer or middle ear and into the inner ear. This can occur when earwax or fluid builds up in the ear canal, or when there is damage to the eardrum or bones in the middle ear. There may also be a birth defect that prevents sound waves from entering the ear to stimulate the acoustic nerve, such as atresia or microtia.

Treatments may include surgery to repair structural abnormalities, a procedure to remove blockages, or the use of a hearing aid, cochlear implant. A cochlear implant is a small electrical machine placed under the skin behind the ear. It translates sound vibrations into electrical signals that brain can interpret as meaningful sound.

When this type of hearing loss occurs, patient may find it difficult to hear soft or muffled sounds. So nurse should use clear and higher pitched sound.

Mixed Hearing Loss

In some cases, a person may be suffering from both a sensorineural and conductive hearing loss. Mixed hearing loss affects both the inner ear and outer or middle ear, and as such, it can lead to a more profound hearing loss.

Treatments will vary depending on the severity of the hearing loss, but in addition to a surgical procedure, hearing aids and cochlear implants may be necessary.

Auditory Neuropathy Spectrum Disorder

Sometimes sound is able to enter an ear normally and reach the acoustic nerve, but there is a problem when the sound is transmitted to the brain. This hearing loss is known as auditory neuropathy spectrum disorder (ANSD).

ANSD can occur due to various reasons. In some cases, the hair cells of the inner ear are damaged and are unable to properly transmit sound information to the brain. Sometimes a genetic mutation is the cause of this hearing loss, and other times damage to the auditory nerve can lead to ANSD.

People with ANSD may seem to have normal hearing sensitivity on a hearing test, but they may struggle to understand spoken words. In some cases, a hearing aid or cochlear implant paired with a hearing assistive technology (HAT) system can help mitigate the negative effects of this hearing loss. However, more severe cases, in which the person has great difficulty understanding speech, may require the use of a visual communication technique, like sign language or a picture exchange communication system (PECS).

Physical exam

A physical exam can help differentiate SNHL from conductive hearing loss. A doctor will search for inflammation, fluid or earwax build-up, damage to your eardrum, and foreign bodies.

Tuning forks

A tuning fork test as an initial screening. In Weber's test a 512 Hz tuning fork stroked softly and places it near the midline of forehead. If the sound is louder in affected ear, hearing loss is likely conductive. If sound is louder in unaffected ear, hearing loss is likely sensorineural. Whereas in Rinne test a tuning fork stroked and places it against mastoid bone behind ear until person no longer hear the sound. Then the tuning fork is moved in front of ear canal until person can't hear the sound. If anyone has SNHL, will be able to hear the tuning fork better in front of your ear canal than against your bone.

Audiogram

During the test, headphones are worn in a soundproof booth. Tones and words will be played into each ear at different volumes and frequencies. The test helps find the quietest sound that anyone can hear and specific frequencies of hearing loss as mentioned earlier.

Precautions

- Use safety equipment if you work in areas with loud noises, and wear earplugs when you swim and go to concerts.
- Keep your headphone volume under 60 percent.
- Consult a doctor before starting a new medication.
- Have regular hearing tests if you work around loud noises, swim often, or go to concerts on a regular basis.
- Avoid prolonged exposure to loud noises and music.
- Seek help for ear infections. They may cause permanent damage to the ear if they are left untreated.

Prevention of Noise Pollution

A variety of approaches may be needed to prevent and control the noise pollution; there are as follows:
- **Carefully planning of cities:** In planning the cities, the following measures should be taken to reduce noise:
  - Division of the cities into zones with separation of areas concerned with industry and transportation.
  - The separation of the residential area from the main street by means of wide green belts. Houses front should lie not less than 15 meters from the road and the intervening space should be thickly planted with trees and bushes.
  - Widening of the main street to reduce the penetration of noise into the dwelling area.

- **Control of the vehicles:** Heavy vehicles should not be routed into narrow streets. Vehicular traffic on residential streets should be reduced. The indiscriminate blowing of the horn and use of pressure horn should be prohibited.
- **To improve acoustic insulation of building:** From the acoustic standpoint, the best arrangement is the construction of detached buildings rather than a single large building or one that is continuous. Installation that produces noise or disturb the occupant within the dwelling should be prohibited. Buildings should be soundproof where necessary.
- **Industries and railways:** Control of the noise at the source is possible in industries. The special area must be earmarked, outside residential areas, for industries, railways, marshaling yards, and smaller installations. When these demands cannot be met, a protective green belt must be laid down between the installations and residential areas.
- **Protection of exposed persons:** Hearing protection is recommended for all workers who are consistently exposed to noise louder than 85 decibels in the frequency band above 150 Hz. Workers must be regularly rotated from noisy areas to comparatively quiet posts in factories. Periodical audiogram check-ups and use of earplugs must be ensured. Muffs are also essential as the situation demands.
- **Legislation:** Many adapted legislation provided for controls that are applicable to a wide variety of sources. Workers have the right to claim compensation if they have suffered a loss of ability to understand speech.
- **Education:** No noise abatement program can be successful without people's participation. Therefore, their education through all available media is needed to highlight the importance of noise as a community hazard.

QUESTIONS

Q.1: Use of stethoscope for listening to sounds for human body.
Q.2: During pregnancy ultrasound examination is advised instead of an X-ray examination.
Q.3: Discuss about the hearing aid and transmission of sound in the ear.

BIBLIOGRAPHY

1. Berglund B, Lindvall T, Schwela D, et al. "World Health Organization: Guidelines for Community Noise". World Health Organization, 1999.
2. Field JM. "Effect of personal and situational variables upon noise annoyance in residential areas". Journal of the Acoustical Society of America, 1993;93(5):2753-63.
3. Kryter, Karl D. The handbook of hearing and the effects of noise: physiology, psychology, and public health. Boston: Academic Press,1994.
4. National Research Council (US) Committee on Disability Determination for Individuals with Hearing Impairments; Dobie RA, Van Hemel S, editors. Hearing Loss: Determining Eligibility for Social Security Benefits. Washington (DC): National Academies Press (US); 2004. 2, Basics of Sound, the Ear, and Hearing. Available from: https://www.ncbi.nlm.nih.gov/books/NBK207834/
5. Park K. Park's Textbook of Preventive and Social Medicine. 20th edition. Jabalpur: Banarsidas Bhanot Publishers, 2009.
6. Passchier-VW, Passchier WF. "Noise exposure and public health". Environ Health Perspect. 2000;108(1):123-31.
7. Paul Davidovits, Waves and Sound, Editor(s): Paul Davidovits, Physics in Biology and Medicine (Fifth Edition), Academic Press, 2019,Pages 173-92. https://doi.org/10.1016/B978-0-12-813716-1.00012-4.
8. Walker JR, Fahy F. Fundamentals of noise and vibration. London: E & FN Spon, 1998.

CHAPTER 15

Electricity and Electromagnetism

Suresh K Sharma, Navjot Kaur

Chapter Outline

- Types of Electricity
- Sources of Electric Current
- Effects of Electric Current
- Effects of Electricity on the Human Body
- Magnetism
- Applications of the Magnet and Magnetism
- Electroencephalography (EEG)
- Electrocardiography (ECG)
- Phonocardiography
- Electromyography (EMG)
- Electromyography Pattern
- Electrostimulation
- Electroconvulsive Therapy (ECT)
- Electronic Cardiac Pacemaker
- Brain Pacemaker
- Defibrillation
- Automated External Defibrillator
- Magnetic Resonance Imaging (MRI)
- CAT Scan

INTRODUCTION

The phenomenon of electricity was known to the ancient Greeks, who observed in 600 BC, that a piece of amber, when rubbed vigorously with a woolen cloth would attract light particles of matter towards it. Gilbert is credited with gaining the term 'electric'. He called these substances that exhibited attraction forces for one another when rubbed, as 'electrics' from the Greek word for amber 'electron'.

A charge is an inherent property of matter. Just as the mass is responsible for the gravitational forces, charge is responsible for electric forces. The three most common particles are electrons, protons, and neutrons. Electrons are negatively charged and protons are positively charged while neutrons are neutral. Charge on an electron repels charge on another electron while it attracts a proton, i.e., similar charges repel each other while opposite charges attract. We can experience by rubbing two solid bodies against each other. If we pass a comb through dry hair, it becomes electrically charged and can attract pieces of paper. A sheet of paper becomes charged when it is passed through a printing machine.

TYPES OF ELECTRICITY

Basically, electricity is classified into two broad categories, i.e. electrostatics or static electricity and electrodynamics.
1. **Electrostatics or Static Electricity:** It is characterized by the accumulation of charges of electricity on the surface of substances.
2. **Electrodynamics:** It is characterized by the flow of electrons through a conductor.

Electrostatics (Static Electricity)

- If a glass is rubbed with a silk cloth and suspended, it will be repelled by a rod similarly treated when the second rod is brought close to the first.
- A hard-rubber rod rubbed with wool is similarly repelled by another hard rubber rod.
- If the glass rod is placed near the suspended rubber rod, however, the two are attracted. These are examples of the production of electricity by friction **(Fig. 15.1)**.
- For example, many of us have at one time or another experienced the shock of static electricity by walking across a thick rug and then touching a metal object such as a door knob or key in a lock.

Theory of Electrification

Static electricity is with respect to the structure of the atom. All atoms are made of a closely packed nuclei having a positive charge and containing neutrons and protons. Around the nucleus are electrons with negative charges.

The electrons are found at various energy levels or in orbits at a distance from the nucleus. In an object such as a copper wire, which is made-up of many copper atoms, it is conceivable that electrons in the outer regions of the atoms might move at random from one atom to another, if an electron leaves the outer region of one atom, another electron must move in from a different atom to maintain the neutrality of first atom **(Fig. 15.2)**. These are called free electrons.

It is generally assumed that non-electrified or uncharged objects possess equal numbers of positive and negative charges. When friction is applied, in the case of the glass rod rubbed with silk, some negative charges (electrons) are apparently transferred from the glass to the silk. This leaves the glass rod with a net positive charge and the silk with an equal net negative charge. Similarly, the hard rubber rod receives negative charges from the wool and leaves

Charges build in static electricity

Fig. 15.1: Static electricity.

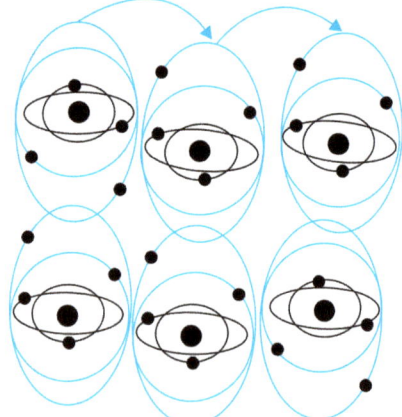

Fig. 15.2: Theory of electrification.

the wool positively charged. It is theorized that free electrons are actually transferred in the rubbing process. If a substance receives extra free electrons from another, the substance is said to be negatively charged. If an object loses free electrons, it is said to be positively charged.

Coulomb's Law

It states that "force of attraction or repulsion between the two charges is directly proportional to the product of the charges and inversely proportional to the square of the distance between them".

$$F = \frac{KQ_1Q_2}{r_2}$$

Mathematically, here Q_1 and Q_2 are the charges on the particles, 'r' is the distance between them, and 'K' is the constant of proportionality which depends upon the medium.

Conduction

A piece of matter of any size contains billions of atoms, and each atom contains a positively charged nucleus and several electrons around it. In gases, the atoms almost do not interact with each other or a negligible interaction is there. In solids and liquids, the interaction is stronger. In some of them, the outer electrons of each atom are weakly bound to it (called free electrons) and have a high conductivity, called conductors. In another type of material, all electrons are tightly bound to their respective atoms or molecules, i.e. there are no free electrons, called insulators. There is one more type of material, that behave like insulators at 0K, but at higher temperatures, few electrons are able to free themselves from atoms and thus conduct electricity, called semiconductors.

We can summarize, that substances that transmit electrons freely are good conductors of electricity. Examples of such good conductors are metals and aqueous solutions of acids, bases, and salts. Out of the metals, silver is the best conductor, however, because of the cost factor, copper is mostly used **(Fig. 15.3)**.

Substances that do not transmit electrons freely are called insulators. A few examples are dry air, rubber, and glass. Dry wood, distilled water and alcohol are intermediate in action and are called poor conductors.

Fig. 15.3: Good conductors.

Fig. 15.4: Bad and semiconductor.

Semiconductors, the substances, those are intermediate with respect to conducting electrons. Very common examples are germanium and silicon mainly used in transistors **(Fig. 15.4)**.

Examples

- Because the water for household use almost always contains some salts in solution. It conducts electricity.
- A frayed, wet electric cord in which the wires are exposed may shock a person touching it.
- Electrocution has occurred from touching a faulty switch or the chain of an electric fixture with wet hands.
- Since the tissues of the human body are bathed by a saline solution, the body itself is capable of conducting electricity. This is the basis for many treatments and diagnostic tests.

Induction

It is also possible to electrify objects by a process known as induction.

- **Process of induction:** In this process, if a negatively charged rod is brought close to an uncharged insulated conductor, the electrons on the side of the conductor nearer the rod are repelled, and move toward the other side of the conductor, leaving the side nearer the rod positively charged. Actually, there is no gain or loss of electrons, but rather a separation of two kinds of charges. If the conductor is then grounded (connected to earth by a wire) or touched with the finger, the electrons pass to ground. In this way the conductor retains the positive charges. For example, lightning rod.
- In the atmosphere, positive charges accumulate on moving "thunder clouds". Under the cloud on the surface of the earth, a corresponding negative charge is induced. As the cloud begins to move toward the earth, the tension between its charges and those on the earth's surface increases. The air becomes ionized, it is no longer a good insulator, and the charges unite with a flash of light and a release of heat energy that is commonly called lightening. A lightning rod is an example of a pointed conductor that extends from damp or wet ground to the air above buildings. The lightning rod causes some of the charge induced in the earth by the charges on the cloud to pass into the air, thus reducing the potential difference between the cloud and earth to a level at which no lightning is produced **(Fig. 15.5)**.

Fig. 15.5: Lightening rod.

Discharging of Charged Bodies

There are three ways in which a charged object may discharge its electricity. These are by spark, by brush discharge, and by conduction. The spark is disruptive and causes a breakdown of the surrounding medium with the emission of radiant energy. It occurs from highly polished spherical knobs that have dry air between them (**Fig. 15.6**).

In a brush discharge, on the other hand, charges accumulate unevenly and are concentrated at projections and sharp points. The air molecules next to these "brush points" become charged with the same charge as is on the points. The air is then repelled from the point since both charges are the same and this actually creates a breeze, moving the air back from the point of discharge.

Electrostatic precipitation: It is used in industry to reduce air pollution and to recover material that would otherwise be lost in smoke. In this procedure, metallic points or small wires that are highly charged by induction from an electrostatic machine are placed in smoke stacks. When the wires are charged, the air in the chimney is repelled and the particles in the smoke is "precipitated out". Lightning rods also act by brush discharge during a storm when no lightning occurs. Discharges may be made also by conduction through a process called grounding. In this procedure, the discharge is practically instantaneous. Grounding is the process of removing the excess charge on an object by means of the transfer of electrons between it and another object of substantial size. When a charged object is grounded, the excess charge is balanced by the transfer of electrons between the charged object and the ground. The earth is said to be a great

Fig. 15.6: Discharge by spark.

Fig. 15.7: Electrostatic precipitation.

reservoir for excess electrons. When an object is grounded, charges either pass from it to the earth or from the earth to it **(Fig. 15.7)**.

Applications of Electrostatics

- In hospitals, static charges may collect on the hands because of friction with the bedclothes. When a woolen blanket or a sheet is rubbed briskly across a bed. Because of this, sparks accompanied by mild shock may form between the nurse's hand and the patient when she touches the patient. The formation of such sparks can be prevented by touching some metal object or water pipe with a flat hand. In this way, excess electrons are conducted to the ground.
- The use of woolen blankets on beds of patients in an oxygen tent and in operating rooms is sometimes forbidden for the same reason. Tests indicate that potential differences between the floor and the operating room table of as much as 10,000 volts may be produced in moving a woolen blanket when it is rubbed briskly over a rubber-covered mattress. The formation of sparks would be extremely dangerous in an atmosphere filled with explosive mixtures of anesthetic such as ether and air.
- The use of silk, nylon, or Dacron uniforms in the operating rooms is forbidden in some hospitals.
- Rubber-soled shoes are not recommended since they insulate the wearer from the floor and cause charges to accumulate on the person.
- Because dry air tends to promote an accumulation of static electricity, high relative humidity in the operating room will help to prevent spark formation.
- It is the practice in some operating rooms to wrap a damp cloth around the feet of the operating room tables to allow for easier passage of the charges from the table to the floor.
- All electrical equipment used in the operating room, including the operating table, should be grounded. Grounding is produced by means of a chain or cable leading from the apparatus to a water pipe or radiator that makes contact with the earth.
- Articles should be checked periodically with conductivity tests which can detect how well one object can conduct away static electric charges that tend to accumulate on its surface.

Electrodynamics

Most practical applications of electricity involve electric current, from your table lamp to power lines transferring energy from power companies to homes and businesses. We use the term 'electric current' or 'simply current' to describe the rate of flow of charge through some space. When charges accumulate on a conducting body, they tend to move and this gives rise to electric current.

We can say that "charge in motion constitutes current and the study of its effects is known as electrodynamics".

The amount of flow of charges depends on the material through which charges are being passed and the potential difference across the material.

Current

Consider two points between which a potential difference exists and suppose they are connected by a copper wire. Free electrons tend to flow from a lower potential point to a higher potential point (opposite to the direction of the electric field). Current is assumed to be opposite to the direction of flow of negative charges and in direction of flow of positive charges **(Fig. 15.8)**.

"The rate of flow of charge in a conductor is known as current".
Mathematically, we can write current

$$I = \frac{Q}{t}$$

Where
- I = current
- Q = change
- t = time

We can visualize the electric current as the number of electrons that pass through any section per second. The practical unit of current is ampere, which is donated by 'A'.

Battery and Electromotive Force

Electromotive force is defined as the electric potential produced by either electrochemical cell or by changing the magnetic field. Electromotive force is the commonly used acronym for electromotive force. A battery is an electrochemical device that maintains a potential difference between its two terminals. The battery's internal mechanism exerts forces on charges of battery material so that positive charges move towards the positive terminal of the battery and negative charges towards the negative terminal of the battery. And thus, creates a potential difference between its two terminals.

Electromotive force is defined as the work done on a unit charge. The free electrons in conductors are the charges constituting electric current in a circuit. In addition to these free electrons, some sort of force is needed to push the electrons along the circuit. This force comes from the potential difference or electromotive force. It is measured in volt.

Fig. 15.8: Flow of charges.

Fig. 15.9: Electronic circuit with resistance.

Resistance

Just as friction opposes the mechanical motion, the opposition to the flow of electric current in an electric circuit is known as resistance (**Fig. 15.9**).

The practical unit of electrical resistance is the ohm. One ohm is that resistance across which a potential difference of 1 volt produces a current of 1 ampere. The resistance of a conductor wire depends on its length, area of cross-section, the nature of the material, and temperature.

To understand EMF and resistance, we can form an analogy between water pipes and electric wires. Just as higher the height of the water tank or more pressure in the pipe, water will flow with more speed; higher potential difference leads to higher current. Suppose if we insert a few pieces of cotton in a pipe, water will flow with a comparatively slower speed now; similarly, the resistance is, depends on the material and opposes the flow of charges.

Ohm's Law

The relationship between resistance, voltage, and current was formulated by Ohm. It is stated as follows:

"The current in a conductor is linearly proportional to the difference of potential between any two points and inversely proportional to the resistance, provided physical conditions such as temperature, pressure, area of cross-section, etc. remain unchanged".

Mathematically, we can write:

$$I = \frac{V}{R}$$

Here 'I', is current in amperes, 'V' is voltage in volts, 'R' is resistance in ohms.

■ SOURCES OF ELECTRIC CURRENT

Since an electric current exists only when electrons move through a conductor. A continuous source of energy must be available to keep the electrons in motion. This energy may be of various types such as radiant, thermal, chemical, mechanical, or magnetic.

Radiant source of electricity: When light rays fall upon a clean metallic surface such as a film of potassium or sodium, electrons are emitted by the surface of the metal. This phenomenon is called the photoelectric effect. In addition to potassium and sodium, lithium, cesium, and selenium have photo-emissive properties. They emit electrons when light falls on their surfaces.

Device: These electrons can be made to form an electric current through a device called a photoelectric cell (**Fig. 15.10**). The cell consists of a tube containing a curved plate of photosensitive metal. This plate is called the cathode of the tube. In addition, there is a rod of

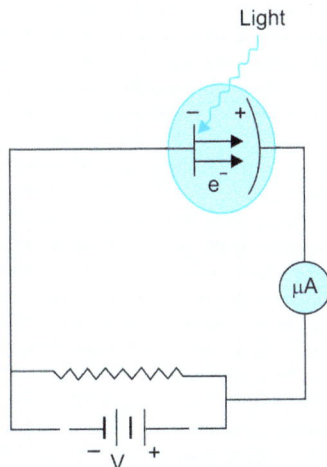

Fig. 15.10: Photoelectric cell.

metal such as copper called the anode sealed within the tube. When the light falls on the plate, it emits electrons. Because electrons are negatively charged objects, they will be attracted to a positively charged object. The metal rod is made positive. Essentially, this produces an electric current.

Uses

- Automatic illumination of buildings
- Traffic signals
- Automatic opening and closing of doors as persons approach them.

Thermal source of electricity: Heat can also be used to develop small amounts of electricity. If a wire loop consisting of a piece of copper joined to a piece of iron is heated at one junction, a current will flow through the loop. Such a loop of dissimilar metals joined at both ends is called a thermocouple **(Fig. 15.11)**.

The flow of electrons continues as long as one junction is at a higher temperature than the other. The thermocouple is used to measure high temperatures. It is sometimes used to control the supply of fuel to a gas furnace. It cannot be used for producing large amounts of electricity continuously. It may be used to detect heat from a distant object. The degree of heat is ascertained by measuring the amount of current produced.

Fig. 15.11: Thermocouple.

Fig. 15.12: Voltaic cell.

Chemical source of electric current: Certain metals placed in a solution of acids, bases, or salts (electrolytes) give off electrons. When two dissimilar metals are separated from one another by an electrolyte, a current will flow, for example, the orthopedic surgeon immobilizing bones with metal plates uses the same type of metal in the plate and in the screws that hold the plate in place. If the precautions were overlooked, the resulting current between two dissimilar metals might be so painful that the plate would have to be removed **(Fig. 15.12)**.

$$\text{Voltaic cell: } Zn^{(-)} \text{ and } Cu^{(+)} \text{ in } H_2SO_4$$

Magnetic and mechanical sources of electricity: Light, heat, and chemical energy can generate electricity, but the amounts are limited. To produce almost unlimited amounts of electricity, a method of making it by utilizing magnetism, specialty a magnetic field, is generally employed. The process can be traced back to two sides. In 1820, Oersted discovered the presence of a magnetic field around a wire coil carrying an electric current, and in 1931, Faraday discovered the flow of electric current when he moved a bar magnet through a wire coil. Faraday also found a flow of electricity as he withdrew the magnet. The motion of the electricity in the coil continued only while the magnet was in a motion and passed into or out of the coil. Thus, it was a comparatively simple method of producing electricity. Examples, generators or dynamo **(Fig. 15.13)**.

■ EFFECTS OF ELECTRIC CURRENT

As other forms of energy can be transformed into electrical energy, vice versa is also true. When an electric current passes through a conductor, a variety of effects may be produced. These effects may be described as radiant, thermal, chemical, mechanical, or magnetic.

Fig. 15.13: Working of generators.

Radiant Effects

- It is the transformation of electric energy into light energy.
- When the electrons in a circuit pass through a tungsten filament of an incandescent lamp, they heat the wire and give off electromagnetic waves of visible light.
- The incandescent filament in a 100-watt lamp produces a temperature of about 4,600 degrees Fahrenheit.
- If the filament were surrounded by air, the metal filament would oxidize and burn up at the temperature produced. For this reason, the air is removed from the bulb and an inert gas that does not support combustion is captured in the light bulb.
- Another example is fluorescent tubes.

Thermal Effects

- The flow of electrons through a conductor such as a special resistance wire produces heat.
- Electric hot plates, irons, toasters, heaters, heating pads, and electric cauterizes operate on this principle.
- Specially made surgical instruments operating on low amperage and high-frequency alternating currents may be used to coagulate tissues and small bleeding vessels during an operation. The current is discharged from the edges of the instrument directly to the tissues, thereby producing heat. These instruments are sometimes employed when it is necessary to prevent hemorrhage as in brain surgery. For example, electric cautery (**Fig. 15.14**).

Chemical Effects

- When a direct current flows through a solution of an electrolyte, chemical changes occur.
- Electrolysis may be used to destroy the follicles of unwanted hair by causing the cells of the follicle to disintegrate chemically. Considerable skill is required to destroy the hair follicle by electrolysis without damaging the skin.
- Under certain conditions, the electric current is found in the circuits of private homes. An institution may be sufficient to cause death. When a person is standing in water, as may

Fig. 15.14: Electric cautery.

happen in a tub or shower, current travels rapidly from the appliance through the person towards the ground. This sudden passage of electricity may overstimulate the vagus nerve to the point of stopping the heart and death may result. Death may also occur from the chemical disintegration of the tissues through which the current passes.

Mechanical Effects

A generator is an apparatus for producing an induced current by rotating a wire loop through magnetic lines of force. A motor might be called a generator in reverse. The electric motor uses electrical energy produced by the generation to produce motion. Electric motors are used in an almost endless list of modern devices such as fans, refrigerators, sewing machines, sanders, polishers, and typewriters, and in the hospital for operating suction machines, centrifuges, and many other therapeutic apparatus. Basically, the motor consists of a rotating coil in a magnetic field. A current is passed through the wire coil of the motion, and this coil, known as the armature, rotates to produce power that can be used for a variety of activities. The motor is an apparatus that transforms electric energy back into mechanical energy. Some motors operate on alternating current only; other operates on direct current only. A motor that operates on both AC and DC is said to be universal. The type of current used by the motor is indicated on a tag attached to the cape of the equipment. Permanent damage may result from the use of the wrong type of current. Equipment in the hospital and home should be checked for this identifying tag before use.

The Electromagnet

- The electromagnet is an example of the inter-dependability of electricity and magnetism. All electric motors are dependent upon on electromagnet for their operation **(Fig. 15.15)**.
- An electromagnet is a combination of a coil of wire and a core of iron or steel. When current passes through the wire coil, these lines of force that pass out in all directions are collected in the core where less resistance is offered them than in the surrounding air. Each molecule of the core acts like an independent magnet and combined, these form a large magnet. By using this technique, magnets with many times the strength of an ordinary magnet can be formed.
- Large electromagnets can be used to raise extremely heavy masses of iron, and still for short distances. Small electromagnets are basic in the operation of an electric bell or buzzer, telegraph equipment, telephones and other electric equipment.

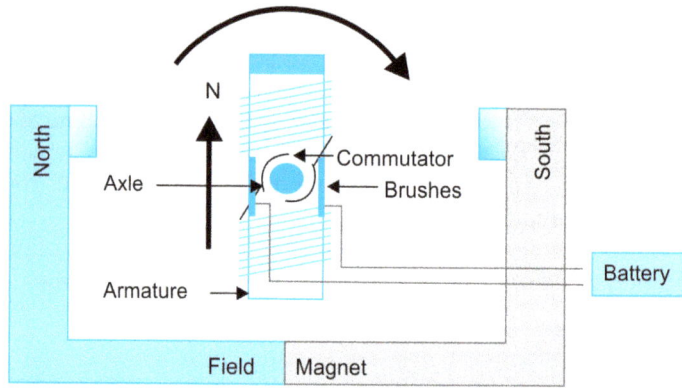

Fig. 15.15: Electric motors.

EFFECTS OF ELECTRICITY ON THE HUMAN BODY

The study of the effects of electricity on the human body helps the health workers to take appropriate decision for appropriate action when human beings are sometimes exposed to shocks accidentally. Electric shocks may be administered therapeutically for diagnosis or for treatment of nervous and muscular disorders. The common effects are:

- The amount of electric current that flows through the body, most of the voltage is believed to cause adverse effects. The amount of current varies directly with the voltage and inversely with the resistance between the points of application of the voltage.
- In most electric accidents contact of the body with the source of electricity is not complete and the contact resistance cuts down the amount of electric current that flows.
- Other things being equal, when contact resistance is low, flow of current is high and vice versa.
- If a person is standing on wet ground or in water so that contact resistance to the ground is low, and if at the same time he is making good contact with the source of voltage above ground, large quantities of current will flow.
- In case, even though the voltage may be low, the current may be large enough to cause death.
- When, on the other hand, contact resistance is high and the person is insulated to some degree from the ground, even though the voltage is high enough to cause a significant flow of current, heat may be generated instead, and surface burns may result.
- The central nervous system is especially susceptible to electric injury. In an electric shock, if current flow through the brain is large, unconscious may occur, retrograde amnesia is experienced and the patient remembers nothing about the accidents.
- Damage to the cranial nerves may produce sensory hallucinations.
- Blindness and deafness may result from permanent damage to the retina and organ of Corti. Death from shock is usually through the cardiac or respiratory arrest.

MAGNETISM

Magnetism was known to the ancient Greek tribe called the magnetes. There is evidence that magnetite or lodestone, a rock that is naturally magnetic, was known to the Greeks in the seventh century BC if not earlier. A European treatise on magnetic behavior was prepared in the thirteenth century who discussed use of lodestone in a mariner's compass. Present-day understanding of magnetic behavior arose from the combined work of many scientists in many countries. The relationship between an electric current and a magnet led Michael Faraday, to the discovery of the electromagnetic effect that is the basis of the dynamo and electric motor. Our present technology is largely built upon the many applications of electromagnetism.

Polarity

An iron or a rod of steel that has been magnetized is called a bar magnet. If such a bar magnet is suspended so that it can turn freely, it will arrange itself with its axis along a north and south line in the absence of other magnetic materials. The same end of the magnet will always turn toward the north. It is called the north-seeking or north pole of the magnet. Similarly, the other end of the magnet is called south-seeking or south pole of the magnet. Opposite poles of a magnet attract each other and similar poles repel each other.

Law of Magnetic Force

Coulomb's law: "The force of attraction or repulsion is directly proportional to the product of the strength of the poles and inversely proportional to the square of the distance between them".

The force in dynes is obtained from the following equation:

$$F = \frac{m_1 m_2}{D_2}$$

If $m_1 = m_2 = 1$ unit pole, d (distance) = 1 cm, then F = 1 dyne.

The unit pole is defined as one that exerts a force of 1 dyne upon another pole of equal strength when the two are 1 cm apart in a vacuum.

Magnetic Fields

- The region around a magnet in which its magnetic effects are apparent is called the magnetic field of the magnet. The magnetic field may be considered to be made of many lines of force that, according to an agreement among physicists are said to pass from the north pole towards the south pole of the magnet outside the magnet.
- When unlike poles are brought close together, some of the lines of force pass out of the north pole of one magnet to the south pole of another magnet and two magnets are attracted (**Fig. 15.16**).
- When like poles are brought close to one another, the lines of force separate the two magnets passing from the south pole to the respective south poles of each magnet (**Fig. 15.17**).

Field strength: "It is defined as the force in dynes acting upon a unit magnetic pole at a specified point". The unit of magnetic field strength happens to be ampere per meter or A/m. It is also represented by 'H'.

Fig. 15.16: Magnetic attraction.

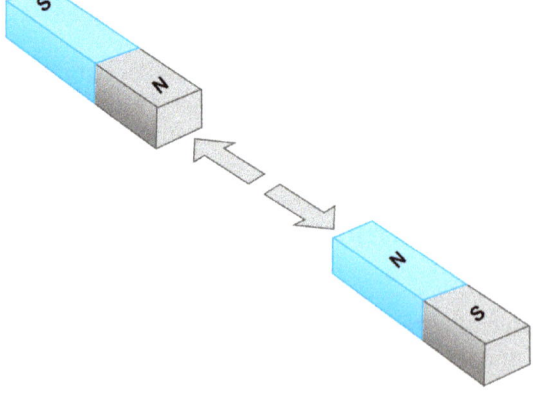

Fig. 15.17: Magnetic repulsion.

CHAPTER 15: Electricity and Electromagnetism

Characteristics of Magnetic Lines of Force
- When a magnet and a steel needle are separated by a piece of glass, the needle is still attracted to the magnet through the glass. Magnetic lines of force can pass through some substances such as glass, wood, zinc, lead and copper without appreciable change. Such substance are said to have low permeability to magnetism.
- When other substances such as soft iron, steel cobalt and pure nickel are placed beside a magnet, they concentrate magnetic lines of force and become magnets themselves. Such substances are said to be highly permeable to magnetism.
- Magnetic lines of force follow the path of least resistance. If a bar of soft iron and a bar of glass are placed next to the same magnet, the lines of force enter the iron because it is more perusable to magnetism than glass.

Magnetic Inductions
- When a piece of iron or steel is rubbed with a magnet or is placed in a magnetic field, it becomes a magnet. Magnets produced in the manner is said to be induced magnets and this produced is called magnetism by induction. Different kinds of iron and steel differ in their ability to retain magnetism. A very soft iron bar placed near the magnet becomes magnetized by induction. When it is taken away from the original magnet, however, it becomes demagnetized.
- Hard steel, on the other hand, can be magnetized by induction also, but it remains magnetized which it is removed from the magnetic field.
- Substances such as iron develop the strong intensity of magnetism. When put in a magnetic field are said to be ferromagnetic. Nickel and cobalt are ferromagnetic.
- Highly magnetic alloys containing two or all three of the ferromagnetic group of metals-iron, nickel, and cobalt are important industrially. There are sometimes called permalloys because they have a high degree of permeability to magnetism.
- Other substances such as aluminum are not ferromagnetic; they are unable to concentrate lines of force in a magnetic field. These substances are weakly magnetic and are said to be paramagnetic.
- Still, other substances that are called diamagnetic tend to move away from strong magnetic fields into weaker ones.
- When a current of electricity passes through a coil of wire because the current loops act as a magnet and set up a magnetic field. If a soft iron rod is placed within the coil while the current is flowing, it becomes magnetized. The magnetic field of the current aligns the atoms in the iron rod. When the current is turned off, the atoms in the rod become disordered. A magnet made in this way is called an electromagnet.

Effect of Temperature on Magnet
- Magnetic properties of the ferromagnetic group of elements seem to be affected by temperature changes. If a bar of nickel is picked up by a magnet and heated, it will fall away from the magnet at about 350°C. Above this temperature, it is not attracted to the magnet. This is also true of iron and steel. A piece of iron will also lose its magnetic properties at a temperature above 800°C.
- It is believed that heat energy increases the internal energy of atoms and random orders of the atoms in the substance. The vigorous random motion destroys the alignment of the atoms as they exit in the magnetized state. The substance cannot exist as a magnet without the orderliness of the atoms.

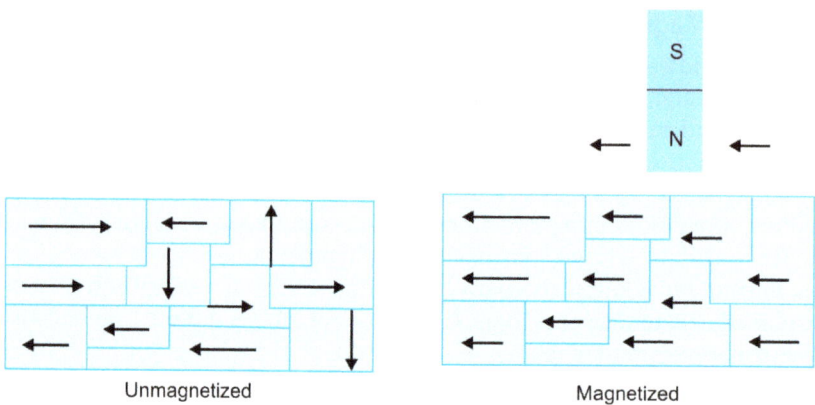

Fig. 15.18: Domain theory.

- **Magnetic moment:** A useful quantity for measuring a magnetic strength is called field force (mmf).
- **Domain theory:** It is a curious fact that if a magnet is cut in two, isolated north and south poles are not produced; rather, each half becomes a complete magnet, again with north and south seeking poles. If cut in half once again four complete magnets are produced. Conceivably, this subdivision could be carried down to the atomic state and each atom would become a magnet **(Fig. 15.18)**.

The domain theory of magnetism refers to a grouping of atoms with similarly aligned magnet moments into a domain. When a substance such as iron is subjected to an external magnetic field the walls of the domains move to increase the number of domains that are in line with external force. Some of the unaligned domains rotate and lineup.

Earth as a magnet: The earth itself acts as a magnet, with one magnetic pole at the north and the other almost directly opposite at the south. The magnetic field of the earth is shaped generally as if it were produced by a huge bar magnet.

APPLICATIONS OF THE MAGNET AND MAGNETISM

- Many devices that are important to our present civilized existence are based on magnetism. Among such devices are the telephone, telegraph, the electric bell, and the buzzer, the generation of electric current, and motors that transform the electric current into useful work **(Fig. 15.19)**.
- Magnets as such have many varied uses. In industries, they are sometimes used to remove small bites of iron or steel from grain or tobacco.
- In the hospital, a bar magnet with a rounded end may be used to remove iron and steel splinters that lodge in the conjunctiva of the eye.
- Large magnets may be used in surgery to remove foreign bodies of iron and steel from regions difficult to reach by other methods.
- A special device that has been reported operates on the basis of a magnetic force; it can be used to detect the presence of and position of metallic foreign substances in the body **(Fig. 15.19)**.
- There are reports of the passing of a catheter around eleven tortuous curves in the neck and cranium into the middle cerebral artery of the brain using a special magnetized catheter and electromagnet. The catheter is guided in the passage by gentle vibrations produced by the electromagnet on the magnet in the catheter under ordinary conditions; this is a difficult, if not possible procedure. The vibrations ease the catheter into the vessels eliminating the friction that would occur between ordinary catheters and blood vessel walls.

Fig. 15.19: Magnetic devices.

ELECTROENCEPHALOGRAPHY (EEG)

* Some action potentials within the body are manifested as surface potentials. The electroencephalogram is an example of a record of electrical activity of surface potentials that result from electrical activity within the body, in this case, the brain is the body part from where electrical activity is recorded.
* By using the electron tube amplifiers that amplify over 10 million times, it has been shown by investigators that the cerebral cortex exhibits rhythmic electric variations of potential. The potentials of the cortex are found to be present at all times except during profound anesthesia and stoppage of blood supply. When the cortex is destroyed, the pattern changes.
* Waves can be led away from the scalp by means of padded electrodes applied to the scalp or by needle electrodes placed into the scalp. One of these is a fine needle connected below the superficial layer of the scalp. Another type is a flat disk-shaped electrode that is fastened to the scalp with a conducting material.
* The waves are the result of action potentials of the neurons of the cerebral cortex.
* A significant property of waves is their frequencies. The range in normal subjects to 1 to 60/sec. A crude classification is as follows **(Fig. 15.20)**:
  * **Alpha waves:** Frequency between 5 and 13/second or less
  * **β-waves (sedation):** 14 to 60/second.
  * **Delta waves (sedation):** 5/sec or less.

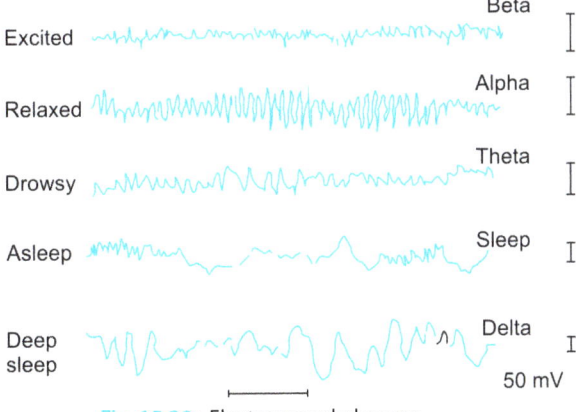

Fig. 15.20: Electroencephalogram.

Classification according to form of wave:
- Spiked
- Flattened
- Serrated

A recording is done graphically or electrically by a cathode ray recording. The recording is called an electroencephalogram (EEG). The waves are evaluated according to their frequencies, voltages, incidences, waveforms and patterns.

Uses of EEG

- In diagnosing epilepsy, tumors, hematoma, trauma, drug addiction, and alcoholism.
- Studies have been made that show that the depth of anesthesia experienced by a patient may be revealed by encephalography.
- In one study, seven levels of brain depression from the normal waking state to a complete absence of electric discharges have been described for ether.

■ ELECTROCARDIOGRAPHY (ECG)

- In this case, a record of surface potentials is made of active heart muscles during the cardiac cycle.
- Several methods are employed today to record ECG.

Process of ECG

Generally, electric charges are carried from the surface of the body to a fine gold-plated quartz fiber. That is supported between the poles of an electromagnet. As current passes through the fiber, it moves, a beam of light that passes across the poles of a magnet and the image of the motion of the fiber is recorded on a film.

In another method, a heated stylus is attached to the moving fiber and the stylus describes the pattern of the electrical activity of the heart on a roll of plastic-coated paper.

Technique

In the technique, generally used, electrodes are placed on the right arm, left arm, and left leg. Other electrodes are placed at various levels of the chest and back. Any two of these electrodes may be connected to a galvanometer at any one time and the voltage of one of them with respect to the other one is recorded. These voltages will be the algebraic sum of the body surface voltages under each the electrodes. The voltages are associated with electrical manifestations of the activities in the cardiac cycle. During the cardiac cycle, when the upper part of the heart is active, the upper extremities will be at a lower electric potential than the lower extremities. The difference in potential is small, but it can be amplified by a triode tube.

During a recording of ECG, the body acts as a container of saline solution, which is a conductor. The recording electrodes that are fixed to the skin with a conducting paste respond to the potential field produced by heart action.

Wave Pattern

ECG represents a series of waves and deflections during a complete cycle. The waves are known as the P wave, QRS complex, and the T wave (**Fig. 15.21**).

- **P wave:** Follows the initiation of a heartbeat by a pacemaker. The wave is produced by the movement of a wave of electrical activity through the atria. This represents the atrial contraction. It represents the electrical activities associated with the spread of the original

Fig. 15.21: Electrocardiogram.

impulse from the sinoatrial node (SA) through the atria. If the P waves were absent or altered, the cardiac impulse originates outside the SA node.

- **PR interval:** This represents the time required for the impulse to travel from the SA node to the atrioventricular node. If this interval is prolonged, a conduction delay exists in the AV node (e.g., first-degree heart block). If the PR interval is shortened; the impulse must have reached the ventricle through a "shortcut." (as in Wolff-Parkinson-White syndrome).
- **QRS complex:** This represents ventricular electrical depolarization associated with ventricular contraction. This complex consists of an initial downward (negative) deflection (Q) wave, a large upward (positive) deflection (R wave) and a small downwards deflection (S wave). A widened QRS complex indicates abnormal or prolonged ventricular depolarization (as in bundle branch block).
- **ST-segment:** This represents the period between the completion of depolarization and the beginning of repolarization of the ventricular muscles. This segment may be elevated or depressed in transient muscle ischemia (e.g., angina) or 'a muscle injury', as in the early stages of myocardial infarction.
- **T wave:** This represents ventricular repolarization (i.e., return to neutral electrical activity).
- **U wave:** This deflection follows the T wave and is usually quite small. It represents the repolarization of the Purkinje fibers within the ventricular. Through the analysis of these, waveforms and time intervals, valuable information about the heart may be obtained.

PHONOCARDIOGRAPHY

The phonocardiography records the sounds of the heart by means of suction microphones that are attached to the chest wall. The pressure waves produced by the sound are connected to electric current, amplified, and recorded in a similar manner to the way in which the electrical impulses are recorded on ECG. In some cases, the electrical impulses are reconverted to sound that can be recorded or heard directly.

ELECTROMYOGRAPHY (EMG)

Electromyography is a study of the electrical activity of the muscle to determine the condition of the muscle and its nerve supply either in a particular disease or following injury. The electrical activity is picked up by needle electrodes that are inserted into the muscle. The needle is insulated except for the tip; consequently, it detects only electric variations in the region of the tip. The electrode voltage is amplified and can be observed directly on the screen of the cathode rays oscilloscope. If a permanent record is desired, the visual image of electric changes that appear on the screen may be photographed. The amplified voltage may also be transmitted to the loudspeaker and heard.

ELECTROMYOGRAPHY PATTERN

- There is a definite EMG pattern for normal contracting muscle. Differences obtained from the normal pattern are interpreted.
- Amplitudes of EMG potential vary in parts of a muscle. Observations are usually made in several parts of the muscle in order to get a representative **(Fig. 15.22)**.
- There are also difficulties of patterns among different muscle. The uterus during labor was the subject of one electromyographic study.
- In addition to records of surface potentials related to action potential, some studies have been made of potential gradients during the formation of neoplasm and peripheral lesions, wound healing and the menstrual cycle.

ELECTROSTIMULATION

Some investigators believe that galvanic stimulation of denervated muscle may help to preserve muscle tissue and prevent atrophy. In fact, galvanic stimulators have been used in treating some patients. The apparatus consists of two small cathodes that are placed on either end of the affected muscle. A small galvanic current generator is connected to a dry cell and the time and the strength of the current are regulated by a stimulator that can be placed in the pocket of the patients where it is easily accessible to him. The patients control the stimulation by a special device on the apparatus.

Fig 15.22: Electromyography.

In addition to artificial muscle stimulation; electrotherapy includes the use of direct current and the application of high frequency current. There have been reports of electrical stimulation of the phrenic nerves to induce respiration.

ELECTROCONVULSIVE THERAPY (ECT)

- ECT is a physical or somatic therapy in which, with the help of two electrodes current is passed through the temporal region in between the two hemispheres of the brain to produce grandmal seizures.
- It has been shown that a small current of electricity applied to areas of the cortex of the brain will produce symptoms manifested as simple muscle twitches. When certain areas, described as epileptogenic areas, exist in an epileptic patient, stimulation of these areas will produce convulsions that may be localized or generalized.
- ECT is a painless form of electric therapy, primarily used for patients with depression, and schizophrenic disorders.
- The patient is prepared by the administration of barbiturate anesthesia and an injection of a chemical relaxant.
- An electric current of 70 to 130 volts is applied for 0.1 to 1 second through electrodes placed on the temporal region. This immediately produces seizures or convulsions **(Fig. 15.23)**.
- The biological effects of the ECT are believed to be achieved by neurophysiological, neuroendocrine and neurochemical changes. However, the catecholamine hypothesis of its mechanism of action is more widely accepted.
- There is no absolute contraindication of ECT. However, it had increased risk in patients with increased intracranial pressure either due to brain tumor, hematoma, hemorrhage, osteoporosis or recent history of fracture or thrombolytic therapy.

ELECTRONIC CARDIAC PACEMAKER

- A device called the electronic cardiac pacemaker maintains normal heartbeats in cases of heart block or arrhythmia that prevents normal transmission of impulses from SA-mode, the natural cardiac pacemaker.
- An electronic cardiac pacemaker may be temporary or permanent.

Fig. 15.23: Electroconvulsive therapy machine.

Fig. 15.24: External cardiac pacemaker.

- Temporary pacemakers are helpful to persons who have a transient blockage of the conduction pathway after a myocardial infarction or cardiac surgery. If the chest wall is opened as during surgery pacing electrodes may be implanted on the epicardium, extended through the chest incision, and connected to an external pacing battery control box. A pacing electrode can also be implanted directly into the right ventricle by passing it through the external jugular subclavian antecubital or femoral vein. In this case, to the electrodes may then be connected to the pacing battery box that is kept near the patient. The temporary pacer is usually tried first with most patients because the device can be removed when necessary relatively simple. In addition, battery can be replaced early if required **(Fig. 15.24)**.
- In cases of irreversible cardiac damage and complete conductive pathway blockage, a permanent pacemaker may be used. The electrode can be implanted through the vein as a temporary one, but here battery box about the size of a pocket watch a smaller is permanently implanted into the subcutaneous tissue of the chest wall or abdomen. These batteries may be of several types of different life expectancies.
- In the types, these pacemakers could be fixed or demand in the input of electric impulses.

■ BRAIN PACEMAKER

- A device consisting of a plate of silicon-covered dacron mesh that contains four pairs of platinum disk electrodes, an internally implanted radio frequency receiver and a pocket-sized external transmitter have been reported beneficial to patients with uncontrolled seizures and spasticity associated with epilepsy, stroke, cerebral palsy and other brain disorders **(Fig. 15.25)**.
- The plates are applied to the cerebellar surface through small occipital and suboccipital craniotomies. Two receivers are implanted in the chest below the clavicles and are connected by subcutaneous leads to the plates. An antenna is placed directly over the receiver and stimulation is controlled by an external transmitter.
- The rationale briefly is that stimulating the cerebellar cortex is inhibitory and assists with the control of skeletal activity. The stimulator contains an automatic timer. The rate, frequency,

Fig. 15.25: Brain pacemaker.

and timing depends on the person's requirement. Generally, the electrodes in each plate are stimulated simultaneously several minutes off the several minutes on.
* A button located in the transmitter that is activated simultaneously rather than alternate stimulation is reported to be successful in preventing or aborting seizures. This technique is still experimental, but if perfected, offers a means for normal life to a person who might otherwise be seriously limited.

■ DEFIBRILLATION

Cardiac defibrillation is the act of administering a transthoracic electrical current to a person experiencing one of the two lethal ventricular dysrhythmias, ventricular fibrillation (VF) or pulseless ventricular tachycardia (VT). A defibrillator is an electric device used to deliver an electrical current (shock) of present voltage to the heart through paddles placed on the chest wall (closed-chest procedure). This current causes the entire myocardium to depolarize completely at the moment of shock, thus producing transient asystole and allowing the heart's intrinsic pacemaker to regain control. The amount of energy required to produce this effect is determined largely by the client's transthoracic impedance or resistance to current flow. Because of this factor, the amount of energy that reaches the heart is less than the amount that the defibrillator is charged to deliver **(Fig. 15.26)**.

The procedure is associated with potential hazards, particularly myocardial damage. The higher the amount of energy or frequency of the shock, the greater the risk of injury. Advances in the equipment now allow measurement of transthoracic impedance. Once impedance is determined, the defibrillator automatically selects the amount of the current. It is expected this mode of defibrillation will reduce the risk of complications.

Fig. 15.26: Defibrillator.

The degree of transthoracic resistance depends on several variables:
- **Energy level:** The higher the energy level that is selected, the more current will follow. Usually, 360 J with monophasic and 200 J with biphasic is delivered during defibrillation.
- **Number and frequency of shock:** The more shocks administrated and the shorter the time between them, the lower the transthoracic resistance.
- **Ventilation phase:** Resistance is lower when there is less air (and therefore a smaller diameter) in the lungs.
- **Paddle size:** The larger the paddle, the lower the resistance.
- **Chest size:** The smaller the distance between the defibrillator electrodes once they are in place, the lower the resistance.
- **Paddle-skin interface material:** Conductive material between the skin and paddle, helping to overcome transthoracic resistance. Exerts, about 25 pounds of pressure on each paddle.
- **Paddle placement:** Place one paddle on the upper chest, to the right of the sternum; place the other paddle on the lower left chest, to the left of the nipple, with the center of the paddle in the midaxillary line. If the client has a permanent pacemaker or internal cardiac defibrillation, place the paddles at least 5 inches away from the generator to avoid damaging it. If a temporary pacing system is in use, disconnect the pacing lead from the pulse generator immediately before defibrillation and reconnect it after the shock.

■AUTOMATED EXTERNAL DEFIBRILLATOR

An automated external defibrillator (AED) is a portable electronic device **(Fig. 15.27)** that automatically diagnoses the potentially life-threatening cardiac arrhythmias of ventricular fibrillation and ventricular tachycardia in a patient, and is able to treat them through defibrillation, the application of electrical therapy which stops the arrhythmia, allowing the heart to reestablish an effective rhythm. AEDs are designed to be simple to use for the layman, and the use of AEDs is taught in many first aid, first responder, and basic life support (BLS) level CPR classes.

Uses

An automated external defibrillator is used in cases of life-threatening cardiac arrhythmias which lead to cardiac arrest. The rhythms that the device will treat are usually limited to:
- Pulseless ventricular tachycardia (shortened to VT or V-tach)
- Ventricular fibrillation (shortened to VF or V-fib)

Fig. 15.27: Automated external defibrillator.

In each of these two types of shockable cardiac arrhythmia, the heart is active, but in a life-threatening, dysfunctional pattern. In ventricular tachycardia, the heart beats too fast to effectively pump blood. Ultimately, ventricular tachycardia leads to ventricular fibrillation. In ventricular fibrillation, the electrical activity of the heart becomes chaotic, preventing the ventricle from effectively pumping blood. The fibrillation in the heart decreases over time, and will eventually reach asystole.

Automated external defibrillators (AEDs), like all defibrillators, are not designed to shock asystole ('flat line' patterns) as this will not have a positive clinical outcome. The asystolic patient only has a chance of survival if, through a combination of CPR and cardiac stimulant drugs, one of the shockable rhythms can be established, which makes it imperative for CPR to be carried out prior to the arrival of a defibrillator.

Mechanism of Operation

Automated external defibrillator is external because the operator applies the electrode pads to the bare chest of the victim, as opposed to internal defibrillators, which have electrodes surgically implanted inside the body of a patient.

Automatic refers to the unit's ability to autonomously analyze the patient's condition, and to assist this, the vast majority of units have spoken prompts, and some may also have visual displays to instruct the user. When turned on or opened, the AED will instruct the user to connect the electrodes (pads) to the patient. Once the pads are attached, everyone should avoid touching the patient so as to avoid false readings by the unit. The pads allow the AED to examine the electrical output from the heart and determine if the patient is in a shockable rhythm (either ventricular fibrillation or ventricular tachycardia). If the device determines that a shock is warranted, it will use the battery to charge its internal capacitor in preparation to deliver the shock. This system is not only safer (charging only when required), but also allows for faster delivery of the electrical current.

When charged, the device instructs the user to ensure no one is touching the victim and then to press a button to deliver the shock; human intervention is usually required to deliver the shock to the patient in order to avoid the possibility of accidental injury to another person (which can result from a responder or bystander touching the patient at the time of the shock).

Depending on the manufacturer and particular model, after the shock is delivered most devices will analyze the victim and either instruct that CPR be given, or administer another shock.

Many AED units have an 'event memory' which stores the ECG of the patient along with details of the time the unit was activated and the number and strength of any shocks delivered. Some units also have voice recording abilities to monitor the actions taken by the personnel in order to ascertain if these had any impact on the survival outcome. All this recorded data can be either downloaded to a computer or printed out so that the providing organization or responsible body is able to see the effectiveness of both CPR and defibrillation.

Automated external defibrillators (AEDs) available to the public may be semi-automatic or fully automatic. Fully automatic units are likely to have a few buttons, often activating as soon as the case is opened, and possibly just one button to shock, or in some cases, this will be performed automatically. The user has no input in the operation of the unit apart from attaching the pads and following the prompts. Health care professionals and other trained responders may use a semi-automatic defibrillator, which is likely to have an ECG readout display, and the possibility to override the rhythm analysis software. This allows trained personnel to provide a higher level of care.

The first commercially available AEDs were all of a monophasic type, which gave a high-energy shock, up to 360–4400 joules depending on the model. This caused increased cardiac injury and in some cases second and third-degree burns around the shock pad sites. Newer AEDs (manufactured after late 2003) have tended to utilize biphasic algorithms which give two sequential lower-energy shocks of 120–200 joules, with each shock moving in an opposite polarity between the pads. This lower-energy waveform has proven more effective in clinical tests, as well as offering a reduced rate of complications and reduced recovery time.

■ MAGNETIC RESONANCE IMAGING (MRI)

Magnetic resonance imaging (MRI), or nuclear magnetic resonance imaging (NMRI), is primarily a medical imaging technique most commonly used in radiology to visualize detailed internal structure and limited function of the body. MRI provides much greater contrast between the different soft tissues of the body than computed tomography (CT) does, making it especially useful in neurological (brain), musculoskeletal, cardiovascular, and oncological (cancer) imaging. Unlike CT, it uses no ionizing radiation but uses a powerful magnetic field to align the nuclear magnetization of (usually) hydrogen atoms in water in the body. Radiofrequency (RF) fields are used to systematically alter the alignment of this magnetization, causing the hydrogen nuclei to produce a rotating magnetic field detectable by the scanner. This signal can be manipulated by additional magnetic fields to build up enough information to construct an image of the body **(Fig. 15.28)**.

Mechanism of Operation and Uses

The body is largely composed of water molecules which each contain two hydrogen nuclei or protons. When a person goes inside the powerful magnetic field of the scanner, the magnetic moments of these protons align with the direction of the field.

A radiofrequency electromagnetic field is then briefly turned on, causing the protons to alter their alignment relative to the field. When this field is turned off, the protons return to the original magnetization alignment. These alignment changes create a signal which can be detected by the scanner. The frequency at which the protons resonate depends on the strength

Fig. 15.28: Magnetic resonance imaging.

of the magnetic field. The position of protons in the body can be determined by applying additional magnetic fields during the scan which allows an image of the body to be built up. These are created by turning gradients coils on and off which creates the knocking sounds heard during an MR scan.

Diseased tissue, such as tumors, can be detected because the protons in different tissues return to their equilibrium state at different rates. By changing the parameters on the scanner this effect is used to create contrast between different types of body tissue.

Contrast agents may be injected intravenously to enhance the appearance of blood vessels, tumors, or inflammation. Contrast agents may also be directly injected into a joint in the case of arthrograms, and MR images of joints. Unlike CT, MRI uses no ionizing radiation and is generally a very safe procedure. Patients with some metal implants, cochlear implants, and cardiac pacemakers are prevented from having an MRI scan due to the effects of the strong magnetic field and powerful radiofrequency pulses.

MRI is used to image every part of the body, and is particularly useful for neurological conditions, disorders of the muscles and joints, for evaluating tumors, and for showing abnormalities in the heart and blood vessels.

■ CAT SCAN

The word "tomography" is derived from the Greek tomos (slice) and graphein (to write). Computed tomography was originally known as the "EMI scan". It was later known as computed axial tomography (CAT or CT scan) and body section roentgenography. Computed tomography (CT) is a medical imaging method employing tomography created by computer processing. Digital geometry processing is used to generate a three-dimensional image of the inside of an object from a large series of two-dimensional X-ray images taken around a single axis of rotation. The machine was developed by physicist Allan MacLeod Cormack and electrical engineer Godfrey Hounsfield.

The CT scan is essentially an X-ray study, wherein a series of rays are rotated around a specified body part, and computer-generated cross-sectional images are produced. The advantage of these tomographic images compared to conventional X-rays is that they contain detailed information about a specified area in cross-section, eliminating the superimposition of images, which provides a tremendous advantage over plain films. CT scans provide excellent clinicopathological correlation for a suspected illness.

- ❖ **Uses:** It is used to diagnose several disorders of a different area of the body:
  - **Head:** CT scanning of the head is typically used to detect:
    - Bleeding, brain injury, and skull fractures
    - Bleeding due to a ruptured/leaking aneurysm in a patient with a sudden severe headache
    - A blood clot or bleeding within the brain shortly after a patient exhibits symptoms of a stroke
  - A stroke
    - Brain tumors
    - Enlarged brain cavities in patients with hydrocephalus
    - Diseases/malformations of the skull
  - **Chest:** CT can be used for detecting both acute and chronic changes in the lung parenchyma, that is, the internals of the lungs. Like emphysema, fibrosis, lung cancer, pneumonia, etc. CT angiography of the chest may be helpful in the detection of pulmonary embolism (PE) and aortic dissection.
  - **Abdominal and pelvic:** CT is a sensitive method for diagnosis of abdominal diseases, especially cancer; can also be helpful in the investigation of abdominal pain to rule out renal stones, appendicitis, pancreatitis, diverticulitis, abdominal aortic aneurysm, and bowel obstruction, etc.

Process

X-ray slice data is generated using an X-ray source that rotates around the object; X-ray sensors are positioned on the opposite side of the circle from the X-ray source. The earliest sensors were scintillation detectors, with photomultiplier tubes excited by (typically) cesium iodide crystals. Cesium iodide was replaced during the eighties by ion chambers containing high-pressure xenon gas. These systems were in turn replaced by scintillation systems based on photodiodes instead of photomultipliers and modern scintillation materials with more desirable characteristics. Many data scans are progressively taken as the object is gradually passed through the gantry. They are combined together by mathematical procedures known as tomographic reconstruction. The data are arranged in a matrix in memory, and each data point is convolved with its neighbors, according to a seed algorithm using Fast Fourier Transform techniques. This dramatically increases the resolution of each voxel (volume element). Then a process is known as back projection essentially reverses the acquisition geometry and stores the result in another memory array. This data can then be displayed, photographed, or used as input for further processing, such as multiplanar reconstruction.

In conventional CT machines, an X-ray tube and detector are physically rotated behind a circular shroud (see the image above right); in the electron beam tomography (EBT) the tube is far larger and has higher power to support the high temporal resolution. The electron beam is deflected in a hollow funnel-shaped vacuum chamber. X-rays are generated when the beam hits the stationary target. The detector is also stationary. This arrangement can result in very fast scans, but is extremely expensive.

The data stream representing the varying radiographic intensity is sensed at the detectors on the opposite side of the circle during each sweep, then computer processes to calculate cross-sectional estimations of the radiographic density, expressed in Hounsfield units. Sweeps cover 360° or just over 180° in conventional machines, and 220° in EBT.

Newer machines with faster computer systems and newer software strategies can process not only individual cross-sections, but continuously change cross-sections ions as the gantry, with the object to be imaged, is slowly and smoothly slid through the X-ray circle. These are called helical or spiral CT machines. Their computer systems integrate the data of the moving individual slices to generate three-dimensional volumetric information (3D-CT scan), in turn, viewable from multiple different perspectives on attached CT workstation monitors. This type of data acquisition requires enormous processing power, as the data is arriving in a continuous stream and must be processed in real-time.

QUESTIONS

Q.1: The electronic device that picks up sound waves and converts them into electric current is called…………..
Q.2: The process in which electric shock is imparted to the chest to normalize heartbeat is called……………
Q.3: Electric switches should not be touched with wet hands.
Q.4: Therapeutic uses of electricity.
Q.5: Why synthetic cloth dresses are not allowed in operation theaters?
Q.6: Why the use of three-pin plugs in electrical connection safe than two-pin plugs?
Q.7: Use of silk or nylon is generally forbidden in operating theaters. Explain
Q.8: Human body is a good conductor of electricity. Discuss

BIBLIOGRAPHY

1. American Red Cross. CPR/AED for the Professional Rescuer (participant's manual). Yardley, PA: StayWell, 2006.
2. Bird J. Electrical and Electronic Principles and Technology, 3rd edition, Newnes, 2007.
3. Bullock TH. Electroreception, Springer, 2005.
4. Close F. The New Cosmic Onion: Quarks and the Nature of the Universe, CRC Press, 2007.
5. Dibner B. Oersted and the Discovery of Electromagnetism. Blaisdell Publishing Company, 1961.
6. Dosdall DJ, Fast VG, Ideker RE. Mechanisms of defibrillation. Annu Rev Biomed Eng. 2010;12:233–258. doi:10.1146/annurev-bioeng-070909-105305
7. Duffin WJ. Electricity and Magnetism, 3rd edition, McGraw-Hill, 1980.
8. Goyal A, Chhabra L, Sciammarella JC, et al. Defibrillation. [Updated 2022 Feb 7]. In: StatPearls [Internet]. Treasure Island (FL): StatPearls Publishing; 2022 Jan-. Available from: https://www.ncbi.nlm.nih.gov/books/NBK499899/
9. Griffiths DJ. Introduction to Electrodynamics, 3rd edition. Prentice Hall, 1998.
10. Hammond P. Electromagnetism for Engineers, Pergamon, 1981.
11. Jackson JD. Classical Electrodynamics, 3rd edition. Wiley, 1998.
12. Morley A, Hughes E. Principles of Electricity, 5th edition, Longman, 1994.
13. Morris SC. Life's Solution: Inevitable Humans in a Lonely Universe, Cambridge University Press, 2003.
14. Naidu MS, Kamataru V. High Voltage Engineering, Tata McGraw-Hill, 1982. Nilsson, James; Riedel, Susan. Electric Circuits, Prentice Hall, 2007.

15. Patel PR, De Jesus O. CT Scan. [Updated 2022 Jan 5]. In: StatPearls [Internet]. Treasure Island (FL): StatPearls Publishing; 2022 Jan-. Available from: https://www.ncbi.nlm.nih.gov/books/NBK567796/
16. Patterson WC. Transforming Electricity: The Coming Generation of Change, Earthscan, 1999.
17. Rothwell EJ, Cloud MJ. Electromagnetics. CRC Press, 2001.
18. Sears F, et. al., University Physics, Sixth Edition, Addison Wesley, 1982. Benjamin, P. A history of electricity (the intellectual rise in electricity) from antiquity to the days of Benjamin Franklin. New York: J. Wiley and Sons. 1998.
19. Simpson B. Electrical Stimulation and the Relief of Pain, Elsevier Health Sciences, 2003.
20. Stewart J. Intermediate Electromagnetic Theory, World Scientific, 2001.
21. Tipler P. Physics for Scientists and Engineers: Vol. 2: Light, Electricity and Magnetism, 4th edition. WH Freeman. 1998.
22. Udupa JK, Herman GT. 3D Imaging in Medicine, 2nd edition, CRC Press, 2000.
23. Wangsness RK, Cloud MJ. Electromagnetic Fields, 2nd Edition, Wiley, 1986.

CHAPTER 16

Nuclear Physics

Suresh K Sharma, Navjot Kaur

Chapter Outline

- Structure of Atom
- Applications
- Clinical Uses of Radioisotopes and Radio Elements
- Radiation Protection Limits
- Instruments Used for Detection of Ionizing Radiation, X-rays

■ INTRODUCTION

You might have exposure to the model of the atom since your school education. The atom can be visualized as a mini solar system in which the nucleus is surrounded by electrons. You may also be aware that the atomic nucleus is a very small and dense object consisting of two types of particles namely proton and neutron. It has taken a long time and a series of classic experiments from the early ideas about atoms to the present-day atomic models.

Nuclear physics is the study of the protons and neutrons at the center of an atom and the interactions that hold them together in a space just a few femtometers across. For example, nuclear reactions include radioactive decay, fission, the break-up of a nucleus, and fusion, the merging of nuclei.

■ STRUCTURE OF ATOM

Thomson's Atomic Model

After the discovery of electrons and protons, the scientists started thinking of arranging these particles in an atom. The first simple model was proposed by JJ Thomson known as Thomson's Atomic model. JJ Thomson proposed that the positive charge is spread over a sphere in which electrons are embedded to make the atom as a whole neutral. The radius of the sphere is of the order of 10-p10 cm, which is equal to the size of the atom. This model was much like raisins in a pudding and is also known as the Thomson plum pudding model. The model could explain why only negatively charged particles are emitted when a metal is heated and never the positively charged particles. It also could explain how the ions and ionic compounds of chemistry are formed **(Fig. 16.1)**.

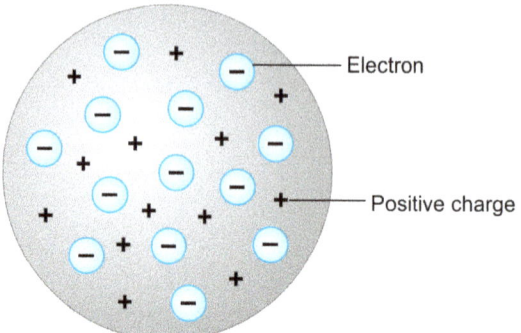

Thomson's plum pudding model

Fig. 16.1: Thomson's atomic model.

Rutherford's Model of an Atom

Thomson's model had some advantages and could explain a few phenomena successfully, but at the same time, it had certain disadvantages too. According to this model, charges are spread over the total volume of the atom, but this was not consistent with the fact that cathode rays pass through the atom almost freely. The atom must have a lot of space for this to happen.

Rutherford did an experiment known as Rutherford's scattering experiment. In this experiment, a piece of a radioactive substance is placed in a lead block. The block is constructed in such a way with slits that only a narrow beam of X-particles could escape. The beam of alpha particles then passes through the thin gold foil to detect alpha particles after scattering, a movable circular screen coated with zinc sulfate is placed around a gold foil **(Fig. 16.2)**.

The following observations were made from these experiments:
- Most of the α-particles nearly pass through the gold foil undetected. It means there must be a very large empty space.
- Some of them get deflected from some angles. It means there is a heavy positively charged mass present in the atom. Moreover, this mass must be occupying a very small space within the atom because only a few particles suffered large deflections.

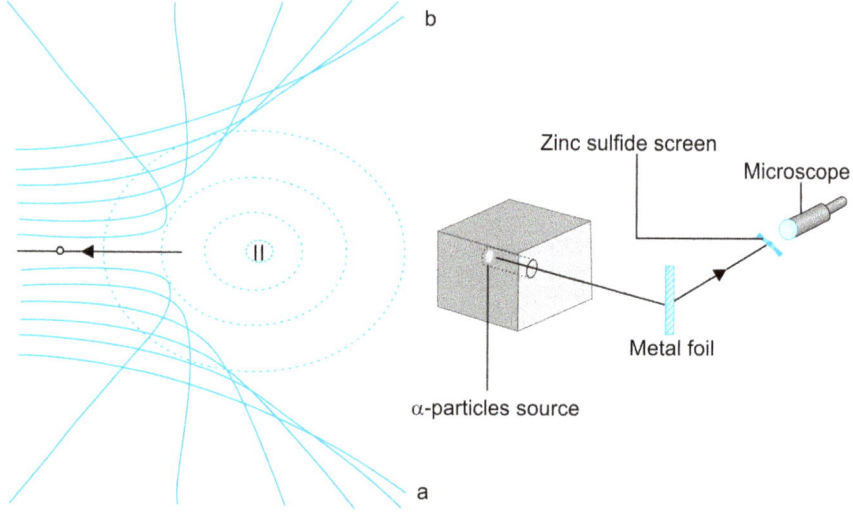

Fig. 16.2: Rutherford's scattering experiment.

- Very few, about one in 20,000 did not pass through the foil at all but suffered large deflections (more than 90%) or even came back suffering a deflection of 180°. It means there is a direct collision with the heavy positively charged mass.

Main Features
- In an atom, the entire mass and the positive charge are concentrated in a very small region at the center known as the nucleus.
- The positive charge of the nucleus is due to protons.
- The mass of the nucleus is due to protons and some other neutral particles each having a mass nearly equal to the mass of the proton. It was called a neutron.
- The nucleus is surrounded by negatively charged electrons which balance the positive charge on the nucleus. Thus, the atom is electrically neutral.
- The electrons are not stationary but are revolving around the nucleus at very high speeds like planets revolving around the sun. Thus, electrons are planetary electrons.
- The electrons and nucleus are held together by electrostatic forces of attraction.
- Most of the space in an atom between the nucleus and revolving electrons is empty.

Failures
- It was shown by Clark Maxwell that a charged body moving under the influence of attractive forces loses energy continuously in the form of electromagnetic radiations. Thus, unlike a planet, the electron is a charged body, it should emit radiations while revolving around the nucleus. As a result, the electron should lose energy at every turn and move closer and closer to the nucleus following a spiral path. Consequently, the orbit will become smaller and finally the electron would fall into the nucleus. In other words, the atom should collapse, but this never happens. Therefore, the model cannot explain the stability of an atom.
- This model does not explain the structure of atoms, i.e. distribution of electrons around the nucleus and their energies.
- It does not explain the appearance of many spectral lines of the hydrogen atom.

Bohr's Model of an Atom
- An atom consists of a small heavy positively charged nucleus in the center surrounded by electrons. The electrons in an atom revolve around the nucleus only in certain selected circular paths called orbits. These orbits are associated with definite energies and are called energy shells or energy levels. These are numbered as 1, 2, 3, 4, etc. from the nucleus. These are alternatively designated as K, L, M, N, shells, etc. (**Fig. 16.3**).
- As long as the electrons remain in a particular path, it does not lose or gain energy. This means that the energy of electrons in a particular energy shell remains constant. Therefore, these orbits are also called stationary states. The term stationary does not mean that electron is stationary, but it means that the energy of the electron does not change with time. This accounts for the stability of an atom.
- Only those orbits are permitted in which the angular momentum of the electron is a whole number multiple of $h/2\pi$ (where h is Planck's constant). An electron like any other moving body in a circular orbit has an angular momentum equal to mvr. Thus, according to Bohr, the angular momentum mvr is a whole number multiple of $h/2\pi$.

$$mvr = \frac{nh}{2\pi}$$

where, $n = 1, 2, 3...$

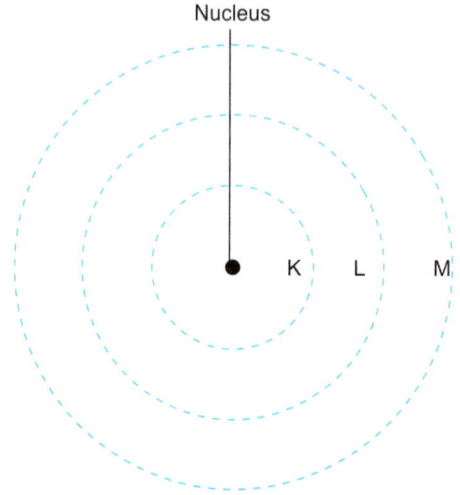

Fig. 16.3: Orbits of an atom.

- The energy is emitted or absorbed only when electrons jump from one energy level to another. When energy is supplied to an atom, its electrons absorb one or more quantum of energy and jump to a higher energy level. This higher energy state of the electron is called its excited state. When the electron jumps back to the lower energy level, it radiates the same energy. The amount of energy emitted or absorbed is given by the difference in the energies of the two energy levels concerned. That is:

$$\Delta E = E_2 - E_1$$

$E_2 - E_1$
Energy absorbed

$E_1 - E_2$
Energy released

Success

- Bohr's atomic model the stability of an atom. According to Bohr, an electron revolving in a particular orbit cannot lose energy. Therefore, emission of radiation is not possible as long as the electron remains at one of its energy levels, and hence, there is no cause of instability in his model.
- Bohr's concept of atoms explained successfully the atomic spectrum of the hydrogen atom. From Bohr's atomic model, it is clear that electrons can have only a certain definite energy levels. When the electron is present as close to the nucleus as possible, the atom has the minimum possible energy and is said to be in the ground state. When energy from some outside source is supplied, it jumps to a higher energy state. This is called the excited state. This excited state is unstable the electrons come back to lower energy levels and energy is emitted in the form of a quantum equal to the difference in energy between the two levels. When this quantum of energy strikes the photographic plate, it gives its impression in the form of a line.

Now:

$E_2 - E_1 = h\nu$

$\nu = E_2 - E_1 / h$

Since

$\nu = \text{frequency} = c/\lambda$

$c/\lambda = E_2 - E_1 / h$

$\lambda = hc / E_2 - E_1$

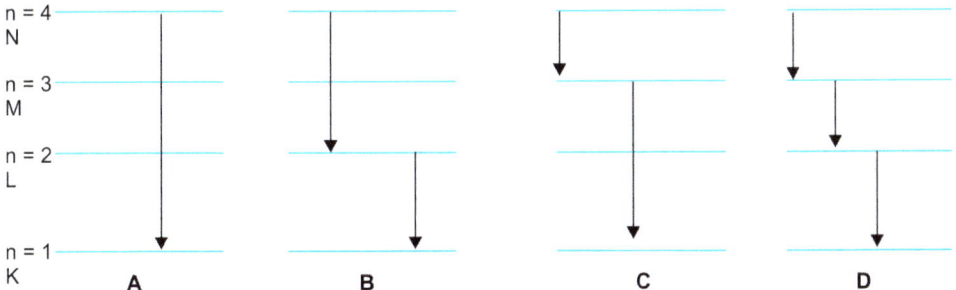

Fig. 16.4 A to D: Simultaneous appearance of a large number of lines in the spectrum of hydrogen.

Since h and c are constants and E_2-E_1 corresponds to definite energy, thus each transition from one level to another will produce light of a definite wavelength. This is observed as a line in the spectrum of the hydrogen atom. If the electron jumps from third to first energy level, then:

$$\lambda' = hc/E_3-E_1$$

Similarly,

$$\lambda'' = hc/E_4-E_1 \quad \text{and} \quad \lambda''' = hc/E_5-E_1$$

Thus different spectral lines in the spectra of atoms correspond to different transitions of electrons from higher energy levels to lower energy levels **(Fig. 16.4)**.

In any sample of hydrogen gas, there are a large number of hydrogen atoms. When energy is supplied by passing electric discharge, the electrons in different atoms absorb different amounts of energy, therefore, they are raised to different energy states. For example, the electrons in some atoms may jump to the second energy level (L) while in others may be raised to third (M), fourth (N), and fifth (O) energy levels, and so on. Now the excited electrons come back from the higher energy levels to the ground states in one or more jumps.

For example, when the electron jumps from all the energy levels higher than n = 1, i.e., n = 2, 3, 4, 5... to n = 1 energy level, the lines obtained fall in the ultraviolet region, these lines are called Lyman series.

Similarly, the lines obtained, when an electron jumps to the second energy level (n = 2) from higher levels (n = 3, 4, 5, 6) fall in the visible region. These are called the Balmer series.

In a similar manner, the transition from higher energy levels to n = 3 series produces the Paschen series. Similarly, Brackett and Pfund series correspond to jumps from higher energy levels to n = 4 and n = 5 energy levels respectively. Thus are summarized below **(Fig. 16.5)**:

Lyman series from n = 2, 3, 4, 5... to n = 1
Balmer series from n = 3, 4, 5, 6... to n = 2
Paschen series from n = 4, 5, 6, 7... to n = 3
Brackett series from n = 4, 5, 6, 7... to n = 4
Pfund series from n = 5, 6, 7... to n = 5

Bohr's theory helped in calculating the energy of the electron in a particular orbit of the hydrogen atom and that is:

$$E_n = 2\pi^2 \, me/N^2h^2$$

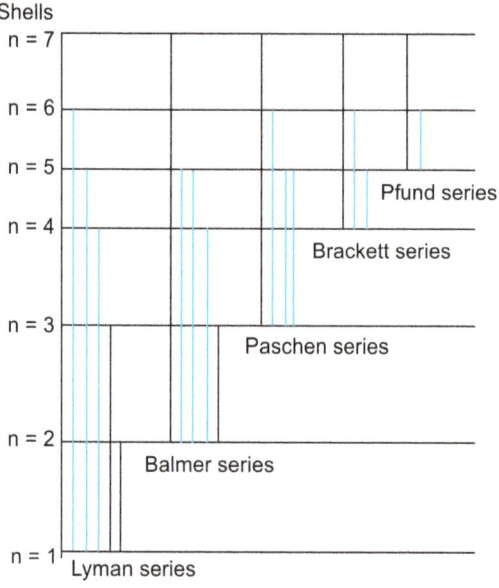

Fig. 16.5: Orbits of an atom.

Weaknesses

- Bohr's model of an atom could not explain the time spectra of atoms containing more than one electron called multi-electron atom.
- Bohr's theory failed to account for the effect of magnetic fields on the spectra of atoms or ions called Zeeman effect.
- Bohr's theory does not provide any clue to explain the shapes of molecules arising out of the directional bonding between atoms.

Applications

Detection of Radioactivity and Monitoring

- To evaluate radiation hazards, periodic readings need to be made in the field around a source or sources of radiation.
- Area monitoring is a term used to describe the periodic or continuous determination of dosage levels in working areas around various radiation sources.
- Each monitoring system uses a detecting element and a device that transcribes the detected radiation into units of measurement. Examples are, Geiger muller counter, the ionization chamber, the scintillation counter, and the proportional counter.
  - *Geiger-Muller counter:* Consist basically of a sealed glass tube in which a gas such as argon is kept at a pressure of above 0.1 atoms, inside the tube is a wire anode electrode and a cathode. A voltage of between 1,000 and 2,000 volts is present between these electrodes. When no radiation is present the gas is not ionized and the current does not flow. A single electron entering the chamber between the electrodes initiates lionization causing the flow of electric current, which is then transformed into an audible click. It is useful for detecting radioactivity in radiation survey work **(Fig. 16.6)**.
  - The ionization chamber is based on the principle that radiation causes ionization in the gas. Two electrodes at opposite potentials are placed in a sealed gas-filled tube. Passage of radiations through the chamber produce ions that are attracted to the oppositely charged electrode. The current produced in this apparatus is read on a meter.

Fig. 16.6: Gigger-Muller counter.

- *The proportional counting chamber.* This differs from the previous apparatus in that, it produces a pulse whose strength is proportional to the energy of the entering ionizing radiations. This apparatus is useful in measuring alpha radiations. It can also distinguish alpha from beta and gamma radiations because of the energy differences between these three kinds of radiations.
- *Scintillation counters:* Contain crystals that liberate light when exposed to radiations. The flashes of light are too faint to be seen and are therefore converted into electrical impulses through the use of a photomultiplier tube. Scintillation counters are useful for rapid counting and for discriminating between different types of radiations that are emitted spontaneously.
  - Some counters are reduced to a pocket-size that can be conveniently carried by persons working in an area where radiations are present.
  - In addition to the counters mentioned, the electroscope is a direct viewing apparatus especially employed for measuring gamma radiations. A useful type is the quartz fiber electroscope. This is sealed in a chamber in which a metalized quartz fiber is mounted so that it is insulated from the inner wall of the chamber. A battery puts an initial charge on the fiber and the fiber is deflected. When the gas in the chamber is ionized, the fiber returns to the initial uncharged position. A microscope is used to view and measure the deflection.

Radioactivity and radiation existed before the development of life on Earth and were essential elements of the environment. We are continuously exposed to natural and artificial radiations. These radionuclides are part of our bones (radium and polonium), muscles (radiocarbon, radiopotassium, and thoron), and other tissues and are emitting ionizing radiation. Nuclear fusion in the sun is responsible for the radiation which is essential for life on Earth. So we are living in a radioactive natural world.

Radioisotopes have many applications in medicine. One of the most important is radioimmunoassay. This is a technique that detects and quantifies minute amounts of components in tissues such as hormones or enzymes. It compares the component's ability to bind with an antibody or other proteins to determine if it is the same component that has been radioactively tagged in the laboratory.

Radioisotopes could be released from nuclear fuel cycles or naturally occurring radioactive substances (NORM) mining activities, as well as an accidental radioactive material released into the atmosphere. Protective actions must be taken immediately. The main goal is to concentrate on radioisotopes' applications and radiological protection.

▪ RADIATION AND RADIOISOTOPES

The basic building block of matter is the atom proposed by John in the atomic theory. As we know the atom is composed of a positively charged nucleus, surrounded by a number of negatively charged electrons and so the whole atom is electrically neutral. The number of protons and neutrons present in the nucleus, called atomic number (Z), is known as mass number (A). An element›s atomic number is the same. However, elements with different mass numbers are called "isotopes". An unstable nucleus will result if the nucleus has either too many protons or neutrons. An unstable nucleus will vibrate continuously and attempt to stabilize itself by radioactive decay. The number of neutrons in a nucleus determines whether it is radioactive or not. Radioisotopes are radioactive elements. They can be produced naturally or artificially by accelerators and nuclear reactors. Rutherford and Soddy discovered that radioactivity was directly linked to the state of the atomic nucleus.

Radioactivity and nuclear reactions can happen at the time of emitting radiation from unstable nuclei. Radioactivity is the spontaneous disintegration of a nucleus to produce different types of nuclei or a lower energy nucleus. This results in the emission of alpha (α), beta (β), and gamma (γ) radiation and known as radioactivity. Henry Becquerel discovered radioactivity in 1896. Rutherford discovered alpha, beta, and their ionizing properties in 1899. Villard discovered gamma in 1900. The nucleus reacts with another particle or nucleus to produce nuclear reactions that result in the emission of radiation. Sometimes, the final product can also be radioactive. These radiations can be either electromagnetic (X-rays or γ-rays), or particle-like α and β. Rutherford discovered the nuclear reactions in 1917.

Radiation Classification

Radiation is divided into two main types based on its ability to ionize matter, ionizing radiation and non-ionizing radiation.

Ionizing Radiation

Radiation that passes through matter and breaks down the bonds between atoms or molecules and removes an electron, is known as ionization radiation. It can pass through living organisms or matter and produce a variety of effects. Radioactive decay, nuclear fission, and fusion are the main sources of ionizing radiation. Particle accelerators and extremely hot objects also produce it. There are two types of ionizing radiation: direct and indirect.

Direct Ionizing Radiation

Directly ionizing radiation deposits heat in the medium by direct Coulomb interaction of the ionizing charged particle and orbital electrons. This can be done to atoms by α, β, protons and heavy ions.

Ionizing radiations such as alpha (α), beta (β), and gamma (γ) except neutron, are created from unstable nuclei in an atom that is undergoing radioactive decay.

Alpha Radiation

There are some naturally occurring heavy nuclei that have an atomic number between 82 to 92 decay by alpha emission, in which the parent nucleus loses mass by 4 units and charges by

2 units and becomes a new atom. An α-particle is a helium nucleus ($_2He^4$) consisting of 2 protons and 2 neutrons. They are positively charged moving with a speed of about 2×10^7 ms^{-1} ionizing the surrounding gas and photographic plate. They can cause fluorescence in ZnS.

The parent nucleus ($_ZX^A$) is transformed by the following equation:

$_ZX^A = {}_{Z-2}X^{A-4} + {}_2He^{4+} + Q$ (energy)

$_{92}U^{238} = {}_{90}Th^{234} + {}_2He^{4+} + Q$ (energy)

Uranium thorium alpha particle.

Beta radiation

These are either fast electrons or positrons. They are formed from weak interaction decay of a proton or neutron in nuclei that contain excess of this nucleon. A neutron-rich nucleus can be transformed into a proton through the emission of beta particles or antineutrino. It can also be transformed into a neutron in nuclei containing rich protons by releasing neutrino or positron. Beta particles are negatively charged moving with speed of 2.97×10^8 ms^{-1}. These radiations have a high penetrating power but less ionizing power than alpha particles. ˇ They can also cause fluorescence in ZnS as alpha particles.

The parent nucleus ($_ZX^A$) is transformed by the following equation:

$_ZX^A = {}_{Z+1}X^A + {}_{-1}\beta^0 + Q$ (energy) [n = p + 0 β⁻ + ν]

$_{90}Th^{234} = {}_{91}Pa^{234} + {}_{-1}\beta^0$

Thorium protactinium beta particle

Indirect Ionizing Radiation

Indirectly ionizing radiation deposits heat in the medium in two steps. The first step sees charged particles being released into the medium. The second step is where the charged particles are released into the medium and deposit energy through direct Coulomb interaction. This can be done with atoms such as photons, electrons, X-rays, gamma rays, and neutrons.

Gamma Radiation

Gamma radiation is the most common form of nuclear excitation and can also occur due to internal conversion. They are electromagnetic rays like light and traveling with the speed of light 3×10^8 ms^{-1} have the highest penetrating powers, electrically neutral and least ionizing powers.

X-ray Radiation

The electron cloud around the nucleus produces X-rays. Roentgen discovered them in 1895. X-rays can be produced in X-ray tubes by fast-moving electrons that are suddenly stopped by the target.

Neutron Radiation

It is a neutral particle and causes ionization indirectly through the emission of gamma rays and charged particles while interacting with matter. These charged particles cause ionization. It is more powerful than gamma radiation and can be stopped with thin concrete or paraffin barriers. They can be produced by nuclear reactions and spontaneous fission within nuclear reactors.

Nonionizing Radiation

Nonionizing radiation refers to electromagnetic radiation that does not produce ionization. It has enough energy to excite, but not to create ions in matter. Nonionizing radiations include radio waves, microwaves, and ultraviolets. While nonionizing radiation is vital for life, excessive exposure can cause adverse biological effects.

Natural and Artificial Radiation Sources

Two important sources of radiation are man-made and natural.

Natural background radiation is the radiation that surrounds us. Every living organism, including man, has been exposed to ionizing radiations from various sources, they come from cosmic rays, primordial radionuclides, such as ^{232}Th, ^{235}U, and ^{238}U, as well as their decay products, as well as single-occurring radionuclides ^{40}K and ^{87}Rb that are found in the earth's crust, soil, rocks, and other materials. Natural radiation originates from three main sources: terrestrial, extraterrestrial, and internal sources (intake of radionuclides or their daughter products).

Terrestrial Radiation Sources

Terra is the Latin word for earth. The radiation that originated from the crust of the earth is known as terrestrial radiation. The sources of terrestrial radiation are the primordial radionuclides (^{238}U and ^{232}Th), which are found in different amounts in soil, rocks, and water. The majority of natural radiation comes from ^{40}K, ^{238}U, and ^{232}Th and their decay products. They undergo radioactive decay series before becoming stable isotopes. These radioactive series are naturally occurring radioactive series that have been around since the formation of the earth. Each series nuclei decay by emitting alpha, beta, and gamma particles to become stable (lead). These radioisotopes, which are chemically bound with minerals in soils and rocks, pose no biological dangers other than radon and thoron. The noble radioactive gas noble radon (a product of uranium decay series) and thoron (a product of thorium decay series) can be inhaled to cause lung cancer. UNSCEAR and WHO report that radon and its progeny are second-leading causes of lung cancer, after smoking tobacco.

^{40}K is easily absorbed by the body through drinking water, eating foods, and breathing air. ^{40}K is absorbed quickly through the stomach tract and into the bloodstream. The ^{40}K rapidly enters the bloodstream, where it is distributed to all tissues and organs, mainly muscles. This isotope delivers approximately 18 millirems (mrem), to the soft tissues and 14 mrem, to the bones each year. ^{40}K may pose both internal and external health risks.

Extraterrestrial Radiations

Extraterrestrial radiations (or cosmic radiations) are high-energy radiations or subatomic particles that originate mainly from stars that come from space and bombard the earth and all living creatures. The cosmic ray radiation is composed of about 85% protons, and 14% of alpha particles (helium ions), that hit the earth's atmosphere and consist of a mixture of charged particles like electrons, and protons, and alpha-particles. There is also a small amount of heavier nuclei. These radiations are extremely energetic and can range from 10^2 MeV to more than 10^{14} MeV. The interaction of cosmic charged particles with the earth's magnetic field and atmosphere results in the formation of the cosmic ray shower, which is typically beta or gamma radiation. Due to variations in elevation and the effects of the earth's magnetic field, the dose of cosmic radiation can vary in different areas of the globe. The upper troposphere is where the cosmic radiations are stronger. The cosmic radiation dose rises with altitude. During flights, crew members receive an additional dose of around 2.2 mSv y^{-1}. The annual cosmic radiation doses around the globe are therefore estimated to be between 0.26 and 2.01 mSv y.

The cosmic radiation interacts directly with the molecules and atoms in the atmosphere. This results in a series of secondary radioisotopes in the form of protons, neutrons, and charged/uncharged particles of different energies. These radioisotopes include ^{3}H, ^{7}Be, and ^{14}C. These cosmogonic radionuclides eventually reach the earth's surface, where they can be incorporated into living organisms. They also contribute to natural radiation exposures. The annual equivalent dose of cosmogonic radionuclides to the earth's surface is 12 mSv (14C), 0.15 mSv (22Na), 0.01 mSv (^{3}H), and 0.03 mSv (^{7}Be). The most significant is ^{14}C.

Internal Sources of Radiation

Radioactive material can enter the body through eating, drinking, and injections (from certain medical procedures, radon/thoron, and their progeny). If inhaled or injected in large quantities, the radioactive material can pose a serious health risk.

Artificial or Manmade Radiation

Human beings are also exposed to radiation from nuclear installations, nuclear explosions, nuclear fuel cycle, radioactive waste releases from nuclear reactor operations, and other industrial, and medical such as diagnostic X-rays, nuclear therapy, and agricultural uses of radioisotopes. It can also be generated by consumer products like TVs, luminous watches, dials, and radioactive materials (gas and coal). This includes the whole sequence of mining, milling, and actual production of nuclear power plants, as well as the residual fallout from nuclear weapons testing and accidents.

Radioisotope Applications

Radioisotopes play a major role in improving human life quality. There are some international organizations such as the International Atomic Energy Agency and International Commission on Radiation Protection to identify the needs and provide the infrastructure to support nuclear technology.

Radiotracer

The first report of the clinical use of radioisotopes occurred in 1937 when radio phosphorus was administered to the patient. Since that time there has been phenomenal growth in the use of radioisotopes for diagnosis and treatment.

Radiotracers are used extensively in medicine, agriculture, and industry as well as in fundamental research. A Radiotracer can be described as a radioactive element or compound that is added to a nonradioactive element to examine the dynamic behavior and chemical, biological, and physical changes in a system. It emits traceable radiation back. There are over 160 radioisotopes used in various fields. Some of the radioisotopes and their applications are presented in the following **Table 16.1:**

Table 16.1: ????		
Radioisotope	*Half-life*	*Applications*
Bismuth-213	45.59 minutes	It is an alpha emitter used in cancer treatment, such as targeted alpha therapy (TAT).
Cesium-131	9.7 days	It emits photon radiation within the X-ray spectrum used in the brachytherapy treatment of malignant tumors.
Chromium-51	28 days	Useful in the diagnosis of gastrointestinal bleeding and labeling platelets.
Cobalt-60	5.27 years	This is used to control the growth of cancerous cells.

Contd...

Contd...

Radioisotope	Half-life	Applications
Iodine-131	8 days	Widely used for treating thyroid cancer, diagnosing and imaging the thyroid and renal blood flow.
Iron-59	46 days	Used in iron metabolism studies in the spleen.
Lead-212	10.6 h	Use in TAT for cancers.
Palladium-103	17 days	This is used to create brachytherapy permanent implant seeds for early-stage prostate carcinoma. Soft X-rays.
Potassium-42	12.36 h	Used to study the distribution of potassium in bodily fluids, and to locate brain tumours.
Radium-223	11.4 Days	This is used to treat prostate cancers that have spread to the bones.
Rhenium-186	3.71 days	This is used to treat bone cancer pain and also for imaging purposes.
Sodium-24	15 h	This is used to study electrolytes in the body.
Ytterbium-169	32 days	Useful for cerebrospinal fluid studies in the brain.
Cobalt-57	272 days	It is used to determine the size of an organ and in vitro diagnostic kits.
Copper-64	13 h	This is used for PET imaging of tumors, and also for cancer therapy.
Fluorine-18	110 minutes	Useful as fluorothymidine FLT.
Gallium-67	78 h	This is used to locate inflammatory lesions and tumors (infections).
Indium-111	2.8 Days	Brain studies, colon transit, and infection.
Iodine-123	13 h	This is used to diagnose thyroid function.
Rubidium-82	1.26 minutes	Convenient PET agent for myocardial perfusion imaging.
Thallium-201	73 h	This is used to locate low-grade lymphomas.

Radiotracer is an essential and advanced diagnostic tool for radiotherapy and medicine.

Diagnostic Purpose

Technetium (^{99}Tc) is the most commonly used radioactivity isotope in the radioactive tracer. To locate brain tumors, inject intravenously ^{99}Tc into the head and scan the head using suitable scanners.

To study the function of malfunctioning thyroid glands, ^{131}I, ^{132}I, and ^{123}I were recently used. Compounds containing ^{131}I are also used to study kidney function. ^{33}P can be used for DNA sequencing. Tritium (3H) has been used in biochemical research as a tracer. ^{14}C is used extensively to track the progression of organic molecules through metabolic pathways.

The most recent advancement is positron emission tomography (PET), which allows for more accurate and precise detection of tumors within the body. A positron-emitting radionuclide (e.g., ^{13}N, ^{15}O, ^{18}F, etc.). It is administered to the patient and accumulates in the target tissues. It emits a positron, which quickly combines with nearby electrons. This causes simultaneous emission of two different g-rays. A PET camera detects these g-rays and gives precise information about their origin. This technique can also be used for brain and cardiac imaging.

Complementary X-ray tomography (CT scans). A radioactive tracer emits gamma radiation or single photons, which a gamma camera can detect. A computer can use these emissions to create an image. CT scans target specific areas of the body like the neck and chest or an organ like the thyroid.

Therapeutic

The most popular therapeutic use for radioisotopes in cancer treatment is ^{60}Co. Sometimes, wires and sealed needles containing radioactive Isotopes such as ^{192}Ir and ^{125}I can be directly inserted into cancerous tissue. As long as the needle/wire remains in place, the radiations from radioisotopes target the tumor. These are then removed after the treatment is completed. This is a common treatment for mouth, breast, lung, and uterine cancers. ^{131}I can be used to treat thyroid cancers and other abnormalities. ^{32}P can be used to treat excess red blood cells in the bone marrow.

For total sterilization of the diets of immunocompromised patients, astronauts, military personnel, adventure sports, and military personnel, higher doses of radiation can be used.

Agricultural Research

Research in agricultural science is focusing on the development of high-yielding plants, oilseeds and other economically valuable crops, as well as the protection of the plant from insects. In order to increase crop variety and improve mutation breeding, irradiated wheat, rice, maize, and cotton seeds are going through profound genetic changes. These crops have higher yields and are more resistant to disease.

The sterile insect technique (SIT) is the best method for controlling pests and insects. To sterilize insects that have been raised in large numbers, radiation is used. This allows them to not produce offspring, but they can still be sexually competitive. It enhances crop production and preserves natural resources with biodiversity.

Food Preservation and Sterilization

According to the WHO, 25–35% of world food production is susceptible to pests, bugs, bacteria, and fungi, causing great economic losses for the country. Irradiating food has many more benefits than traditional methods. Food irradiation is not recommended by all radiations. Only three types of radiation are recommended including ^{60}Co, ^{137}Cs and X-rays. Food products are subject to intense controlled radiation to kill pests, bugs, and parasites. This not only extends shelf life but also decreases nutrition by degrading vitamins A, B_1 (thiamin), and C.

Radiated potatoes can be kept at a higher temperature, around 15° Celsius by inhibition of bulbs or tubers. This will not only save energy but also prevent sweetening from potatoes that is often caused by low temperatures.

These fruits, all types of mangoes, can be irradiated at the hard mature pre-climacteric phase at 0.25–0.75 kGy to delay the ripening process for about 7 days. This will improve shelf-life up to 30 days, at 12–14°C in modified environments.

Poor handling and processing conditions can lead to spices becoming contaminated with microbial pathogens and insect eggs while being transported. Semi-processed and processed foods can be contaminated with microbes and pathogens. This can lead to spoilage and pose a risk to consumers. A 10 kGy dose will result in near sterility, or commercial sterility, while still retaining the natural properties of spices.

Industrial Use

Industry uses radioisotopes to check for blocked pipes and detect oil leakage. A small amount of radioactive ^{24}Na can be placed in an enclosed ball that is allowed to move through pipes with water. A detector is used to monitor the radioisotope-containing moving ball. The obstruction is indicated if the ball's movement stops. Radioisotope ^{24}Na mixed with oil in underground pipes is another example. Radioisotopes can also be used to monitor fluid flow, and filtration, detect leaks, and gauge engine wear.

Industries need to monitor their production processes in order to ensure quality and control. Quality control devices that use the unique radiation properties of radiation are used to monitor production. These devices are known as nuclear gauges. They are more useful at extreme temperatures, in harmful chemical processes, molten glass, and metals. They are used to measure thicknesses of sheet materials such as metals, textiles, and paper, and to inspect the integrity of welds and metal parts across many industries..

Radioisotope Exposure Effects

Radiation that passes through the material causes the bonds to break down by removing an electron from one or more atoms or molecules. This can cause physical, chemical and biological changes. Ionizing radiation concentrates large amounts of energy in highly concentrated areas of irradiated material. This energy can cause damage by interaction with nuclei and orbiting electrons. This energy interaction can alter the material structure, causing changes in the mechanical properties of bulk materials. Radiation-induced degradation technology (RIDA) is a novel application for developing viscose and pulp, paper, pharmaceutical production, food preservation, and natural bioactive agents industries.

Radiation Effects on the Body

Health effects refer to the harmful effects of radiation exposure on human health. A trail of ionized molecules and atoms are the result of all physical interactions between incident radiation and cells. Radiation interacts directly with the DNA of sensitive sites in the tissue to cause damage through breaking chemical bonds. Interaction of primary radiation with the DNA of the tissue produces chemically active free radicals through ionization. The figure below shows both direct and indirect damage to DNA caused by radiation.

It is caused by the chemical radicals that are generated by radiation and interact with water molecules. Indirect action accounts for about 80% tissue. Because they can travel far enough to cause chemical changes in critical areas of biological structures, free radicals are crucial. Free radicals can cause chemical damage by destroying DNA.

DNA is a double-helix structure. If radiation/free radicals only break one strand, the damage can be easily repaired using the opposite strand as a template. Double strand breakage makes it impossible to repair the cell. This can lead to mutations, or changes in the DNA code that cause cell death or cancer. These molecules can be repaired by natural biological processes to a certain degree, but this depends on the severity of the damage.

Radiation damage can have long-term or short-term effects. Acute radiation effects are those that result from prolonged exposure to radiation for a short time. A chronic effect, or delayed effect, is a small amount of radiation that has been exposed for a longer time. If the dose is greater than 500 mSv, then deterministic effects can be severe. The severity of effects are shown in **Table 16.2:**

Table 16.2: ???		
Effective dose	Time of exposure	Effects
<1 Sv	Weeks Very short period	Reduction of white blood cells Recovery is good
About 2 Sv	1 h within one week 3-4 weeks	Nausea, headache, or vomiting 50% decreases in lymphocytes, 50% decreases in thrombocyte levels It is possible to recover quickly
3 Sv	From hours to days After few days Within one week or more	Radiation sickness can cause nausea, vomiting, and fatigue as well as loss of appetite, infection, infections, dehydration, and hair loss. The patient may feel better Recovering well
4 Sv	Few weeks	Intestine mucous membrane and bone marrow tissue have been damaged
5–6 Sv	—	There is a strong chance of death
>6 Sv	—	It is unlikely that you will survive for more than a few weeks.
>10 Sv	Within 2 weeks	Death will result from the irreparable damage to the mucous membranes of the intestines.
50 Sv	Within hours Within one day	Loss of consciousness and damage to the central nervous system could result in death.

The delay in the time between exposure and the observed health effects is due to chronic exposure. These health effects can include cancer, as well as other outcomes like cataracts and benign tumors.

To minimize radiation exposure for medical professionals, it is possible to follow as low as reasonably practicable (ALARA) or to use personnel shielding options (e.g. two-piece wraparound aprons and thyroid shields) to reduce scattered X-ray levels. Dose limits are not applicable to patients who are exposed for medical reasons. Medical radiation is not subject to dose limits. Instead, doctors use the diagnostic reference level (DRL), which is a reference value for medical radiation.

Radiation exposure risk must be reduced by minimizing medical radiation exposure. Furthermore, ionizing radiation-related examinations must be optimized to reduce radiation exposure. Justification refers to the medically justified and clinically useful examination. Optimization refers to the use of doses as low as possible in order to achieve the diagnostic task.

Public exposure control is usually achieved by controlling radiation at the source, rather than in the surrounding environment. The ICRP recommends that the dose limits not exceed 1 mSv y^{-1} (excluding normal background radiation). In exceptional circumstances, however, a higher dose limit can be permitted for a single year, provided that the average of 5 years does not exceed 1 mSv y^{-1}.

The following parameters can be used to control occupational exposure:

Distance: To reduce radiation exposure, the distance between the source worker and the worker should be great.

Time: Radiation dose is directly proportional to the amount of radiation received. The radiation dose should therefore be kept as short as possible.

Shielding: Different materials can be used depending on the type of radiation. High-atomic numbered elements for gamma radiation are used because the rate at which energy is lost is directly proportional Z^5. High absorption cross-sections and low-atomic number elements are used to shield neutrons. Hydrogen and hydrogen-based materials work well for neutron shielding. We can use plastic to create a barrier that protects against high-energy beta radiation.

■ RADIATION PROTECTION LIMITS

The normal exposure of individuals resulting from all relevant practices should be subject to dose limits to ensure that no individual is exposed to a risk that is judged to be unacceptable.

Table 16.3: Dose limitations.

Part of the body	Occupational exposure	Public exposure
Whole body (Effective dose)	20 mSv/year averaged over 5 consecutive years; 30 mSv in any single year	1 mSv/y
Lens of eyes (Equivalent dose)	150 mSv in a year	15 mSv/y
Skin (Equivalent dose)	500 mSv in a year	50 mSv/y
Extremities (Hands and feet) Equivalent dose	500 mSv in a year	-

For pregnant radiation workers, after the declaration of pregnancy 1 mSv on the embryo/fetus should not exceed.

The Nuclear Regulatory Commission (NRC) and the Environmental Protection Agency (EPA) have established three layers of radiation protection limits to protect the public against potential health risks from exposure to radioactive liquid discharges (effluents) from nuclear power plant operations.

Layer 1:3 mrem per year ALARA (As Low as in Reasonably Achievable) Objective- Appendix 1 to 10 CFR Part 50

The NRC requires that nuclear plant operators must keep radiation doses from gas and liquid effluents as low as reasonably achievable (ALARA) to people offsite. For liquid effluent releases, such as diluted tritium, the ALARA annual offsite dose objective is 3 mrem to the whole body and 10 mrem to any organ of a maximally exposed individual who lives in close proximity to the plant boundary. This ALARA objective is 3% of the annual public dose limit of 100 mrem.

The NRC selected the 3 mrem and 10 mrem per year values because they are a fraction of the natural background radiation dose, a fraction of the annual public dose limit, and an attainable objective that nuclear power plants could meet. Power plants that meet these objectives are considered to be ALARA in reducing exposures to the general public from nuclear power plant effluents.

Nuclear power plant operators must monitor the authorized releases (effluents) from their plants. If a given nuclear power plant exceeds half of these radiation dose levels in a calendar quarter, the plant operator is required to investigate the cause, initiate appropriate corrective actions, and report the actions to the NRC within 30 days from the end of the quarter.

Layer 2:25 mrem per year standard—10 CFR 20.1301 (e)

In 1979, EPA developed a radiation dose standard of 25 mrem to the whole body, 75 mrem to the thyroid, 25 mrem to any other organ of an individual member of the public. The NRC incorporated these EPA standards into its regulation in 1981, and all nuclear power plants must now meet these requirements. These standards are specific to facilities that are involved in generating nuclear power (commonly called the 'uranium fuel cycle'), including where nuclear fuel is milled, manufactured, and used in nuclear power reactors. EPA determines the basis of the standards by comparing the cost-effectiveness of various dose limits in reducing potential health risks from operations of these types of facilities. EPA assumes the standards would be able to meet for up to four fuel cycle facilities at one location. Notably, the NRC's ALARA objectives are lower than these EPA standards.

Layer 3:100 mrem per year limit—10 CFR 20.1301 (a) (1)

The NRC's final layer of protection of public health and safety is a dose limit of 100 mrem per year for individual members of the public. This limit applies to everyone, including academics, universities, and medical facilities that use radioactive material.

The NRC adopted the 100 mrem per year dose limit from the 1990 recommendations of the International Commission on Radiological Protection (ICRP). The ICRP is an organization of international radiation scientists who provide recommendations regarding radiation protection-related activities, including dose limits. The basis of the ICRP recommendation of 100 mrem per year is that a lifetime of exposure at this limit would result in very small health risk and is roughly equivalent to background radiation from natural sources.

Basic Three Factors for Radiation Protection (Working Personnel and Public)

Time
- Exposure to radiation source is directly proportional to the time
- Reduce the period of exposure to radiation to reduce the dose received from the source.

Distance
- Increase distance from source to decrease exposure rate.
- $I_1 d_1^2 = I_2 d_2^2$ (Inverse-square law)
- Double the distance from the source; dose-rate falls to ¼ the original value.
- Halve the distance from the source; the dose-rate increases to 4 times the original value.
- More the distance from the source—The lesser the radiation

Shielding
- Use an appropriate shielding material or protection devices
- Shielding reduces exposure rate
- Use large shielding thickness (High-Z materials e.g., Lead, Steel, Concrete, etc.)—to reduce the exposure rate of gamma/X-ray radiation.

INSTRUMENTS USED FOR DETECTION OF IONIZING RADIATION, X-RAYS

Ionizing radiation, such as X-rays, alpha rays, beta rays, and gamma rays, remains undetectable by the senses, and the damage it causes to the body is cumulative, related to the total dose received. Therefore, workers who are exposed to radiation, such as radiographers, nuclear power plant workers, doctors using radiotherapy, workers in laboratories using radionuclides, and some HAZMAT teams are required to wear instruments that can keep a record of their exposure, to verify that it is below legally prescribed limits. Ionizing radiations can be measured or monitored by Dosimeters, Geiger counters, and scintillation counters.

- **Dosimeters:** Dosimeters measure an absolute dose received over a period of time. Ion-chamber dosimeters resemble pens and can be clipped to one's clothing. Common types of wearable dosimeters for ionizing radiation include:
  - Quartz fiber dosimeter
  - Film badge dosimeter
  - Thermoluminescent dosimeter
  - Solid-state (MOSFET or silicon diode) dosimeter
    - Film-badge dosimeters enclose a piece of photographic film, which will become exposed as the radiation passes through it. Ion-chamber dosimeters must be periodically recharged, and the result logged. Film-badge dosimeters must be developed as photographic emulsions so the exposures can be counted and logged; once developed, they are discarded. Another type of dosimeter is the TLD (Thermoluminescent Dosimeter). These dosimeters contain crystals that emit visible light when heated, in direct proportion to their total radiation exposure. Like ion-chamber dosimeters, TLDs can be re-used after they have been 'read'. Common types of wearable dosimeters for ionizing radiation includes.
- **Geiger counters:** Geiger counters are used to detect ionizing radiation (usually beta particles and gamma rays, but certain models can detect alpha particles). An inert gas-filled tube (usually helium, neon, or argon with halogens added) briefly conducts electricity when a particle or photon of radiation makes the gas conductive. The tube amplifies this conduction by a cascade effect and outputs a current pulse, which is then often displayed by a needle or lamp and/or audible clicks. Modern instruments can report radioactivity over several orders of magnitude.
- **Scintillation counters:** A scintillation counter measures ionizing radiation. The sensor, called a scintillator, consists of a transparent crystal, usually phosphor, plastic (usually containing anthracene), or organic liquid (see liquid scintillation counting) that fluoresces when struck by ionizing radiation. A sensitive photomultiplier tube (PMT) measures the light from the crystal. The PMT is attached to an electronic amplifier and other electronic equipment to count and possibly quantify the amplitude of the signals produced by the photomultiplier.

QUESTIONS

Q.1: Radioiodine is given to patients with hyperthyroidism. Explain.
Q.2: Which measures are taken to reduce exposure to radioactivity in hospitals?

Q.3: Use of radioisotopes in cancer therapy. Discuss.
Q.4: Use of film badges by radiographers. Explain.

BIBLIOGRAPHY

1. Beyer HF, Shevelko VP. Introduction to the Physics of Highly Charged Ions. CRC Press, 2003.
2. Choppin, Gregory R. Liljenzin Jan-Olov Rydberg Jan. Radiochemistry and Nuclear Chemistry. Elsevier, 2001.
3. Demtröder W. Atoms, Molecules and Photons: An Introduction to Atomic, Molecular- and Quantum Physics (1st edition). Springer, 2002.
4. Fowles GR. Introduction to Modern Optics. Courier Dover Publications, 1989.
5. Gangopadhyaya M. Indian Atomism: History and Sources. Atlantic Highlands, New Jersey: Humanities Press, 1981.
6. Goodstein DL. States of Matter. Courier Dover Publications, 2002.
7. Harrison ER. Masks of the Universe: Changing Ideas on the Nature of the Cosmos. Cambridge University Press, 2003.
8. Jevremovic T. Nuclear Principles in Engineering. Springer, 2005.
9. Knoll G. Radiation Detection and Measurement. John Wiley and Sons, 1999.
10. L'Annunziata MF. Handbook of Radioactivity Analysis. Academic Press, 2003.
11. Lequeux J. The Interstellar Medium. Springer, 2005.
12. Levere TH. Transforming Matter: A History of Chemistry from Alchemy to the Buckyball. The Johns Hopkins University Press, 2001.
13. MacGregor MH. The Enigmatic Electron. Oxford University Press, 1992.
14. Manuel O. Origin of Elements in the Solar System: Implications of Post-1957 Observations. Springer, 2001.
15. Mazo RM. Brownian Motion: Fluctuations, Dynamics, and Applications. Oxford University Press, 2002.
16. Moran BT. Distilling Knowledge: Alchemy, Chemistry, and the Scientific Revolution, 2005.
17. Myers R. The Basics of Chemistry. Greenwood Press, 2003.
18. Padilla MJ, Miaoulis I, Cyr M. Prentice Hall Science Explorer: Chemical Building Blocks. Upper Saddle River, New Jersey USA: Prentice-Hall, Inc., 2002.
19. Pfeffer JI, Nir S. Modern Physics: An Introductory Text. Imperial College Press, 2000.
20. Scerri ER. The Periodic Table. Oxford University Press, 2007.
21. Shultis JK, Faw RE. Fundamentals of Nuclear Science and Engineering. CRC Press, 2002.
22. Siegfried R. From Elements to Atoms: A History of Chemical Composition. DIANE, 2002.
23. Woan G. The Cambridge Handbook of Physics. Cambridge University Press, 2000.
24. Zaider M, Rossi HH. Radiation Science for Physicians and Public Health Workers. Springer, 2001.
25. Radiological Protection Principles. Available from https://www.aerb.gov.in/english/radiation-protection-principle. Cited 29-05-2022

CHAPTER

Electronics in Nursing

Suresh K Sharma, Rakhi Gaur

Chapter Outline
- Principles of Electronics
- Capacitors
- Transistors
- Transducers
- Common Electric Equipment Used in Patient Care

■ INTRODUCTION

The use of electronics can be observed in most of the basic and advanced healthcare practices. Advancement in science in technology has brought the boom in the use of electronics in healthcare practices. One can observe the use of electronic thermometers for recording patient's temperature, and electronic blood pressure monitoring devices. Patient bedside automatic monitors can automatically detect the vital signs, ECG, oxygen saturation, carbon-dioxide saturation, apnea status of patients, etc. These monitors are frequently observed in intensive care units (ICU) and operation theatres (OT). Recently, the use of advanced ventilators and robots in healthcare practices are new examples of the use of electronics in nursing.

Electronics is that branch of physics and technology that deals with the electrical circuits involving active components such as diodes, transistors, etc. Active components of an electrical circuit control the electron flow and are able to amplify weak signals, e.g. battery, transistor, etc. Most electronic devices use semiconductor components to control electron flow. Before semiconductor and solid-state devices, vacuum tubes were the prime electronic components. Electronic circuits can be divided into two categories:

- **Analog Circuits:** Analog circuits use continuous voltages. They perform amplification, etc. on continuous signals.
- **Digital Circuits:** Digital circuits are those electronic circuits that work on a number of discrete voltage levels. They are the basis of digital calculators, computers, and all modern electronic instruments.
    - *Diode:* A diode is a two-terminal electronic device, made of semiconductor materials, which have a non-linear resistance. Its prominent feature of it is to allow an electric current in one direction while blocking an electric current in opposite direction.

- Diodes are the basic building blocks of all electronic circuits. Today, most the diodes are made of silicon or otherwise germanium.

PRINCIPLES OF ELECTRONICS

Principles of electronics can be understood by the explanation of the following aspects of electronics.

Vacuum Tubes

In 1883, Thomson Edison an American inventor, noticed in working with his early incandescent lamps that a small current would pass between the hot filament of the lamp and an additional electrode sealed inside the tube when the additional electrode was made positive. The phenomenon did not occur when the electrode was made negative. This was due to the escape of electrons from the surface of the metal. The escape of electrons from the surface of hot metal is known as thermal electron emission or thermionic emission.

Phenomenon

In the tube, this thermionic emission will result in a cluster of electrons around the emitting hot metal and makes the escape of other electrons difficult. By placing a valve in the form of a positive charge plate in the tube, the negatively charged electrons move toward the positive plate, making room for additional electrons to escape from the hot filament. This action results in a flow of electrons or an electric current. If the tube is evacuated of air, the electrons will flow more rapidly from the emitting filament to the positively charged plate.

Types of Vacuum Tubes

- **Diode tube:** The simplest type of vacuum tube is known as a diode because it contains two electrodes. It consisted of a hot filament at one end of the tube from which electrons "boil off" by thermionic emission into the tube. At the other end of the tube is a metal plate that is charged positively. Because the metal plate is positively charged, the electrons that are negatively charged pass from the filament to the plate. The plate can also be negatively charged. When the plate is negatively charged there is no flow of electrons. A third element can be added to the diode tube to make it into a triode tube **(Fig. 17.1)**.

Fig. 17.1: Diode tube.

Fig. 17.2: Triode tube.

- **Triode tube:** An American inventor Lee de Forest developed the triode tube by introducing a third electrode called the grid to the diode tube is usually made of a mesh screen and is placed between the other two electrodes that is between the cathode and the plate. The grid acts as a control and modifier of the flow of electrons in the vacuum tube **(Fig. 17.2)**.
  - When the grid is made positive, it speeds the movement of the negatively charged electrons through it on their path towards the positive metal tube. When the grid is negatively charged, it slows the speed of the electrons towards the positively charged metal plate. In this way, the grid acts as a regulator and small changes in the electric charge of the grid produce great changes in the flow of electrons through the tube. Because of this structure, the triode tube can be used to amplify a very small current.
- **Multi-element tube:** In addition to diode and triode tube, multi-element tubes have been developed. The simplest of these is the tetrad tube which is another element called a screen is inserted between plates and grid.
- **Pentode tube:** Adding still another element, a suppressor grid between plate and screen produces a pentode tube.

Uses

A vacuum tube may be used to produce electrical oscillations to "magnify" weak oscillations millions of times or to control oscillations. Electronic computers, radar, and patient monitoring systems are important applications of the vacuum tube.

■CAPACITORS

A capacitor is a device that stores electrical energy in an electric field. It is a passive electronic component with two terminals. Or a combination of two conductors placed near each other is called a capacitor. These two conductors can be of any shape, e.g. circular, rectangular plates or cylindrical, but generally two parallel conducting rectangular plates are used. These plates are separated by a thin sheet of insulating material called the dielectric. A capacitor is used in a variety of electronic devices to produce even voltages. Its prime objective is to store charges.

A simple example of such a storage device is the parallel-plate capacitor. If positive charges with total charge +Q are deposited on one of the conductors and an equal amount of negative

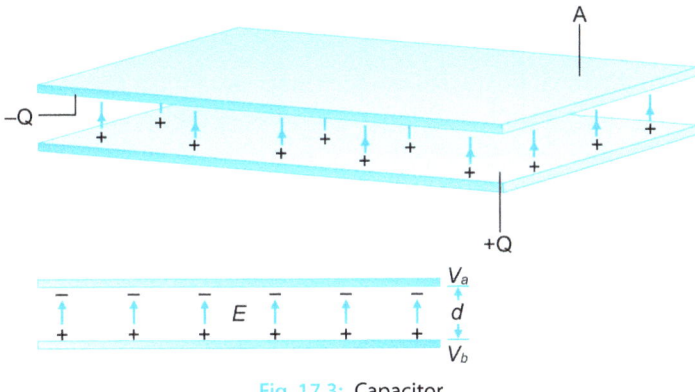

Fig. 17.3: Capacitor.

charge –Q is deposited on the second conductor, the capacitor is said to have a charge Q (**Fig. 17.3**)

Working

There is no direct flow of current through the capacitor because of the insulation between the two parallel conducting plates. When placed in a circuit, one plate becomes charged positively and the other negatively. The charge on the positive plate is called the charge on the capacitor and the potential difference between plates is called the potential of the capacitor.

For a given capacitor, the charge Q on the capacitor is proportional to the potential difference V between the plates, i.e.,

$$Q \alpha V$$
$$Q = CV$$

The proportionality constant 'C' is the capacitance of the capacitor. It depends on the shape, size, and distance between the plates of the capacitor and the medium between them. Its SI unit is Farad.

Capacitors store charges, and when a certain force is reached they pass across the insulator, neutralize each other and break the circuit. After this event, charges rebuild on the plates, and the process repeats (**Fig. 17.4**).

Diagrammatic Presentation

- These are the two plates of a capacitor.
- The plate on the capacitor that attaches to the negative terminal of the battery accepts electrons that the battery is producing.

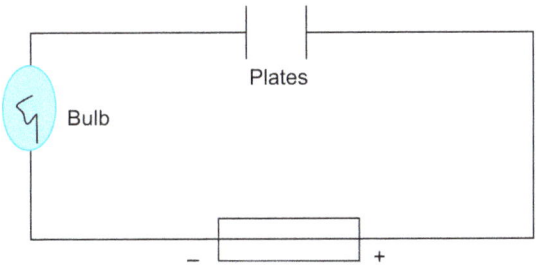

Fig. 17.4: Diagrammatic presentation of a capacitor.

- The plate on the capacitor that attaches to the positive terminal of the battery loses electrons to the battery.
- Once it is charged the capacitor has the same voltage as of the battery.
- Here you have a battery, a light bulb, and a capacitor. If the capacitor is big, what you will notice is that when you connect the battery, the light bulb will light up as current flows from the battery to the capacitor to charge it up. The bulb will get progressively dimmer and finally go out once the capacitor reaches its capacity. If you then remove the battery and replace it with a wire, the current will flow from one plate of the capacitor to the other. The bulb will light initially and then dim as the capacitors discharge until it's completely out.
- **Uses of capacitors:** Capacitors are used for several purposes.
    - *Timing:* For example, with a 555 timer IC controlling the charging and discharging.
    - *Smoothing:* For example, in a power supply.
    - *Coupling:* For example, between stages of an audio system and to connect a loudspeaker.
    - *Filtering:* For example, in the tone control of an audio system.
    - *Tuning:* For example, in a radio system.
- **Storing energy:** For example, in a camera flash circuit.

■ TRANSISTORS

Although the vacuum tube made many electromedical apparatus possible, scientific researchers searched for a device to transmit and amplify current that was smaller than a vacuum tube.

Properties

- Transistors are solid-state semiconductors.
- They are like triode tubes.
- They differ from the vacuum tubes in several ways:
    - Require little input.
    - Last indefinitely.
    - Considerable amplification.
    - They are superior to vacuum tubes when space, and power are primary factors.
- They can be powered by a battery instead of a house current and because of their size, the instrument can be miniature. For example, hearing aids.

■ TRANSDUCERS

In some of the physiologic phenomena measures and records are by nature non-electric for example, sound, heat, or motion. An intermediate instrument is needed in such situations to convert that physical quantity into the equivalent electric quantity and measure accordingly.

Parts and Working

The transducer is an apparatus that converts other forms of energy into electric energy so that they can be measured.

Before explaining the use of the transducer, it is necessary to point out that a purely electronic system, an arrangement of electron vacuum tubes or transistors by itself would be of no use in communications. The system must include apparatus to receive stimuli and emit responses. The stimulus-receiving and response giving devices are input and output transducers **(Fig. 17.5)**.

- ***An input transducer*** may be a microphone or a photoelectric cell. Since the transducer is an energy-converting device, the microphone converts sound energy into electric energy.

CHAPTER 17: Electronics in Nursing

* ***The output transducer*** is sometimes known as a reproducer because it recreates the stimuli in their original form, but usually on a large scale or in a form more conveniently perceived by the observer.

Fig. 17.5: Working of the transducer.

■ COMMON ELECTRIC EQUIPMENT USED IN PATIENT CARE

Thermionic Thermometer

One instrument that changes heat to electric energy is the thermionic thermometer **(Fig. 17.6)**.

Working Principle

Temperature-measuring instrument consists of two wires of different metals joined at each end. One junction is placed where the temperature is to be measured, and the other is kept at a constant lower (reference) temperature. A measuring instrument is connected to the electrical circuit. The temperature difference causes the development of an electromotive force that is approximately proportional to the difference between the temperatures of the two junctions. Temperature can be read from standard tables, or the instrument can be calibrated to display temperature directly **(Fig. 17.7)**.

Uses

* It depends on its action on a crystal that conducts an electric current. The electric resistance of the crystal varies with changes in temperature.

Fig. 17.6: Thermionic thermometer.

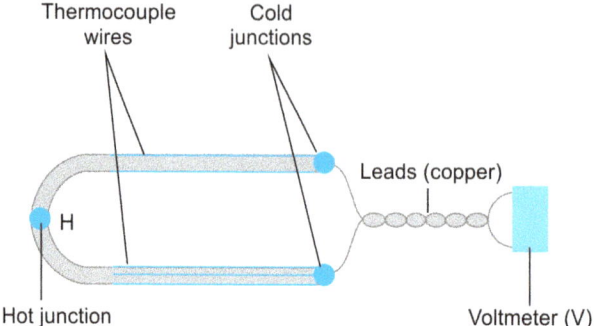

Fig. 17.7: Working of thermionic thermometer.

- It is used for obtaining temperatures internally or on the surface of the body.
- The unit is equipped with a variety of probes for obtaining temperatures.
- The thermionic thermometers offer greater accuracy than clinical mercury thermometer can be located up to 1,000 ft from the unit and registers the temperature in about 5 seconds.

Patient Monitors

Patient monitors consist of one or more transducers that are attached to the patient to pick up physiologic information.

Working

As stated, the transducer changes the physiologic information into electrical energy, which is then passed through electronic circuits. These circuits amplify the electrical impulses and may transform them into mechanical energy in the form of a moving stylus that records the patient's pulse temperatures, respiration and blood pressure on a graph **(Fig. 17.8)**.

Other monitors are equipped with flashlights or ring bells if the patient is exceeding certain physiological limits that have been programmed into the circuits.

Fig. 17.8: Electronic monitors.

Uses

- An apparatus has been reported that during surgery, pick-up impulses from the patient and convert them into lighted numbers on a visible panel where they can be seen readily by a surgeon, nurse, and anesthetist.
- Cardioscope, delivers a picture of cardiac activity on a screen in the form of a light flick.
- Fetal monitors report the condition of the fetus during pregnancy, labor, and delivery.

Cathode Ray Oscilloscope

It is an important aid to the biophysicist, physiologist, and clinician in the study of the electric potentials in the human body.

Functioning

The basic operation on which the instrument functions is a stream of electrons that are liberated from a hot filament or cathode. The electron stream then passed through an anode at a high potential and strikes a fluorescent screen at the end of the tube. Whenever an electron strike a fluorescent screen a spot of light appears **(Fig. 17.9)**.

Use

The electron stream is deflected from pursuing a straight path by an amplified current, that is received from the part of the body under study. This action current is connected to a pair of horizontal plates that deflect the electrons vertically and vice versa. The picture produced on the screen is a pattern of these deflections as the beam sweeps horizontally across the screen. The light pattern formed may be studied immediately or a photograph may be recorded for future study.

Electron Microscope

- It depends upon the properties of the electron for its operation.
- Ordinary microscopes cannot be used to view objects less than 0.000039 cm in diameter which is the same in magnitude as the shortest wavelength of visible light.
- Electrons possess a wave property similar to that of light waves. The wavelength emitted depends upon the voltage with which the electrons are accelerated. Under certain conditions, the wavelength may be 0.05A. This is so much shorter than the shorter wavelength of visible lights (3,900A) that such minute objects as bacteriophage particles have been seen with the aid of the electron microscope.

Fig. 17.9: Cathode ray oscilloscope.

Fig. 17.10: Electron microscope.

- The electron beam is provided by an electron gun. It contains an anode with a small opening to allow the electrons to pass through. The anode is grounded while the filament is at a negative voltage of 50,000 or more. There is also a doughnut-shaped coil of wire that acts on electrons like a convex lens, bending them on the object. The electrons beam is altered by the material by being stopped, retarded, or scattered. The electron beam is then passed through another electron lens that corresponds to the objective of the optical microscope. A third lens magnifies the image that is then focused on a fluorescent screen where it may be seen or photographed **(Fig. 17.10)**.
- Difference between electron microscope and ordinary microscope:
  - Stream of fast-moving electrons instead of light rays.
  - Coils of wire in place of lenses.
  - A fluorescent screen or photographic plate instead of an eyepiece.

Diathermy

- The passage of an electric current through tissues will cause heating. To obtain a significant amount of heat with ordinary low-frequency currents, it would be necessary to use a large amount of current so that the tissue would be destroyed. High-frequency current however may be passed through tissues for a heating effect without causing damage. Diathermy is a means of producing heat in tissues of the body by use of high-frequency electric currents.
- The heat is generated by induction, which means it is produced without actual contact of the electrodes carrying the current within the tissues.
- Diathermy uses electromagnetic waves of higher frequencies than infrared radiations

Uses

- Diathermy has been reported effective in traumatic and inflammatory conditions of the skeleton for relief of bronchitis and pain of pleurisy.

❖ Ultra high-frequency diathermy may be used for inducing fever. This reaction known as electro pyrexia is of value in the treatment of general paresis.

Application of Electronics in Nursing

1. **Application in assessment:** Many electronic equipments are used for assessment and routine check-up of health conditions such as digital and thermionic thermometer for temperature, BP monitor for measuring blood pressure and pulse, and auscultation and recording of heart and lung sounds with a digital stethoscope. Assessment of glucose level in blood with glucometer for diabetes and hemoglobin for anemia also level of oxygen in the blood is assessed through oximeter.
   - To assess the heart condition through ECG and mental condition with EEG is possible by electronics.
❖ **Application in continuous monitoring:** Monitors are providing continuous data regarding vitals inwards, ICU, and operation rooms to take early necessary action if the condition is about to deteriorate. Nowadays, smartwatches and mobile technology is providing continuous data related to the health and fitness of a person, this may be used for tracking and monitoring especially to geriatric and specially-abled persons.
   - Electronic fetal monitoring measures the response of the fetus's heart rate to contractions of the uterus. It provides an ongoing record. As a nurse, we should be able to read and review the electronic recording of the fetus's heartbeat. A pair of belts are wrapped around the abdomen of mother. One belt uses Doppler to detect the fetal heart rate. The other belt measures the length of contractions and the time between them.
❖ **Application in treatment and follow-up:** Medication dispenser for the elderly people to have in time medication with the correct amount of doses.
   - The pacemaker is used to resolve the missing heartbeat or slow heartbeat by generating electrical pulses and bringing the heart back to working condition as a nurse, we should know the normal and abnormal ECG patterns with the pacemaker.
   - Neural stimulator relieves the pain signals between the spinal cord and the brain by generates electrical impulses and soothes the body quickly. As a nurse, we should be able to identify malfunction early as miss firing or hyper-firing.
   - Triaxial accelerometer and many other sensors are being used to monitor the activity level of patients. Many sensors are being used in physiotherapy to track and correct the exercise patterns so we should know the proper positioning and use of them.
   - During surgery, the anesthesia machine is maintained the levels of gases like oxygen, air, nitrous oxide, and isoflurane. For this purpose, sensors are required to control temperature, humidity, and pressure. There is a water lock to prevent seepage of water in a machine that should be monitored regularly and changed periodically, and a nurse should know the functioning basics so malfunctioning is identified early.
   - As nursing person, we should know the changing technologies and proper use them, in the near future, we will be surrounded by so many electronic sensors to help us from assessment to implementation and evaluation of care with adequate follow-up and feedbacks.
   - Automated IV pumps control the dosages and drips given to patients. Software and medical tech allow nurses to change the drip amounts and medication doses so patients aren't waiting for changes. There are IV pumps for nutrition that give needed meals at the right times. Additionally, there are self-pumps that allow patients to increase a controlled amount of pain medication for themselves. Automated IV pumps help speed up nursing processes and can be crucial if there is a need for immediate adjustment. Changing

medication through an automated process also removes elements of human error that could present issues for clinical patients and hospitals.
- Electronic health records (EHR) are replacing older paper filing methods. Electronic health records allow nursing experts to document care provided to patients and retrieve information that can help prioritize care. Additionally, information entered into computer systems can then be accessed by the care team, including doctors and even patients themselves when necessary.
- Telehealth is a valuable, newer element in healthcare. Hospitals and clinics allow patients to virtually video chat with a doctor or nurse to describe their symptoms or show doctors things like rashes or bumps. This helps patients with a quick diagnosis without leaving the comfort of their own home. They can find out if they need to come in for further testing or diagnosis, get a prescription for medicine, or get medical advice.
- Telehealth saves both patients and doctors money and time. Similarly, it prevents sick patients from coming to public places and exposing other patients. This technology is changing the way clinics operate and how patients are cared for.

■ QUESTIONS

Q.1: Describe about vacuum tubes.
Q.2: Discuss about common electronic equipment used in patient care.

■ BIBLIOGRAPHY

1. Bullock TH. Electroreception, Springer, 2005.
2. Flitter HH, Rowe HR. An Introduction to Physics in Nursing. St Louis: The CV Mosby Company, 1995.
3. Gomber KL, Gogia KL. Fundamental Physics. Ambala: Paedeep Publishers, 2004.
4. Goyal RP, Tripathi SP. Oncise Physics, New Delhi: Selina Publishers, August 2007.
5. Jackson MB. Molecular and Cellular Biophysics. New York: Cambridge Publication, 2006.
6. Lal S. Principles of Physics. Ambala: Paedeep Publishers, 2004.
7. Mielczarek EV, Greenbaum E, Knox RS. Biological Physics. New York. American Institute of Physic, 1993.
8. Morris SC. Life's Solution: Inevitable Humans in a Lonely Universe, Cambridge University Press, 2003.
9. Margaret Scisney-Matlock, Donna Algase, Susan Boehm, Patricia Coleman-Burns, Deborah Oakley, Ann E. Rogers. SeonAe Yeo, Erica Young, and Mei-yu Yu. Measuring Behavior: Electronic Devices in Nursing Studies .Applied Nursing Research, Vol. 13, No. 2 (May), 2000: pp 97–102

Index

Page numbers followed by *f* refer to figure and *t* refer to table.

A

Abdomen 274
ABO blood groups 64
Absorption 240
Acceleration 148
   average 148
   instantaneous 148
   stress 150
   types of 148
Accidents, inertia in 150
Accommodation, power of 207
Acetaldehyde 69
Acetaminophen 77
Acetyl
   CoA 129
   number 122
Acid 33
   acetic 35, 113
   action on
      bicarbonates 34
      carbonates 34
      certain metals 34
      hydroxides 34
      indicators 34
      oxides 34
      tissues 34
   antidotes for 34
   arachidonic 114
   aspartic 85, 89
   basic properties of 34
   bile 118, 120
   boric 34, 35
   butyric 113
   caproic 113
   caprylic 113
   carbonic 34
   citric 35
   classification of 34
   deoxyribonucleic 62
   fluids 33
   glutamic 85, 89
   glycochenodeoxycholic 120
   glycocholic 120
   hyaluronic 65
   hydrochloric 34
   hypochlorus 35
   inorganic 34
   lactic 35
   linoleic 114
   linolenic 114
   nitric 34
   number 122
   oleic 114
   organic 34, 35
   palmitic 113
   phosphatidic 123
   properties of 34
   propionic 113
   pyruvic 129
   reaction with 35
   ribonucleic 13
   salicyclic 35
   sour taste 34
   stearic 113
   sulfuric 34
   tartaric 35
   taurochenodeoxycholic 120
   taurocholic 120
   to nurses, functions of 34
   uric 106
Acid-base balance, maintaining 38
Acoustic insulation 252
Activation energy, lowering of 42
Acyl
   carnitine 126
   esters 62
Adipose tissue 124
Adrenocortical hormone 118
Aerobic glycolysis pathway, steps of 66
Agricultural research 295
Air 203
   force of 162
   pressure 220
Alanine 85-87, 102
Albumins 92
Alcohol 11, 77, 117
Alcoholic fermentation 69, 69*f*
Aldosterone 27
Allosteric inhibitors 45
Alpha radiation 290
Alpha-keto acids, amination of 105
Alpha-ketoglutarate, formation of 74
Amino acid 12, 50, 84, 86, 87, 97
   activation of 99
   basic structure of 85*f*
   catabolism of 101
   classification of 85
   essential 85
   functions of 90
   metabolism of 101
   non-essential 85
   part of 84
   properties of 90
   proteinogenic 84
   sequence of 99
   standard 90
   transfer of activated 99
Aminoacyl synthetases 99
Amino group 90
Ammonia 23
   transport 102
Ammonium hydroxide 35
Amphibolic pathway 66
Amplitude 238, 238*f*
Anabolic pathway 66, 100
Anaerobic glycolysis 70
   pathway 68, 69*f*
Analog circuits 302
Anode sealed 261
Anomalous expansion 22
Anomers 61
Antibody 8
Anticoagulant activity 108
Antidiuretic hormone 27
Antisense strand 99
Aphakia 208
Apolipoprotein 124
Apoprotein 124
Apoptosis 13
Applanation method 231
Aqueous humor 207
Archimedes' principle 156*f*
   applications of 156
Arginine 85, 89
   hydrolysis of 104
Arginosuccinate
   cleavage of 104
   synthesis of 103
Arterial pressure 229
Arthritis 196
   management of 184
Artificial radiation sources 292
Asparagine 86, 89, 102
Astigmatism 208, 209
Atmospheric pressure 221, 223
   applications of 223
   instrument for measuring 223
   lower 21
Atom 284
   orbits of 286*f*, 288*f*
   spectra of 287
   structure of 283
Atomic nucleus 290
Atomic number 290
Audiogram 251
Audiometry 245
Auditory neuropathy spectrum
   disorder 250
Automated external defibrillator 276,
   277, 277*f*, 278
Automated IV pumps 311

B

Back pain 184
Backward jerk 162
Bad and semiconductor 256*f*
Balanced traction 180*f*
Balloon system 232
Balmer series 287
Basal metabolic rate 171
Base 35
   antidotes for 36
   examples of 35, 35*t*
   functions of 36
   of support 158
   on polarity 86
   properties of 35
Basic life support 276
Bath
   normal 197
   sitz 197

Index

Battery and electromotive force 259
Becker bolt 232
Beta radiation 291
Bicarbonate 27, 39, 107
   level 33
   system 37
Bile salts 120
   common primary 120
Biochemistry 3, 4
Biological methods 228
Biomedical importance 111, 114
Biophysics 133, 135
   atomic physics 138
   center of gravity 137
   electricity 137
   force 137
   gravity 136
   heat 137
   light and sound 137
   meaning of 136
   measurement 136
   molecular physics 138
   motion 136
   pressure 137
   specific gravity 137
   work and energy 138
Bismuth-213 293
Bitter taste 35
Blood
   constituents of 107
   nitrogenous constituents of 107
   route 53
   transfusion 166
   vessel walls 268
Blood clotting 108
   regulation of 114
Blood glucose 80
   factors maintaining 76
   level
      decrease 77
      increase 76
   regulation 75
Blood pressure 220
   cuff 229
Blood sugar
   causes of low 81
   levels 4
   regulation, mechanisms of 75, 75f
Blurred vision 80
Body
   alignment 158
   balance 158
   buffers in 37
   chemical reactions 31
   endocrine functions of 54
   energy content of 169
   mass of 153
   parts of 164
   pressure 221
   radiation effects on 296
   water distribution 23
Body cells 8
   and organs, functioning of 27
Body fluid 20
   compartments 24
   distribution 24f
Body mechanics 173
   principles of 173
Body temperature
   internal 194
   regulation of 193
Bohr's atomic model 286
Bohr's model 285
Bohr's theory 287
Boiling point 189
Bones
   constituting 176
   normal position 178
Bony parts 164
Borax 23
Bowel diseases 53
Boyle's law 226
Brachial muscles 174
Brackett and Pfund series 287
Brain pacemaker 274, 275f
Breathing 171
Bronchoscopes 214
Buffer systems, primary 37
Buffering capacity 108
Buoyancy results 155
Buoyant force 155f
Burger's capillary glass tube method 229

C

Calcium 30, 107
   common sources of 31t
   functions of 30
   hydroxide 23, 35
   requirement of 30t
   sources of 30
Cancer treatment 295
Capacitor 304, 305f
   parallel-plate 304
   uses of 306
Capillary tube 186
Carbamino reaction 90
Carbamoyl phosphate
   formation of 103
   synthesis of 103
Carbohydrate 58, 59, 82, 111, 130f, 171
   absorption of 50
   basics of 53
   biomedical importance of 58
   classification of 59
   complex 58, 59f
   digestion 48
      description of 49t
      goal of 49
      process of 49f
   functions of 64
   lipid and proteins 130
   metabolism of 64, 66f
   simple 58, 59f
Carbon 58
   dioxide 69
Carboxylic group, reactions to 90
Carcinogens 11
Cardiac glycosides 118
Cardiac pacemaker 279
   external 274f
Cardiac tissue 18
Cardiolipin 123
Cardiovascular disease 120, 179
CAT scan 279
Catabolic pathway 65, 100
Catalytic function 108
Catalyzing enzyme 100
Catheters, ordinary 268
Cathode ray oscilloscope 309, 309f
Cations 27
Celiac disease 53, 56
Cell 168
   active 13
   and tissue growth 96
   animal 7
   biochemistry and 3
   body's 30
   components of 5, 6
   contents 25
   cytoplasm 66
   death 13
   division 6, 17f
   eating 14
   foreign 8
   gonad 11
   human 8, 30
      body 5
   inclusion 18
   live 32, 135
   membrane 6-8
   nerve 243
   of malignant tumors 217
   photoelectric 261f
   powerhouse of 12
   prokaryotic 5, 6t
   red blood 247
   sensory 159
   size 6
   structure of 5
   types of 5
   voltaic 262f
   wall appendages 6
Cellular metabolism 136
Cellular respiration 13
Cellulose 65
Celsius and Fahrenheit scale 192f
Celsius fahrenheit 193
Center of gravity 152, 153f, 158
Centimeter-gram-second 139
Central nervous system 18
Central venous pressure 230
Centrifugal force 167, 167f
Centrifuge 159
   devices, motion in 149
Centrioles 16
   functions of 16
   structure of 17f
Centripetal force 166, 166f, 167
Cephalins 123
Cerebral cortex, occipital region of 198
Cerebral edema 29
Cerebral palsy, case of 159
Cerebrosides 124
Cerebrovascular disease 81
Certain lifestyle factors 54
Cervical traction 179
Cesium-131 293
Chain elongation 100
Chain synthesis, initiation of 100
Chain termination 100
Charged bodies, discharging of 257
Charges, flow of 259f
Charles's law 226
Chemical
   effects 263
   influences 54
   properties 22

Chemokinesis 116
Chemotaxis 116
Chest
    physiotherapy 157
    size 276
    wall 274
Chloride 27, 32, 107
    functions of 32
    sources of 33
Cholesterol 7, 118, 119
    blood level of 119
    chemical structure of 119f
    features of 119
    functions of 119
    occurrence of 118
    source of 118
Choroids 206
Chromatin 9
Chromium-51 293
Chromoproteins 92
Chromosomes 9, 16
Chylomicrons 124
Ciliary muscle 206
Circadian disorder 213
Circadian rhythm 212
Circular motion, forces in 166
Circulatory problem 179, 180
Cisterns 10
Citric acid, formation of 74
Citrulline, formation of 103
Claustrophobia 179
Clinical thermometer 193
Clofibrate 77
Closed-chest procedure 275
Clothing and gloves, protective 47
Cobalt-57 294
Cobalt-60 293
Cochlear implant 250
Coil carrying 262
Combustion, heat of 190
Competitive inhibitors 44
Component's ability 289
Compound lipids, description of 112t
Computed axial tomography 279
Computed tomography 278
Concentration gradient 50
Condensation, heat of 190
Conduction 186, 255
Conductors, applications of 187
Confusion 29
    signs of 196
Conjugated proteins, kinds of 92t
Constructive interference 241f
Contusions, management of 184
Convection 187
Copper 107
Copper-64 294
Cornea 206
    thickness of 248
Coronary artery disease 80
Corpuscle's theory of light, failures of 199
Cosmic radiation 292
Coulomb's law 255, 265
C-reactive protein 108
Creatinine 4
Cristae 12
Crystalline 209
Crystals 18
Current 259

Cyclopentano phenanthrene ring 118f
Cysteine 85-87
Cystic fibrosis 79
Cystine 85
Cystoscopes 214
Cytoplasm 6, 18
Cytoskeleton 18
    functions of 18
Cytosol 5, 9

D

Dairy foods 31
Dalton's law 227
De novo synthesis 127
    steps of 128f
Deamination 101
    minor oxidative of 101
Defibrillation 275, 276f
Delirium 29
Deoxy sugars 62
Derived units 138
Destructive interference 242f
Device 260
Dextran 65
D-galactose, chemical structure of 61f
D-glucose, chemical structure of 61f
Diabetes 53, 79, 80
Diacylglycerol 121
Diapause 212
Diathermy 248f, 310
Dielectric 304
Diffraction 240
Diffuse reflection 202
Digestive enzyme 22, 54
Digestive failure 55
Digestive juices, part of 32
Digestive organs, exocrine functions of 54
Dihydroxyacetone phosphate 68
Diode 302
    tube 303, 303f
Disaccharide 48, 59, 62, 63
    components of 63t
    description of 63t
Discharge by spark 257f
Disease condition 196
D-isomer 51
    chemical structure of 60f
Distant vision, least distance of 207, 208
Diurnal rhythm 211
D-mannose, chemical structure of 61f
Domain theory 268, 268f
Doppler effect 244
Dosimeters 300
Dressing 194
Drying oils 121
D-xylose test 55
Dynamic contour tonometry 231

E

Ear
    inner 243
    middle 244
Earthworms 211
Eating habits 54
Echocardiography 248

Echoencephalography 248
Ecu-de-cologne 188
Electric 253
    bell 264
    cautery 263f
    equipment 264, 307
    motors 264f
    resistance, unit of 260
Electric current 259, 262, 275
    chemical source of 262
    effects of 262
    flow of 262
    sources of 260
Electricity 253
    flow of 262
    magnetic and mechanical sources of 262
    on human body, effects of 265
    phenomenon of 253
    radiant source of 260
    thermal source of 261
    types of 254
Electrification, theory of 254, 254f
Electrocardiogram 270, 271f
Electrocardiography, process of 270
Electrochemical gradient 8
Electroconvulsive therapy 273
    machine 273f
Electrodynamics 254, 258
Electroencephalogram 269f
Electroencephalography 269
    uses of 270
Electrolyte 20, 28
    disorders, common causes of 33
    type of 28t
Electromagnet 264
Electromagnetism 253
    applications of 265
Electromyography 272, 272f
Electron 254
    beam 310
        tomography 280
    jumps 287
    microscope 309, 310f
    motion of 199
    transfer of 257
    vacuum tubes 306
Electronic
    application of 311
    cardiac pacemaker 273
    circuit with resistance 260f
    devices, variety of 304
    equipment 300
    health records 312
    monitors 308f
    principles of 303
    use of 302
Electrostatic 254
    applications of 258
    precipitation 257, 258f
Electrostimulation 272
Emitting ionizing radiation 289
Endocrines 212
Endocytosis 8
Endoplasmic reticulum 7, 10, 11, 13
    functions of 11
    structure of 10f
Energy 161, 169, 234
    calorie 169
    conservation of 171

Index

conversion factor 169t
heat 194
in body 170
kilogram calorie 169
kilowatt-hour 169
kinetic 169, 170f, 229, 235
light 198
nucleus, lower 290
of electrons 285
of single quantum 201
potential 169, 170f, 235
quanta of 201
transformation 169
types 169
values, typical 171t
Environment preparation, use in 195
Environmental conditions 193
Enzyme 8, 16, 41, 55, 93, 96, 108
    activating 99
    aldolase 68
    cardiac 46
    characteristics of 41
    classification of 45
    concentration 44
    diagnostic applications 46
    digestion and absorption 41
    enolase 68
    function of 41, 46
    gastric 46
    in other body fluids 46
    liver 46
    lysosomal 15
    measuring 48
    mechanism of action 42
    nonfunctional 46
    phosphofructokinase 67
    phosphoglycerokinase 68
    phosphoglyceromutase 68
    pyruvate kinase 68
    specificity of 45
    status of 44
    triose phosphate 68
Enzyme action
    induced fit theory of 43f
    key and lock theory of 43f
    mechanism of 42f
Enzyme activity
    effect of
        heavy metals 44
        inhibitors 44
        metals 44
        radiation 44
        water 44
    factors affecting 44
    pH of medium 44
    secretion of 54
    substrate concentration 44
    temperature 44
Epimers 61
Epinephrine 77
Equilibrium vapor pressure 190
Erythrocytes 77
Esterification 62
Estrogens 119
Euglena 211
Eukaryotic cell 5, 6t
    structure and components of 6f
Evaporation 188
Exercise
    active 194
    severe 194

Exocytosis 8
    process of 76
Exposed persons, protection of 252
External work 171
Extracellular compartment 20
Extracellular fluid 8, 25
Extraterrestrial radiations 292
Eye 207, 208
    action of 207
    color to 206
    lens 207
    near point of 208
    proteus 211
    short-sighted 209
    structure of 206, 207f
Eyeball 208

■ F

Far sightedness 209
Fast fourier transform techniques 280
Fat 111, 130f, 171
    and oils, characterization of 121
    digestion and absorption of 48
    metabolism 113
    tissue 124
Fatty acid 113, 114, 124
    activation of 125, 125f
    beta-oxidation of 126
    classification of 113
    de novo synthesis of 127
    essential 114
    esters of 120
    free 53
    functions of essential 114
    long-chain 53, 113
    metabolism of 125
    monounsaturated 114
    oxidation 125
        enzyme of 125
        steps of 126, 127f
    pathway 128f
        mitochondrial transportation of 126f
    polyunsaturated 114
    saturated 113, 113t
    short-chain 113, 121
    synthesis 127
        energetic of 129
    transport of 125, 126
    unsaturated 114, 114t
Fetal heart monitoring 248
Fiber 49
Fibrinogen 107
Fibrous proteins 93
First aid treatment 48
    consumer exposure assessment 48
    eye contact 48
    inhalation 48
    skin contact 48
First atom 254
First class lever 174, 174f
Flagella 8
Flagellum 8
Fluid 224
    balance 25, 97
    friction 165
    mosaic model 7
    normal balance of 32
Fluorine-18 294

Food 171
    preservation 295
    sterilization 295
    types, selected 171t
Foot, lever action of 175, 175f
Force 161, 163
    changes 161
    characteristics of 161
    magnetic lines of 267
Forearm
    lever action of 176, 176f
    lower raised 176
Foreign bodies 268
Formaldehyde 90
Freezing point 188
Frequency 238
Frequent urination 80
Friction
    opposes, force of 162
    principles of 165
Frictional force 164
Fructose 49
Fumarate, formation of 74
Functional isomers 60, 61f
Fundamental units 138, 140
Fusion 290
    heat of 189

■ G

Gallbladder, disease of 54
Gallium-67 294
Gamma radiation 291
Gangliosides 124
Gastritis 53
Gastrointestinal infections 53
Gastrointestinal organs, anatomical defect in 54
Gastrointestinal structure 53
Gastrointestinal tract 53
Geiger counters 300
Geiger-Muller counter 288
Gemfibrozil 77
Gene expression 136
Generate electricity 262
Generators, working of 263f
Genetics, molecular basis of 3
Gestational diabetes 78
    abnormal results for 78
Giardia lamblia 55
Gigger-Muller counter 289f
Glacier meltwater 21
Globulins 92
Glucocorticoids 77
Gluconeogenesis 66, 71
    pathway, steps of 71f
    significance 72
    site of 71
    substrates for 72
Glucose 49, 171
    6-phosphate 129
    free 70
    tolerance test 4, 77
        indications of 78
        results, interpretations of 78
    transporter 4 50
Glutamine 85, 86, 89, 102
    formation 104
    synthesis 101
Glutelins 92

Glycemia 76, 77
  abnormal values of 77
Glyceraldehyde phosphate 68
Glycerol 117
  source of 117
  uses of 117
Glycine 85-87
Glycogen 9, 18, 64, 65
Glycogenesis 66, 72, 76
  significance 72
  steps of 72
Glycogenolysis 65, 70, 75
  pathway, steps of 70, 71f
  steps of 70
Glycolipid 7, 112, 123
  classification of 123, 124t
  functions of 124
  name of 124
Glycolysis 65, 66, 68
  cycle, steps of 66
  energetics of 70
  pathway, steps of 67f
  reactions 9
  site 66
Glycoprotein 7, 92
  function 136
  structure 136
Glycosides 62
Goldmann tonometry 231
Golgi apparatus 7
Golgi complex 11, 14
  functions of 11
  structure of 12f
Good conductors 255f
Good solvent 22
Gout 105
  causes of 105
  laboratory study 106
  prevention of 107
  prognosis 106
  progression of 107
  signs of 106, 106f
  symptoms of 106, 106f
  treatment of 106
Gravitational force 165
  acts 161
  on human body, effects of 157
Gravity 151, 157
  application of principles of 157, 182
  edema due to 158f
  fluid movement to 157
  force of 162
  horizon of 159
  IV fluid administration with 158f
  outside, line of 158
  principles of 155, 157
  specific 151, 152t
Growth-stimulating hormones 212
Guinea pigs 211

■ H

Hamburger's red corpuscle method 228
Handling enzyme preparations, precautions of 46
Headaches 29, 80
Health and illness, biochemical basis of 4

Healthcare practices 184, 248
Healthy human body 221t
Hearing 243
  aids 244
  assistive technology 251
  threshold of 242
Hearing loss 249
  conductive 250
  interpreting 246t
  mixed 250
  sensorineural 250
  types of 250
Heart rhythms 31
Heat 184
  and electricity, poor conductor of 22
  and temperature 185
  measurement of 185
  nature of 184
  on matter, effects of 188
  principles, application of 195
  specific 191
  transfer of 186
  transmission, modes of 188f
Heavier nuclei, amount of 292
Helium ions 292
Hemoglobin 96
  system 37
Hemolysis 228
Heparin 65
Heteropolysaccharides 65
Hexokinase 45
Hexoses 62
Hill's method 229
Hip and lever representation 177f
Histidine 85, 91
Histones 92
Homopolysaccharides 65
Hormonal proteins 97
Hormone 8, 76, 212
  aldosterone, action of 28
Human beings, mechanical efficiency of 173t
Human body 20, 24f
  buffer action in 37
  electrolyte of 27
  functions of water in 25
  normal values in 28t
  pressure in 221
  proportion of water in 24f
Human health effects 249
Humidity 190
  absolute 190
  importance of relative 191
  maintain 195
  relative 190, 191
  specific 191
Hydraulic carjacks 226
Hydrocephalus 214
Hydrogen 58
  atom 287
  ions 39
  spectrum of 287f
Hydrolysis 22, 121
Hydrolytic enzymes 14
Hydrostatic pressure 224
Hypercalcemia 33
Hyperchloremia 33
Hyperglycemia 79, 80
  in diabetes, signs of 80

  prevention of 81
  risk factors for 79
  secondary cause of 79
  symptoms of 80
  treatment of 80
Hyperkalemia 33
Hypermagnesemia 33
Hypermetropia 208
  corrected 209f
Hypernatremia 29, 33
Hyperopia 208
  axial 208
  common-simple 208
  curvature 208
  index 208
  positional 208
Hyperphosphatemia 33
Hyperthermia 196
Hypocalcemia 33
Hypochloremia 33
Hypocholesterolemic agent 114
Hypoglycemia 81
  causes of 81
  diagnosis of 82
  prevention of 82
  risk factors of 81
  severe 82
  symptoms of 81
  treatment of 82
Hypokalemia 33
Hypomagnesemia 33
Hyponatremia 33
Hypophosphatemia 33
Hypothermia 196
  mild 196
  severe 196

■ I

Ice glacier 21
Image, formation of 205f, 206f
Immune
  protection 96
  response 3
Impulses 96
Inclined plane 181, 181f
Indium-111 294
Induced fit theory 43
Induction 256
  process of 256
Industrial use 295
Industries and railways 252
Infective agents 55
Infrared radiation 214, 310
Inorganic acids, types of 34t
Insulin resistance 77
Intensity 239
Intensive care units 302
Interstitial fluid 25
Intestinal parasites 55
Intestinal tuberculosis 55
Intestine, obstruction of 248
Intramuscular injection 196
Intra-abdominal pressure 231
Intracellular compartment 20
Intracellular fluid 24
Intracranial pressure 231
  measuring 232
Intraluminal process 54

Index

Intramuscular injection 168
Intraocular pressure 230
  measuring 231
Intravenous glucose tolerance test 77
Intravenous injection 168
Inulin 65
Invasive methods 232
Iodine number 122
Iodine-123 294
Iodine-131 294
Ionization chamber 288
Ionizing radiation 290
  detection of 300
  direct 290
  indirect 291
  types of 290
Ions and ionic compounds 283
Iris 206
Iron 107
Iron-59 294
Isocitrate, formation of 74
Isoleucine 85-87, 91
Isomerism 60

J

Jaw, lever action of 175, 175f
Jelly paste 248
Joint
  and muscles, stiffness of 196
  disease, treatment of 247
  problems 179

K

Kelvin scales 193
Ketogenesis 129
Ketone bodies 129
  metabolism of 129
Kidney 39
  disease of 54
  parenchyma of 15
Krebs cycle 12

L

L isomers 60
Lactic acid fermentation 69, 69f
Lactose 63
  properties of 63
Ladd device 232
L-alanine 86
Lamina terminalis 26
L-arginine 86
L-asparagine 86
L-aspartate 86
L-cysteine 86
Lead-212 294
Lecithin 123
Length, units of 140
Lens 205, 208
  absence of 208
  and images 205
  basic features of 205f
  concave 206f, 210f
    diverging 206
  converging 208
  convex 205f, 209f
  features of 205
  focal length 205, 208
  optic axis 205

optical center 205, 207
principal axis 205
principal focus 205
Leucine 85-87, 91
Leukocytes 91
Leukotrienes 116
  chemical structure of 116f
  functions of 116
  occurrence of 116
Lever 173
  second class 174, 174f
L-glutamate 86
L-glyceraldehyde 60
L-histidine 86
Life, building block of 5
Light 198, 201
  application of principles of 218
  biological effects of 210
  corpuscular theory of 198
  diffuse and smooth reflection of 203f
  electromagnetic theory of 199
  exercise 194
  form of quantum 200f
  in real life, refraction of 204
  in therapy, uses of 213
  nature of 198
  particle 199f
  quantum theory of 200
  rays of 201
  reflection of 202, 202f, 203
  refraction of 202, 202f, 203, 204f
  therapy 213
  wave theory of 199
Lightening rod 257f
Linear momentum 163
Lipid 18, 111, 113, 117
  absorption of 53
  aggregates, emulsification of 120
  classification of 112
  compound 112
  derived 112
  description of simple 112t
    description of 52t
  digestion 52
  digestive process of 52f
  energy source 111
  functions of 111, 113
  insulating material 111
  profile 4
  rich membrane 12
  simple 112
  solubilization of 120
  structural component 111
  transport of 120
  types of 7
Lipofuscin 18
Lipoproteins 92, 112, 118, 124
  functions of 124, 125
  high-density 125
  intermediate-density 125
  low-density 125
  type of 124
  very-low-density 124
Liquid
  molecules of 189
  scintillation counting 300
  water, density of 22
L-isoleucine 86
L-isomer 84

chemical structure of 60f
  types 51
Liver
  action back 177
  action hip joint 176
  disease of 54
  parenchyma of 15
  role of 113
  synthesizes 113
L-leucine 86
L-lysine 86
L-methionine 86
Lock and key theory 42
Locomotion, effect on 210
Long-day animals 211
Lower fixed point 186
Lower pressure, region of 186
L-phenylalanine 86
L-proline 86
L-serine 86
L-threonine 86
L-tryptophan 86
L-tyrosine 86
Lumbar puncture 232
Lumbar vertebra, fifth 177
Luminous bodies 198
Lunar periodicity 211
Lunar rhythms 211
Lungs 38
  role of 38fc
L-valine 86
Lying quietly 194
Lymph 25
Lymphatic route 53
Lysine 85, 89, 91
Lysosome 7, 14
  functional polymorphism of 14
  functions of 15
  primary 14
  secondary 14
  structure and functions of 15f

M

Machine
  efficiency and mechanical advantage of 172
  principles of 172
Macromolecules 111
Macrovascular complications 80
Magnesium 30, 31, 107
  functions of 31
  hydroxide 35
  sources of 31
Magnet and magnetism, applications of 268
Magnetic attraction 266f
Magnetic devices 269f
Magnetic fields 266
Magnetic force, law of 265
Magnetic inductions 267
Magnetic moment 268
Magnetic repulsion 266f
Magnetic resonance imaging 278, 279f
Magnetism 265
  theory of 268
Magnetized state 267
Maintenance and spillage 47
Malabsorption syndrome 54
  causes 55

Index

clinical manifestations 55
diagnosis 55
management 56
Malate, formation of 74
Maltose 63
properties of 63
Manometer 227
Mass and weight 153
unit of 140
Mass number 290
Matrix 12
Measurement, units of 162
Mechanical advantage 173
Mechanical effects 264
Medical radiation 297
Medical treatment 159
Medicine, visible light in 213
Melatonin 212
Melibiose 63
Melting points 188, 189f
Membrane proteins 93
Meningitis 250
Mercury
advantages of 186
column 225
thermometer, construction of 186
Metabolic activities 26
Metabolism 125, 130f
effect on 210
interrelationship in 129, 130
Metallic foreign substances 268
Metalloproteins 92
Methionine 85-87, 91, 100
Metric and English systems,
conversion between 143t
Micelles 120
Microfilaments 18
Microtubules 18
Microvascular complications 80
Microvilli 8
Mitochondria 12, 13, 126
central cavity of 12
functions of 12
membrane 12
structure of 13f
Mitosis 16
Mitotic spindle 17
Molecular oxygen 15
Monoacylglycerol 120
Monoamine 86
Monosaccharides 59, 60, 60t, 62
chemical reactions of 61
primary categories of 60t
Motion 145, 149, 162, 164, 167
applications of 149
circular 147
during walking 149
first law of 162
inertia of 163
oscillatory 147
rotational 147
second law of 164
sickness 149
third law of 164
translatory 147
types of 147
Mouth 51
Movement therapy 159
Mucoprotein 92
Mucosal process 54

Multi-element tube 304
Muscle 289
contract 207
contraction 31
ischemia, transient 271
Musical sound 242
Musocal abnormality 55
Mutarotation 62
Myocardial damage 275
Myopia 208, 209
corrected 210f

N

Natural radiation 292
sources 292
Nausea 29
Near vision 207
Neonate and old person, use in care of 195
Nephropathy 80
Nerve
fibers 159
generation 96
impulse 198
Neural plasticity 159
Neural stimulator 311
Neurons 77
Neuropathy 80
Neurotransmitters 8
Neutral fats 112, 120
Neutron radiation 291
Neutrophils 116
Newborn baby loses 188
Newton's first law 162, 164
Newton's law 151, 162
Newton's second law 163, 164
Newton's third law 164
Nicotinamide adenine dinucleotide 45
Ninhydrin reaction 90
Nitrogen residue, utilization of 101
Noise 242, 249
pollution 249
prevention 249, 251
sources of 249
Non-competitive inhibitors 44
Noninvasive methods 232
Non-oxidative deamination 101, 102
Nonspore-forming bacteria 195
Norum's disease 119
Nuclear division, types of 16
Nuclear fission 289, 290
Nuclear membrane 9
Nuclear physics 283
Nucleic acids, role of 99
Nucleolus 10
Nucleoproteins 92
Nucleus 6, 9
functions of 10
parts of 9
structure of 9f
Nutrients 8
Nutrition, chemistry of 3
Nutritional importance, based on 85

O

Ocular pathologic conditions 208
Ohm's law 260
Oligosaccharides 59, 64
Operation

mechanism of 277, 278
theatres 302
Optical isomers 61
Optical phenomena 201
Oral glucose tolerance test 77
Oral thermometer 193, 193f
Organ pressure 221
Organelles 5, 9
Organic acids, types of 34t
Organum vasculosum 26
Orthostatic hypotension 149
Osmotic pressure 227
applications of 229
biological methods 228
measurement of 227, 228f
mechanical methods 227
physical methods 228
Osmotic regulation 108
Ossicles 243
Osteoporosis 179
Otoscope 214
Oxaloacetate, regeneration of 74
Oxidation 62, 121
Oxidative deamination 101, 102f
Oxidative phosphorylation 69
Oxidoreductases 45
Oxygen 58
Oxytocin stimulates uterine 97

P

P wave 270
Pacemaker 270, 311
temporary 274
Paddle placement 276
Paddle size 276
Paddle-skin interface material 276
Pain 196
temporarily reduce 178
Palladium-103 294
Pancreas, destruction of 79
Pancreatitis 53
Parathyroid
gland 30
hormone 30
Parent nucleus 291
Pascal's law 224
applications of 225
working applications of 225f
Paschen series 287
Patient handling and gravity 158
Patient monitors 308
Pentode tube 304
Pentoses 62
Peptide 93
bond formation 90
Peptidyl transferase complex 98
Peptones 93
Peripheral vascular diseases 81
Peroxisomes 15
functions of 16
structure of 16f
Person's auditory system 250
Personal cleanliness 47
Personal protective equipment, use of 47
Person's circadian rhythm 212
Pesticides 11
Pfeffer's method 227
Phagocytosis 14

Index

Phenylalanine 85, 86, 88
Phonocardiography 271
Phosphate 39
   buffer system 38
   esters 62
Phosphatidylcholine 123
Phosphatidylethanolamine 123
Phosphatidylinositol 123
Phosphatidylserine 123
Phospholipid 7, 112, 122
   bilayer 7
   classification of 122, 123t
   functions of 122
   name of 123
   properties of 122
   types of 122f
Phosphoproteins 92
Phosphorus 32
   functions of 32
   sources of 32
Photoelectric effect 200f
Photokinesis 210
Photomultiplier tube 300
Photon 201
Photoperiodicity 211
Photoperiodism 211
Photosensitivity 211, 218, 218f
   reactions 218
Physical barrier 8
Physical exercise, amount of 25
Physical quantity, measurement of 138
Physical work 170
Physics, language of 168
Physiologic information 308
Pigmentation effects 211
Pigments 18
Pinnotheres maculatus 210
Pinocytosis 14
Pitch 243
Planck's constant 285
Plasma 12, 25, 107
Plasma membrane 5, 7, 8
   appendages of 8
   basic structure of 7f
   formation of 7
   functions of 8
Plasma protein 108
   functions of 108
   levels 4, 108
   system 37
Plasmalogens 123
Pneumatonometry 231
Pneumonia 195
Polarity 265
Polonium 289
Polymorphism, stages of 14
Polyribosomes 13
Polysaccharides 9, 48, 59, 64, 76
   types of 65t
Postmucosal events 54
Potassium 27, 29, 107
   common sources of 29t
   functions of 29
   hydroxide 35
   sources of 29
Potassium-42 294
Power 171
Precursor 114
Pregnancy 179

Presbycusis 250
Presbyopia 208, 209
   cause of 209
Pressure
   amount of 227
   and fluid mechanics 220
   applications of 232
   diastolic 229
   measurement of 229
   systolic 229
   typical 221t
   volume of 227
Principal focus 205
Printing machine 253
Proctoscopes 214
Progesterone 119
Prolamins 92
Proline 85, 86, 89
Prostaglandins 114
   chemical structure of 115f
   classification of 115
   functions of 115
   occurrence of 115
Protamines 92
Protein 7, 13, 53, 84, 91, 93, 96, 130f, 171
   absorption of 51
   biosynthesis 100
   catalytic 93
   chemical properties and structure of 91f
   classification of 91, 93
   conjugated 91
   contractile 93
   defense 93
   derived 91
   digestion 50
      and absorption of 48
      description of 51t
   digestive process of 50f
   factories 13
   functions of 96
      classification of 93t
   genetic 93
   globular 93
   hormonal 93
   in ligaments 196
   in vitro 135
   integral 8
   kinds of 92, 92t
   mechanical support 96
   metabolism of 100
   modification of 11
   molecules 168
   peripheral 8
   simple 91
   storage 93
   structure of 93, 94, 94f, 95, 95f, 96f
   synthesis 97, 97f, 99
      process of 98
   transport 93
   type 93
Protozoa 247
Psoriasis 211
Psychological factors 54
Psychological influences 54
Pulley 178, 178f
   classification 178
   fixed 178

   function of 178
   movable 178
Pulse 236
Pumping blood 171
Putting weights 227

Q

QRS complex 271
Quanta 200

R

Radiant effects 263
Radiation 188, 289, 290
   artificial 293
   classification 290
   internal sources of 293
   manmade 293
   nonionizing 291
   protection limits 298
Radioactive substances, naturally occurring 290
Radioactivity and monitoring, detection of 288
Radiocarbon 289
Radioimmunoassay 289
Radioisotope 290
   applications 293
   exposure effects 296
Radiopotassium 289
Radiotracer 293
Radium 289
Radium-223 294
Rancidity 121
Rapid eye movement 213
Rarefaction 237
Ray
   reflection of 240f
   refraction of 241f
Reaction 90
Red blood corpuscles, fate of 228f
Reflection 240
   irregular 203
   law of 202
   regular 203
   types of 203
   uses of 203
Refraction 203, 240
Renal function tests 4
Renal glycosuria 78
Renal tubules 39
Reproduction and gonads, influence on 211
Residual body 15
Resistance 260
Respiratory 180
   problem 179
   protection 47
Rest and motion 146
Retina 206, 207, 209
Retinopathy 80
Rhenium-186 294
Rheumatoid arthritis 179
Ribonucleoprotein particles 13
Ribosomal proteins 13
Ribosomal RNA 13
Ribosome 6, 7, 11, 13
   70s 13
   80s 13

Index

free 13
functions of 14
structure of 14f
types of 13
Richmond screw 232
Road traffic accident 150
Rocking motion 243
Rough endoplasmic reticulum 10
Rubidium-82 294
Russell traction 181, 181f
Rutherford's model 184
Rutherford's scattering experiment 284f

S

Saccharides 59
Salts 36
    incompatibility of 36
    neutralization 36
Saponification number 121
Saponins 118
Scalar and vector quantity 146f
Scalar quantity 141, 145, 146, 146t
Scalars and vectors 145
Scintillation counters 289, 300
Sclera 206
Scleroproteins 92
Screw 182
Semi-automatic defibrillator 278
Septicemia, disease of 54
Serine 85, 86, 88
    albumin 107
    cholesterol 4
    electrolytes level 4
    enzyme levels 4
    globulin 107
Seven colors
    consists of 204
    spectrum of 204
Sex hormones 118, 119
Shadow, casting of 201f
Shock 277
    electrical 275
    frequency of 276
Short sightedness 209
Silver chloride 36
Simple diffusion 53
Simple machines 172
Simple passive diffusion 51
Simply current 259
Sinusitis 184
Siphon 224, 224f
Skeletal activity, control of 274
Skeletal traction 179
Skin
    cancer 211
    disorders 211
    dry 196
    to skin contact 195
    traction 179
Sleeping 194
Slugs 211
Small intestine 51
Small molecules 5
Smooth endoplasmic reticulum 11
Snell's law 204
Soapy feeling 35
Sodium 27, 107
    common sources of 28t

functions of 28
hydrogen ion exchange channel 39f
hydroxide 23, 35
sources of 28
tetraborate 23
Sodium-24 294
Solid passing, friction of 165
Solid water, density of 22
Solidification, heat of 190
Soluble protein release factors 98
Sound
    characteristics of 242
    echo of 203
Specular reflection 202
Speech
    audiometry 246
    reception threshold 246
Speed 147
Spherical knobs 257
Sphingomyelins 123
Sphingosine 117
    chemical structure of 117f
Spill clean-up 47
Spindle fibers 16, 17f
    functions of 17
Sponging 197
Spontaneous biochemical reactions 41
Sprains, management of 184
Stability and gravity 158
Starch 65
    and glycogen 48
Stated in Newton's words 164
Static electricity 254, 254f
Steam inhalation 197
Stereoisomers 60, 61
Sterile insect technique 295
Sterilization, use of heat for 195
Sterilizers 195, 197
Steroid 77, 117
    hormones 11, 77
    types of 118t
Sterols 117, 118
Stethoscope 244, 245f
Stomach 51
Storage granules 14
Structural elements 114
Sublimation 190
Substance 191
    alcohol 152, 191
    aluminum 152
    atom of 201
    blood 191
        plasma 152
    gold 152
    ice 191
    iron 152
    lead 152
    mercury 152, 191
    organic 111
    platinum 152
    pure water 152
    stable 21
    thermal capacity of common 191t
    water 191
    whole blood 152
Succinate, generation of 74
Succinyl CoA, formation of 74
Sucrose 62-64

properties of 64
Sulfate esters 62
Sulfolipid 112
Swimming 194
Symbalophone 245

T

T wave 271
Telegraph equipment 264
Telehealth 312
Telephones 264
Temperature
    characterizes 185
    on magnet, effect of 267
    scales 192
Template strand 99
Terrestrial radiation sources 292
Testosterone 119
Tetroses 62
Thallium-201 294
Thermal effects 263
Thermal energy, relative expenditure of 194t
Thermionic thermometer 307, 307f
    working of 308f
Thermocouple 261f
Thermography 215, 215f
Thermometer 186f
Thermometric substance 186
Third class lever 174, 174f
Thomas splint traction 180f
Thomson's atomic model 283, 284f
Threonine 85, 86, 88
Thrombolysis 108
Thromboxanes 115
    chemical structure of 116f
    classification of 115
    functions of 116
    occurrence of 116
Time, units of 141
Tissue
    action on 35
    diseased 279
Tomography 279
Tonometry 231
Torricelli's experiment 222, 222f
Torricellian vacuum 222
Total body fluid, distribution of 25f
Traction 178
    balanced 180
    contraindications 179
    purpose of 178
    risks and contraindications 179
Traction fixed 180
Transamination 101, 101f
Transcellular fluid 25
Transducer 306
    input 306
    output 307
    parts and working 306
    using 230
    working of 307f
Transistors 306
    properties 306
Transmethylation 90
Transmission 240
Transthoracic impedance 275
Transverse wave motion 236, 236f
Trehalose 63

Triacylglycerol 120, 121
Triaxial accelerometer 311
Tricarboxylic acid cycle 73
   significance 73
   site 73
   steps of 73, 73f
Triglycerides 119, 120
Triode tube 270, 304, 304f
Trioses 62
Trisodium phosphate 23
Tryptophan 85, 86, 88, 91
Tumors, evaluating 279
Tuning forks 251
Tympanic membrane 239, 243
Tyrosine 85, 86, 88

U

U wave 271
Ultrasonic sound waves 247
   adverse effects of 247
   production of 247
Ultrasound 248
   diagnosis, method of 248
   diathermy 247
   uses of 247
Ultraviolet radiation 216
   dangers and precautions 216
   uses 216
Undressing 194
Uniform bore 186
Uniform circular motion 166
Unit
   concept of 138
   Joule 185
   of length, multiples of 140t
   of mass, multiples of 141t
   systems of 139, 139t
Uranium decay series 292
Urea 4
   cycle 101, 102
      steps of 103, 103f
   formation of 102
Uridine diphosphate glucose 72
Urine 33
   nitrogenous constituents of 107

V

Vacuum tubes 303
   types of 303
Valine 85-87
Valsalva maneuver 231
Vapor
   heat of 190, 196
   pressure 189, 189f
   tension 228

Vasopressin 27
Vector 146t
   quantities 145
Vehicles, control of 252
Velocity 148, 167
   average 148
   change 162
   instantaneous 148
   types of 148
   uniform 148
   variable 148
Venous and arterial systems 231
Ventilation 195
   phase 276
Visible light, application of 214f
Vision 198
   and corrections, defects of 208
   physics of 206
Visual information 213
Vitamin
   A 119
   B injections 56
   B12, absorption of 55
   chemistry of 3
   D 118, 119
      deficiency 33, 55
   E 119
   K 119
Vitreous humor, thickness of 248
Vocalization 243

W

Walking fast 194
Walking slowly 194
Walking upstairs 194
Washing soda mixture 23
Water 20, 25, 203
   and fluid balance 26f
   boiling point of 21
   consumption, amount of 25
   distilled 21
   equal volume of 151
   freezing point of 21
   hard 23, 23t
   heat capacity of 22
   input, regulation of 26
   intake, sources of 26
   loss, sources of 26
   man-made sources of 21
   molecules 168
   output, regulation of 27
   properties of 21
   pure 21
   rain 21
   soft 23, 23t

   sources of 21
   surface 21
   types of 23
   underground 21
Wave
   alpha 269
   delta 269
   elastic 235
   electromagnetic 236, 310
   light 199f
   mechanical 235, 237
   mechanism of propagation of 235, 235f
   non-mechanical 236
   pattern 270
   phenomenon 240
   pressure 236
   sound 234, 237
   theory of light, failures of 200
   types of 235
Wave motion 234
   longitudinal 236, 237f
   types of 236
Wavelength 239f
Waxes 112
Weber's test 251
Wedge 182
Weight and measurements, conversion of 142t
Weight loss 80
Whipple's disease 55
Wire coil 264
Work 161, 168
   measurement of 168

X

X-ray 216, 300
   radiation 291
   slice data 280
   tomography, complementary 294
   types 217
   units 217
   uses 217

Y

Yeast 41
Ytterbium-169 294

Z

Zero acceleration 162
Zinc 107

EU GSPR Authorised Reprsentative
Logos Europe, 9 rue Nicolas Poussin
1700, La Rochelle, France
Phone: +33 (0) 6 67 93 73 78
E-mail: contact@logoseurope.eu

www.ingramcontent.com/pod-product-compliance
Ingram Content Group UK Ltd.
Pitfield, Milton Keynes, MK11 3LW, UK
UKHW050429150426
5217IPUK00019B/1309